Living with Voices

Living with Voices

50 stories of recovery

Prof Marius Romme
Dr Sandra Escher
Jacqui Dillon
Dr Dirk Corstens
Prof Mervyn Morris

PCCS BOOKS
Monmouth

in association with
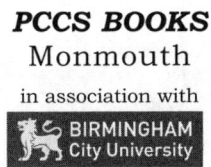

First published 2009 by PCCS Books, Ross-on-Wye

PCCS Books Ltd
Wyastone Business Park
Wyastone Leys
Monmouth
NP253SR
UK
Tel +44 (0)1600 891 509
www.pccs-books.co.uk

In association with Birmingham City University

This collection: © Marius Romme, Sandra Escher, Jacqui Dillon,
Dirk Corstens and Mervyn Morris, 2009

Preface © Michaela Amering
Introduction © Marius Romme and Mervyn Morris
 Chapters 1, 2, 3, 6, 7, 8, 9 © Marius Romme; Chapters 4, 5 © Sandra Escher
The fifty stories © the authors

All rights reserved.
No part of this publication may be reproduced, stored in a retrieval system,
transmitted or utilised in any form by any means, electronic, mechanical,
photocopying or recording or otherwise without permission in writing from the publishers.
The authors have asserted their rights to be identified as the authors of this work
in accordance with the Copyright, Designs and Patents Act 1988.

Living with Voices: 50 stories of recovery

A CIP catalogue record for this book is available from the British Library

ISBN 978 1 906254 22 3

Cover designed in the UK by Old Dog Graphics
Printed in the UK by Short Run Press, Exeter

CONTENTS

Preface: Recovery is Reshaping our Clinical and Scientific   i
Responsibilities
Prof Dr Michaela Amering

Introduction   1
Marius Romme and Mervyn Morris

1   Important Steps to Recovery with Voices   7
Marius Romme

2   The Disease Concept of Hearing Voices   23
and Its Harmful Aspects
Marius Romme

3   What Causes Hearing Voices?   39
Marius Romme

4   Accepting Voices and Finding a Way Out   48
Sandra Escher

5   Making Sense of Voices: The relationship between   54
the voices and the life history
Sandra Escher

6   Metaphors and Emotions   63
Marius Romme

7   Hearing Voices Groups   73
Marius Romme

8   Psychotherapy with Hearing Voices   86
Marius Romme

9   Medication   95
Marius Romme

Introduction to the Fifty Stories   101
Mervyn Morris

The Fifty Stories   104

Ami Rohnitz	104	*John Exell*	212
Andreas Gehrke	108	*John Robinson*	218
Antje Müller	112	*Johnny Sparvang*	222
Audrey Reid	118	*Jolanda van Hoeij*	225
Caroline	124	*Karina Carlyn*	230
Daan Marsman	126	*Lisette de Klerk*	234
Debra Lampshire	130	*Marion Aslan*	238
Denise Bosman	134	*Mieke Simons*	244
Don Dugger	139	*Mien Sonnemans*	248
Eleanor Longden	142	*Odi Oquosa*	251
Elisabeth Svanholmer	147	*Olga Runciman*	253
Fernand Chappin	153	*Patsy Hage*	260
Flore Brummans	157	*Peggy Davies*	265
Frank Dahmen	161	*Peter Bullimore*	267
Frans de Graaf	163	*Peter Reynolds*	273
Gavin Young	169	*Riny Selder*	277
Gina Rohmit	171	*Robert Huisman*	280
Hannelore Klafki	176	*Ron Coleman*	283
Helen	180	*Ronny Nilson*	289
Mrs Hutten	186	*Rufus May*	292
Jacqui Dillon	188	*Ruth Forrest*	296
Jan Holloway	194	*Sasja Slotenmakers*	301
Jeanette Brink	198	*Sjon Gijsen*	307
Jeannette Woolthuis	203	*Stewart Hendry*	309
Jo	209	*Sue Clarkson*	314

Appendix: The invitation to participate in this study   319

Acknowledgements   324

References   338

Contributors   343

Names Index   345

RECOVERY IS RESHAPING OUR CLINICAL AND SCIENTIFIC RESPONSIBILITIES

PROF DR MICHAELA AMERING
DEPARTMENT OF PSYCHIATRY AND PSYCHOTHERAPY
MEDICAL UNIVERSITY OF VIENNA

Voice hearers have been an essential force among the pioneers of the recovery movement, who have created the concepts and a language for recovery. As authors of the groundwork for the movement they have developed and impacted not only alternatives, but also international mental health system transformation efforts and specific models of recovery-oriented practice.

From their work we know that much of recovery is lived outside clinical settings, but also that important challenges concern the roles and responsibilities of clinicians in supporting and assisting people with mental health problems in their efforts towards making full use of their health and resilience, and achieving their goals in life. Self-determination and individual choice of flexible support and opportunities, promoting empowerment and hope, and assistance in situations of calculated risk are the new indicators of the quality of services. In contrast to a deficit model of mental illness, recovery-orientation includes a focus on health promotion, individual strengths, and resilience. A shift from demoralising prognostic scepticism towards a rational and optimistic attitude towards recovery, and broadening treatment goals beyond symptom reduction and stabilisation, require specific skills and new forms of co-operation between practitioners and service users, between mental health workers of different backgrounds, and between psychiatry and the public. New rules for services, for example user involvement on all levels and person-centred organisation of care, as well as new tools for clinical collaborations, for example shared decision-making and psychiatric advance directives, are being complemented by new proposals regarding more ethically consistent anti-discrimination and involuntary treatment legislation, as well as participatory approaches to evidence-based medicine and policy.

Recovery demands all our best efforts in terms of human rights, patients' rights, scientific and clinical responsibility and service, in the interest of those of us who might become patients and those who have. We learn from those who are using services; those who have used services (ex-users), and those who define themselves through overcoming harmful experiences in the support system (survivors). Alliances between people with and without lived experience of mental health problems and of mental health services have been successful but need more support, as do those who work on the development of alternatives outside the traditional system.

The American 'National Coalition of Mental Health Consumer/Survivor Organizations' notably captures their commitment to enriching the field with the 'full range of lived experiences' in their proposition: 'We are the evidence!' This bodes well for the emerging evidence base for recovery-orientation, including an urgent call for a partnership approach which allows all experiences and all forms of evidence to be used at all levels. Co-operative and co-ordinated efforts with (ex-) service users, carers, their spokespeople and public health advocates offer formidable chances to reduce stigma, discrimination and social exclusion, which are currently seriously limiting efforts towards recovery. While the task appears huge, the combination of the wisdom and energy of the user movement and the current need of many clinicians and academics in psychiatry world-wide to overcome reductionistic and uninspired conceptual frameworks might just work in favour of substantial changes now.

LITERATURE

Amering, M & Schmolke, M (2009) *Recovery in Mental Health. Reshaping scientific and clinical responsibilities.* London: Wiley-Blackwell.

Wallcraft, J, Schrank, B & Amering, M (2009) *Handbook of Service User Involvement in Mental Health Research.* London: Wiley-Blackwell.

INTRODUCTION

MARIUS ROMME AND MERVYN MORRIS

This book demonstrates that it is entirely possible to overcome problems with hearing voices and to take back control of one's life. It shows a path to recovery by addressing the main problems voice hearers describe – the threats, the feelings of powerlessness, the anxiety of being mad – and helps them to find their way back to their emotions and spirituality and to realising their dreams. This book also holds true for those who have been given a diagnosis of schizophrenia. This is the third book in a series regarding the experience of hearing voices. It proves the value of our 'accepting' and 'making sense of' voices approach, for which it provides an evidence base.

The first book, *Accepting Voices* (Romme & Escher, 1993) gave a new analysis of the experience of hearing voices outside the medical model. It explained the principles of accepting voices using the stories of hearers who became patients, and hearers who never came into contact with mental health services but who, nevertheless, coped very well with their experience. Accepting voices means accepting the reality of the voices for the voice hearer; it means becoming interested in the different aspects of the experience and in the relationship between the voices and the events of the hearer's life.

The second book, *Making Sense of Voices* (Romme & Escher, 2000a), is a manual for mental health professionals in which a systematic approach to working with the voice hearer and voices is described. In the Appendix to this book is the Maastricht Interview Schedule, an interview schedule that explores the different aspects of the experience. Learning to cope with the voice-hearing experience is explained as a process in which three phases can be distinguished: the 'startled' phase, during which anxiety and a feeling of being overwhelmed dominate; the 'organisation' phase, in which interest in the experience is developed and the voice hearer starts to look for more information; and the 'stabilisation' phase, where a person recovers his/her own potential and capacities. Each phase requires a different approach both from the voice hearer and the professional.

At the heart of this book are the stories of fifty people who have recovered from the distress of hearing voices. They have overcome the disabling social and psychiatric attitudes towards voice hearing and have also fought with themselves to accept and make sense of the voices. They have changed their relationship with their voices in order to reclaim their lives. Ron Coleman neatly formulates this in his book *Recovery: An Alien Concept*? 'Live your life, not your voices' (Coleman, 1999).

All the people in this book describe their recovery; how they now accept their voices as personal, and how they have learnt to cope with them and have changed their relationship with them. They have discovered that their voices are not a sign of madness but a reaction to problems in their lives that they couldn't cope with, and they have found that there is a relationship between the voices and their life story, that the voices talk about problems that they haven't dealt with – and that they therefore make sense.

Although research has shown that most people who hear voices do not seek help, the stories in this book are those of voice hearers who became (often for a long time) psychiatric patients. They were afraid of their voices, overwhelmed by them and felt powerless. Accepting their voices was thus a courageous and a difficult step for them. In this book you will find described in the stories the process by which voices hearers, each in their own unique way, managed to get control, lost their anxiety and were no longer overwhelmed. It tells how they learnt to accept their voices, to change their relationship with them, and started to cope with the problems in life. They succeeded because of their own inner strengths, their will and capabilities, as well as through the help of others.

From the stories it will become clear that for voice hearers, accepting their voices, and relating them to their own life, is the only way to recover from the distress their voices bring. Stimulating people to follow this road is the only way to help them overcome their distress. It also becomes clear that, rather than extinguishing the voices, it is more helpful to change one's relationship with them.

To the voice hearer we want to say that in order to take one's life back into one's own hands, one has to make choices, one needs others to relate to and one has to build up one's 'self' again. In order to stop being a victim and become a victor one also needs opportunities and learning in real-life situations – a process clearly described by Ron Coleman (1999) and by many of those in this book.

WHAT DOES RECOVERY MEAN TO VOICE HEARERS? SOME EXAMPLES

Stewart: *Things have worked out and now I am on my feet. In the past it was a problem just to get out of bed; walking down the road was a big issue, thinking people were talking about me. Getting on the bus was a big problem, a major problem, but now I am really just getting on with day-to-day life. Once I'd started to make a bit more of my life and began to work, that was a big thing for me as well, a sort of sense of worth. I sometimes think about lost time and opportunities but generally I look forward. I remember the first time I really had the experience that they'd [the voices] stopped; it was weird, like I could hear a pin drop.*

Mrs Hutten: *Now I have got back what I wanted to be and wanted to have. I have the feeling to be who I am. I am still married, have friends and doing the catering work I like, and I have become quite self-supporting. I also do not take medication anymore, and don't visit services anymore.*

Debra: *I began to venture out from my home, continued my education, went to university, made friends and gained employment. Instead of having a life totally consumed by voices I began now to devour my ordinary life. It was several years later that I decided to work in the field of mental health as an advisor and educator. I was approached by a clinician who wanted to start up therapy groups for voice hearers. I have found my niche. I have had the opportunity to take what was a catastrophic event and turn it into a positive life-affirming vocation. I am surrounded by people who are as passionate and as committed to working with people, to enhance their well-being and lives, as I am. I have found where I belong.*

Jeannette W: *In therapy I learned you have the right to be there. I don't have to vanish. I started to think 'What will I do with the rest of my life?' I started training. Now I am not only a professional by experience but also a therapist by training.*

Johnny S: *I have a part-time job, minimal home support which will soon cease altogether, and I'm presently zooming up the national chess ratings. I have a hectic social life, have great contact with my family and relatives again, and am always busy helping other voice hearers. In Aarhus we are a small group of voice hearers who've started a local network in an office with a telephone helpline.*

Hannelore: *If this approach had existed at the time when I had these severe life crises, I would have saved myself this psychiatric treatment. Since I became active* *in the German network I haven't been in psychiatry, haven't taken psychopharmaca and haven't got a new diagnosis.*

With these fifty reports we hope to convince other voice hearers and professionals that hearing voices must not be seen as an isolated, individual experience. There is always an interaction between voice hearer and society, voice hearer and family, voice hearer and mental health professional. In this book you will see how a positive approach towards the experience from everyone involved can make a world of difference to the voice hearer. In these stories it becomes evident that recovery from the distress of hearing voices is only possible when the voices become accepted as a human capacity that can have a function in the person's life, and can be used to help voice hearers develop themselves.

A lot of research starts from the position of researchers sitting behind a desk and – by being philosophical, strategic, and objective – working out how to confirm their theory through formulating a researchable question. There are other researchers who start at the other end and try to falsify a theory. We think the best research in this field is to formulate the problem from the experience point of view, to observe experiences in a systematic way. We therefore also involve people who hear voices in the research process as user researchers. Another difference in our approach is that we involve voice hearers who have never become ill and from whom we can learn what is important in the process of living with the experience.

From understanding the perspective of the voice hearer, we have observed that the attitude of mental healthcare researchers and professionals is one of regarding voices not as a source of information, but as a sign of a 'non-existent' reality; it is this attitude that disables people from finding more adequate and helpful information about this experience.

Mental health care should start from the experience of the voice hearer. Effective care should follow the same process as the voice hearers who have recovered. It begins with accepting the undeniable presence of the voices, proceeds to the necessary change of relationship with them, then to finding a fulfilling role in society again, and ultimately to recovery from the distress associated with the voices. In various ways the voice hearers in this book have shown this to be the pathway to recovery.

With the fifty stories in this book we hope to help you realise not only how important the voices are in the process of recovery, but also the problems that lay at their roots. All the people in this book have had not only serious problems in coping with their voices, but also serious other problems related to their voices.

As you read the stories you will see certain themes emerge. For example, voice hearers who have taken their lives back into their own hands, not only have they recovered themselves but have also used their experience to help other voice hearers with their own recovery process and, further on, have made a career in this area. There are stories of voice hearers who have specially profited from hearing voices groups, which they have facilitated and also learnt from, developing greater self-awareness, self-acceptance and self-worth. There are stories highlighting people who have taken their lives back into their own hands through individual therapies, who haven't got involved in the hearing voices movement (or perhaps only tangentially) but have nevertheless found their own recovery path. And there are stories of people who have recovered from distress with their voices and sometimes even lost them, yet have still experienced difficulty from the original problems that lay at the root of their voice-hearing experience.

When starting with the study for this book we, as editors, asked for the cooperation of those people we knew well who had recovered from their distress with their voices. We have come to know many voice hearers through our practice, projects and studies. We also have many contacts from the international network 'Intervoice' and through our relationship with the English, German and Danish Hearing Voices Networks. As well, we have been helped by trustworthy others who have also worked along the lines of accepting and making sense of voices, including psychiatrists Dirk Corstens and Phil Thomas, mental health nurse Trevor Eyles, and social worker Geir Fredrikson. We were most helped by the voice hearers themselves; Jacqui Dillon completed a great number of interviews; quite a number of others wrote their own stories and, last but not least, all the voice hearers who so openly told their stories.

We initially contacted many people by letter asking for their cooperation, explaining the purpose of the study and giving an interview schedule that provided information about our interest in accentuating the recovery process in our approach (see Appendix). Our initial request was for people to write their own stories and this resulted in some very fine narratives, but not enough to meet our target of fifty. We therefore took the step of offering to work with people and we interviewed many of the people whose stories are to be read in this book. We edited the interviews down to a maximum of four A4 typed pages, focusing on what was said about recovery, but keeping the words used by the voice hearer in the interview. We have thus lightened the touch of the editorial process in order to remain as authentic as possible to the way people have expressed themselves. There is more discussion about the editing and organisation of the stories at the start of that section of the book.

The stories will involve you wholly and emotionally as well as giving a lot of information. After reading them it may well be difficult to know what to do with the information. Voice hearers might be able to identify with one or a few of the stories and develop their own ideas about themselves on the basis of that identification. Professionals may feel at a bit of a loss, so for them we have tried to further organise the information. We have formulated nine questions and then answered them with the clearest examples from the fifty stories. Thus, preceding the stories are nine chapters, each with the title of one of the questions we formulated (these can be found as the chapter headings in the table of contents). Because of the complexities of editing and translating the stories, the examples of text taken from the fifty stories may show some minor variations from the text in the stories themselves.

The fifty stories are presented in alphabetical order by the first names of the author, partly to make finding individual stories easier but mainly because we want to be clear that each story carries equal weight, though each may well have a different significance to the reader.

CHAPTER 1

IMPORTANT STEPS TO RECOVERY WITH VOICES

MARIUS ROMME

The stories in this book demonstrate that recovery means 'taking life back into your own hands'. Ron Coleman (1999) expresses this as: 'living your own life, not the life of your voices'. We selected fifty people from different countries who were either known by or recommended to us, because they have recovered. Not only had they seriously suffered from their voice hearing, often they had also received long-term traditional psychiatric care that had not helped. Most of them were diagnosed with schizophrenia. They found an alternative way, outside the traditional psychiatric system. In these stories recovery is shown to mean functioning well and being independent in the circumstances people have chosen for themselves. It means finding a purpose in life – a personal and social recovery – not a clinical recovery where eradicating the voices is the main issue in the recovery process. The stories are good examples of how getting rid of voices is neither necessary, nor that important. Many of the fifty people kept their voices but changed the relationship in a way that the relationship became helpful. Some people got rid of the original negative voices and found positive helpful ones. All got rid of the distress from their voices because they changed their relationship with them. Most do not use medication anymore, but some still take low doses because it helps them with their emotional response. The use of medication will be discussed in Chapter 9.

WHY A RECOVERY APPROACH AND NOT A CURE APPROACH

Voice hearers become ill, in the sense of becoming dysfunctional, as a result of not being able to cope with their voices *and* the problems that lie at their roots. Why? Because these problems are hard to live with and knock people out of emotional balance, both personally as well as in their relationships with important others. They didn't find psychiatry helpful because in psychiatry hearing voices is seen as a result of a disease, and not as a reaction to problems in life that make people feel powerless. The person's problems are thus neglected and seen as irrelevant, making the solving of their life problems more problematic. Voice hearers in psychiatry are mostly approached only in relation to their symptoms, and not as people with problems and possibilities. We describe in Chapter 2 the conditions in traditional psychiatry that fail to help voice hearers to recover.

Ron Coleman (1999) explains the difference between a recovery approach and a cure approach. We see in the stories in this book that a recovery approach is more satisfactory then a cure approach because hearing a voice is not a sign of pathology but a signal of existing problems. How do we know that? From repeated epidemiological studies it became obvious that hearing voices (as well as experiencing delusions) is found in the normal population, and more frequently in people without a diagnosable psychiatric illness than people with a psychiatric diagnosis. Tien's study (1991) shows a ratio of 2/3 to 1/3 regarding voices. Whilst this research outcome indicates that hearing voices is not in itself a sign of mental illness, how do we know it is a reaction to emotional problems?

Our own studies (Romme & Escher, 1989, 1993, 2000a, 2005) and that of Read et al. (2005a – a literature review of 180 studies) show that there is a causal relationship between trauma and hearing voices. Since this major review in 2005, five large-scale studies, including one prospective study, have been published. All of these have found the presence of a significant dose effect between the numbers of traumas experienced and an increased risk of experiencing psychotic phenomena. Other studies have shown a relationship with emotional neglect (Ensink, 1992; Honig et al., 1998). Because of these causal relationships we conclude that hearing voices is a signal of existing problems that are themselves a consequence of these traumatic experiences and emotional neglect. Another indication is that we find references to the traumatic experiences in the characteristics of the voices and what they say to the voice hearer.

WHAT IS RECOVERY?

To recover, voice hearers learn to cope with the social and emotional consequences of their original problems. In the recovery process they will recognise the relationship between their voices and their emotions and what has happened to them. They also get a better view of the power relationship between themselves and their voices. The anxiety, powerlessness, guilt feelings, etc., are metaphors of the power relationship in the traumatic situation and the emotional neglect period. In the recovery process, they will take back power and will express their own power in relation to their voices and their problems. They also create choices that make it possible to take responsibility for their life and emotions, and by doing so heighten their self-esteem. Gradually they discover that voices are expressing emotions, and these emotions are those the voice hearer experienced as the result of the traumatic situation. The recovery process is one of turning points in the relationship with the voices, with the person becoming more powerful and independent. This is what we see as the approach that leads to recovery. It doesn't make sense to attempt to cure signals of problems, and it's not an approach that is particularly successful either because the traumatic background is not recognised and the emotions involved are not coped with. Voices are the stories of threatening emotions; emotions of the person twisted by terrible experiences, hopelessness, feelings of guilt, aggression and anxiety. In the stories of this book you will read again and again about the relationship between trauma, emotional neglect, other stressful problems and hearing voices, because of the overwhelming emotions related to these traumas.

Ron Coleman (1999) is a well-known voice hearer who recovered from the distress related to his voices. He has very clearly described his personal recovery process. He tells about his recovery and shows us four important elements:

- Involve others: because you need to get direction, hope, support and friendship
- Work on the self: self-esteem, self-confidence, self-awareness and self-acceptance
- Make choices: become responsible for your own decisions and find a purpose in life
- Take ownership: learn to own your voice-hearing experience

Each of these is important and we found them all in many of the stories; not so much as steps but as elements to attend to during the whole of the recovery process.

Reading these stories illustrates that there are many more interesting and important steps to make on the road to recovery. For this chapter we have selected those influences and actions that were described as important and also reported repeatedly. We've organised this information below under headings and will illustrate each with examples from the stories' texts. As already mentioned, the role of medication in this process is described in a separate chapter. The role of hearing voices groups is also described in its own chapter, and the role of psychotherapy is also covered separately. Here we focus on recovery process issues.

ISSUES IMPORTANT IN RECOVERING FROM THE DISTRESS WITH VOICES

1. Meeting someone who takes an interest in the voice hearer as a person
2. Giving hope, by showing a way out and normalising the experience
3. Meeting people who accept the voices as real; being accepted as a voice hearer by others, but also by oneself
4. Becoming actively interested in the hearing voices experience
5. Recognising the voices as personal and becoming the owner of one's voices
6. Changing the power structure between you and your voices
7. Making choices
8. Changing the relationship with your voices
9. Recognising one's own emotions and accepting them

1. Meeting someone who takes an interest in the voice hearer as a person
It seems very important to meet someone who takes an interest in the voice hearer as a person. Voice hearers have often experienced negativity from others because of their hearing voices. In psychiatry as well as in society at large hearing voices is seen as a sign of madness and is not accepted. This does not encourage hearers to be open about their voices. The roots of the problems are also often experienced as something shameful, so voice hearers need an approach that is positive for their self-esteem. This is a necessary first step to forming an alliance with them and stimulating them to open up.

Most voice hearers talk about this:

Don tells his therapist in an evaluation: *I was spoken to as a person, I became an identity. You were interested in a theatre play I had written. Before that I was treated as a patient; lived in no-man's-land; there was a cessation of my feelings. When you lowered my medication I woke up and became clear in my mind.*

Eleanor: *I went back to Bradford and my new psychiatrist was Pat Bracken and that was a massive help. The very first time I met him he said to me: 'Hi Eleanor, nice to meet you. Can you tell me a bit about yourself?' So I just looked at him and said 'I'm Eleanor and I'm a schizophrenic.' And in his quiet, Irish voice he said something very powerful; 'I don't want to know what other people have told you about yourself, I want to know about you.'*

Stewart: *During this time* (he was in a care home when 16 and was told that with his diagnosis of schizophrenia he should not have many expectations for his life, like a job, relationships etc.) *there was a social worker, who saw what it was like for me, and eventually found me somewhere more suitable. She* was much more informal and friend-like and treated me more like a person. She also gave me an alternative idea about what my future might be like.

Ron: *Any recovery journey has a beginning, and for me the beginning was my meeting with Lindsay Cooke my support worker. It was her who saw beneath my madness and into my potential. It was her faith in me that kick-started my recovery.*

2. Giving hope, by showing a way out and normalising the experience

Meeting someone who takes an interest in the voice hearer as a person is often combined with that person who gives an alternative and gives hope. Voice hearers tell about this as an important combination at the start of their recovery. I have split these steps because they are such important conditions for voice hearers to make a start. In traditional psychiatry it is difficult to meet this approach because of the existing prejudices about hearing voices. Many voice hearers in this book start their recovery by meeting somebody who expresses interest in them as a person and gives hope by showing a way out, as when **Ron** tells:

It was her (my support worker) who encouraged me to go to the hearing voices self-help group in Manchester at the start of 1991. It was she, not I, who believed that a self-help group would benefit me.

It is not necessarily a mental health professional, as with **Stewart** it can be another voice hearer:

My recovery started when I met another service user who worked for a charity. It was a real eye-opener because she was also a user but she had a job, a partner, a house, all things I was led to believe I couldn't have, things that were beyond me.

Or it can be a carer as with **Antje**:

I was at a point in my life where I said to myself this cannot be life. My conclusion was to bring it to an end definitively. My mother was very worried, and then she saw Hannelore, the coordinator of the German [hearing voices] network on TV. My mother got the address and went there, participated in a group and after that told me about it. But I really did not want to know. She left a flyer called 'Accepting Voices' on the desk by my bed. She put it down and I said: 'You can take it with you, I'm not interested'. When she had left my room I became interested and I read it. I was very surprised that a psychiatrist was writing in a different way about voices ... At that time I also had a new doctor, and she was different. She was the first who asked if anything had happened to me at the start of my hearing voices.

Similarly **Hannelore** tells about the start of her recovery:

Then came the change in this carousel of isolation, admission and always new medicines. I then met an involved social worker who didn't simply see me as this seriously ill woman but who talked to me, as if I was a normal person; for the first time after a long time I felt taken seriously. That was the reason I gradually started to talk about my voices with her. She was one of the first in Germany in the beginning of the nineties who approached hearing voices differently.

Debra tells about a friend when she reports:
I reached a point when I felt I could no longer continue the quest. I had no option but to kill myself, and then I would no longer be tormented; I would be free. But whilst the desire to gain peace was overwhelming the will to live was stronger, so with the help and assistance of a friend I decided to have one last crack at getting the voices under control.

'Normalising' the experience is for some a better term then 'accepting', and we've particularly observed this with people who've suffered sexual abuse, and whose voices had the characteristics of the abuser. For them, accepting might sound as though they have to accept the abuser, and accept everything the voices say; but this isn't what 'accepting' means, and might lead to confusion because of this kind of interpretation. Several stories demonstrate the importance of meeting people who have normalised their experience.

Mien: *My psychotherapist told me I was not mad but that they [the voices] were related to my past, and that it is a rather normal experience you can talk about with others. It helped me to realise voices express what is happening with you. It is something that belongs to me.*

Eleanor tells about her new psychiatrist: *He told me about the philosophy of Marius Romme and Sandra Escher and about the Hearing Voices Network – that this is just normal human experience – and the importance of conceptualising it in your own way.*

3. Meeting people who accept the voices as real

Being interested in the person by asking about what has happened in their life and being open enough to talk about the voices is one way of showing acceptance of the voices. The stories illustrate that it is a requirement *sine qua non* for recovery to meet people who accept the voices as a reality for the voice hearer, as well as accepting voices as a reality oneself.

Ron writes about this: *Anne Walton, a fellow voice hearer who, at my first hearing voices group asked me if I heard voices. When I replied that I did, she told me that they were real. It doesn't sound like much but that one sentence has been a compass showing me the direction I needed to travel and underpinning my belief in the recovery process.*

Flore, who has mainly recovered with the help of a self-help group, talks about the start of her recovery:

Psychiatry didn't give me anything (for 35 years). This changed when I met a psychiatrist who became angry with me because she saw that I was wearing several masks. This was good because I was drugged and just let everything happen. The second change was because of a nurse who was nagging me to follow a self-help group. I went there and discovered that I could be who I was, and that has helped me much.

Jan tells about her meeting the accepting voices approach:

When I first saw Marius and Sandra speaking I was really blown away because they were flying in the face of what most people at that time were saying; that the voices didn't make any sense. Instinctively I knew they [Marius and Sandra] were right, and I had wanted to work that way for 11 years but that was trained out of me. We were told it was dangerous to talk to people about their voices. Therapy enabled me to look at what was going on in my life that had led to the start of me hearing voices.

Acceptance in a broader perspective

Acceptance may have a wider impact than normalising.

Karina: *What helped me was the support I got from the Hearing Voices Network, feeling a part of something and being accepted for who I was. I felt the support I got from the people at the Red House was invaluable.*

Sue gives us a broader view about how acceptance of the voices can open ways to recovery.

As far as acceptance was involved:
  I accepted my voices as real
  I stopped trying to get rid of them, but accepted them as personal
  I became conscious of my ownership of my voices
  I stopped looking for a cause outside myself
  I looked for solutions in myself
  I explored what had happened in my life that might have a relationship with my voices
  I accepted those emotions which I did not like and could not easily master

This wider perspective also leads to acceptance of self.

Sasja formulates it: *You realise the consequences of hearing voices much later. You have to change yourself also, whether you like it or not. I don't like change. Now I am more philosophical but before I wanted to control everything.*

This happens at the end of or after recovering, but is part of ongoing personal development.

4. Becoming actively interested in your experience of the voices

Accepting the voices as a real experience opens the door to their meaning and their relationship with one's own life. This holds for the voice hearer as well as the professional working with voice hearers. When one just sees hearing voices as a symptom of an illness there is not much reason to go into detail about their background in daily life. Discovering the relationship between voices and life experiences gives the hearer a motive to become actively interested in themselves, and the professional a new direction to becoming more helpful. Being actively interested also leads to hearers learning more through reading about voices, talking and exchanging experiences with others.

Eleanor says: *I spoke to Julie Downs [coordinator of the English Hearing Voices Network] on the phone and started reading about the Hearing Voices Network and thought 'whoa; may be I can be part of this'.*

Ami tells: *I came across advertising on a billboard that somebody would give a lecture about hearing voices, a lecture given by Liz Bodil [Karlsson] [who promoted accepting voices in Sweden]. This was the turning point. She also sold books. That book 'Accepting Voices', I read in one night. I just felt this is for me. This described my experience and also said there is a reason for voices.*

Jacqui: *I read a vast amount of material and became better informed of the many ways to understand human experience. I researched the phenomenon of dissociation and began to appreciate the extent to which I had utilised this capacity in my own survival. I also read a lot of attachment theory. Discovering the work of Judith Herman in 'Trauma and Recovery' had a profound effect on me. Suddenly my own experiences were put in a wider perspective. I was not alone in feeling outraged by the damage done by society, in pathologising survivors of abuse.*

5. Recognising the voices as personal

This active interest can be taken in many directions. We see that, at the start, many people are interested in where the experience comes from, especially professionals who like to focus on this question because they often have great difficulty in accepting voices. It is, of course, commonsense to be interested in what they say, because it is the main characteristic of hearing voices: They *say something*, and what *they tell* is where the interest should be focused. There are many more characteristics of the voices that tell about the person's life. Voices can be recognised as personal because of: what they say (Gina); because of the characteristics of the voices (Lisette, Daan); because of what triggers the voices (Daan); because of the emotions they represent (Antje, Sue); because of the demons they represent (Eleanor, Peter B); or in a broader sense (Mien, Johnny S, Hannelore). For these relationships see also Chapter 5 'Making Sense of Voices'.

Gina first explored in psychotherapy what had happened to her before she started hearing voices, and recognised that what had happened had made her powerless. She had lost her friend, her work and lived in a crime-ridden area. Thereafter she and her therapist explored what was personal about her voices:

When I went out, the voices sometimes said to me 'She is going out again'; and that felt like criticism. It was none of their business because I had no work so I could go out. But then I realised that I had the same thought myself. There were more examples: When the voices said 'See how awful she looks'; it happened on days when I felt myself pretty awful. But they always made such exaggerated statements. By exploring this I started to realise that in a certain way the voices expressed my own thoughts. It is rather strange, but they are your own thoughts about an emotion.

Lisette: *My voice is a male voice and has the name of Stefan. My therapist made it explicit to me that there was a resemblance between my voice and my stepfather. When she was telling me that, I got a flashback and saw my stepfather. I understood that whilst they were not the same, my voice resembles his voice and the voice asks me to do the same things as my stepfather asked me to do like 'don't eat so much or you'll get fat'.*

Daan tells: *I thought I was bad because the voices called me all sorts of names. Later I realised that the voices were related to the physical abuse because they have the characteristics of those who abused me. Then I noticed that the voices became more or less intrusive depending on the situation I was in. They became bad when there were conflicts in the house. So they were a kind of mirror of my living situation.*

Antje: *In therapy I worked through the book of Ron Coleman and Mike Smith. We very soon came to the content of the voices, the relationship between my emotions and the way the voices spoke. When I became angry and did not express my anger, they became angry at me. A theme about my parents, especially my father, came into focus. In this way I started to think about myself and began to realise that experiences in my life hang together with the voices.*

Sue: *The relationship with my voices has always been related to suppressed emotions. Whenever I have experienced traumatic experiences in my life, my voices seemed stronger.*

Eleanor: *I began slowly to realise that yes, he is a demon, but he was a personal demon. His demonic aspects were the unaccepted aspects of my self-image.*

Mien: *The ugly voice told me the sexual abuse was a punishment because I was lazy and stupid. But in psychotherapy I got more insight into myself. I understood that voices have everything to do with how I feel myself. Those voices express what has or is happening to me.*

Johnny S: *This was a turning point for me* [he had followed a course on accepting hearing voices] *as I began to relate my past life experience to the voices.*

6. Changing the power structure between you and your voices

This seems to be a necessary prerequisite for recovery. It consists of different aspects and is a process in itself. Steps can be:

(a) Reorganising the way of coping by, for instance, giving the voices a certain time in the day to talk, and then for the rest of the day telling them 'not now, but at the agreed-upon time'.

Stewart: *I was already able to talk back to my voices with my thoughts, but I learnt to make a specific time of day, the evening, when I would focus, and simply tell the voices 'later' if they came at another time.*

Audrey: *When I started working on my voices I gave them time slots. The red voice and another voice would come in the evening. The blue voice more often came at the weekend.*

Jacqui: *I had mantras that I repeated to counter the terror, and that helped to rebuild my belief in myself. If a voice kept saying to me: 'You are a bad mother', I would say, 'I love my daughter and she loves me'. If a voice kept saying 'You are doomed. You will die a horrible death', I would say, 'I am safe now and I am free'. I would repeat these words of power over and over.*

(b) Freeing oneself from the victim role:

Eleanor: *So after seeing that my mum is trying, Pat Bracken is trying, his team is trying, my sister is trying, my dad's trying; I asked: 'Who's not trying here?' The only person not fighting for me was me. It was a real wake-up call. I sat in my front room, I looked in the mirror and I looked pretty bad. Part of me was saying, 'Look, look at yourself,' not in an aggressive way. But this little compassionate part of me was saying: 'Look, is this what it's come to? Are you going to do something about it?' I'd got to the absolute lowest and I couldn't go any lower. It was at that moment that I suddenly thought, right; you are going to do something about this. I realised that the psychiatric system made me a victim, but it was me who was keeping up that victim role. I knew then that what I had to do was take on this voice because it was him who was running the show. He'd say 'jump' and I'd say 'how high?'*

Hannelore wrote: *I have freed myself from the victim role. For this Ron Coleman was and still is a great example for me.*

Jeannette W: *In therapy I learned to say to myself, 'You are responsible for the extent you feel hurt'. It is not only the one who hurts you, but also how heavily you take it to heart.'*

(c) Address the demons of your past:
Peter B: *He [a trainer in the Hearing Voices Network] just said: 'You have to address the demons of your past'. And, when I looked at my life, the demon of my past was my abuser. I still regularly used to see her in Sheffield, walking on the street. When I saw that girl I would run away in real fear. Then one day I decided I would listen to what this guy had said to me. I would not run away. When I saw her down the street my first idea was to run. My heart was beating, but I kept eye contact. I kept walking closer to her. She turned her eyes and looked the other way. I then felt I had altered the balance of power. I did not have to fear her anymore. It was actually meaningless.*

(d) Challenging the power of the voices:
Eleanor tells: *I realised that the fear I felt had created this vicious circle of avoidance and isolation. I tentatively began to test out what the voices claimed. One night he said: 'I want you to cut off your toe and if you don't I'll kill your family'. It was the hardest thing I've ever had to do but I said 'Just do it'. It was a terrible night but nothing happened, so I realised he hadn't much power.*

Debra: *I concluded that the demons had made a mistake in choosing me. I was not up to the task and, if they had made a mistake in picking me, then perhaps they were not as infallible or as powerful as I initially believed. I decided to test this out. I decided that I would set the demons some tasks. I gave them the simple task to wash the dishes unaided. They were unable to achieve this, and so the seed of doubt as to their actual power was sown.*

(e) Taking back power:
Debra: *I realised that the only power the voices had was the power I gave them. They needed me to perform tasks and speak to certain people; without me they were impotent. I approached the voices as I would approach any relationship, and began to put parameters around how and when they could contact me.*

Eleanor, after she had challenged the power of her voices, says: *I began to put boundaries in place, saying things to him like 'Do not talk to me before eight o'clock in the evening because I will not talk to you'.*

Jeanette B: *One day my voices told me I had gone too far, I should be punished. I would die the coming night and fall into the hands of the devil. Although I was very afraid I fell asleep and woke up still alive. This was a turning point, I realised they spoke nonsense, and since then I have systematically closed them out and started to concentrate on my own thoughts.*

Flore: *Before I listened to the voice and just did as he said. I learned that I had my own opinion, my own mind, I did not have to follow the voice.*

Sue: *I accepted my voices as real. I looked for solutions in myself. I reclaimed my personal power.*

Lisette: *I think what was most important for me, and gave me power over my voice, was that I was bold enough to become conscious of what had happened in former days [sexual abuse]. That was not easy because when I started talking about the voice, I became really afraid. It was nice of my therapist to say that my anxiety was no reason for her to stop.*

Audrey: *One of the things I did was to support Aud junior [child's voice] to confront the blue voice [voice of abuser]. It took quite a lot, supporting her to stand up to him and to tell him that what he did was wrong. He did back off and she became stronger. That was a really big breakthrough and took a huge amount of power away from that blue voice.*

7. Making choices

Making choices is important for recovery on different levels during the whole process. Very basic choices such as: to stay alive (Jeannette W); to find people as friends to belong to (Frank); to develop oneself (Debra); to do voluntary work to raise self-esteem and self-worth (Karina, Mien, Flore, Riny, Jolanda); to become self-employed (Stewart); to find a purpose in life (Peter B).

Jeannette W had made a number of suicide attempts without success and tells: *My first choice was staying alive, which had consequences, for instance looking after myself. The next choice was to find out that I was OK. Because my therapist found me OK, I started to think 'Why do I have such high demands on myself; what is so bad about me?'*

Frank: *I joined the self-help group and did a study for the network. I didn't think long about it because I knew I needed friends, because I didn't want to become isolated.*

Debra: *I decided I needed to take the risk of inviting real people into my world and cautiously and clumsily this became my new quest. I eventually got to the stage where I began to venture out from my home, continued my education, went to university, made friends and gained employment.*

Karina: *Doing voluntary work helped improve my self-esteem and gave me a focus and something to do. Being creative helped me, gave me a really important focus, and gave me a belief in myself and an outlet for self-expression.*

Stewart: *Another turning point for me was that I wanted to go self-employed. I decided to take the risk of stopping my disability allowance. Once I'd started to make a bit more of my life and I began to work, that was a big thing for me as well, a sort of sense of worth. I think because my self-esteem started to rise a bit more, it gave me a purpose rather than just sitting around drinking cups of tea!'*

Peter B: *When I kind of challenged the dominant voices, I needed some more focus in life, and I actually contacted the Hearing Voices Network in Manchester. They invited me over to meet them, I went and I just felt this is what my life needed to be. I have come through a hell of a lot, so I like to put something back into it. I got involved with more training and started doing some writing. I got a purpose again.*

8. Changing the relationship with your voices

It seems very important in the recovery process to change the relationship with one's voices, and therefore looks like another *sine qua non* requirement. Below are some examples of how voice hearers have managed in a more special way to change their relationship with their voices.

Antje says: *A shaman therapist taught me to talk friendly and slowly to my voices, and ask them to go to the place they belong. After three or four weeks, talking three or four times a day to the voices in this friendly, slow way, they slowed down and became quieter. This made it possible to let the voices I'd heard for so many years vanish.*

Andreas writes: *I realised that the continuous chain of hatred in the relationship between me and my voices needed a breakthrough. Only when I acknowledged that many things the voices were telling me were true did I become able to forgive them. Only when I asked the angry voices to forgive me did I become less depressed.*

Debra writes: *I decided that everything I was doing so far was not working for me, so doing the exact opposite made sense to me. First I changed my attitude towards them. Instead of bowing to their every whim, I embraced them as friends* *and welcomed their intrusions, greeting them with kindness and respect. As a consequence my fear reduced, which in turn alleviated the distress I felt; now when I heard a voice my anxiety level didn't increase. I also began exploring other areas of my life and discovered what role the voices played in my life; the need to feel connected to someone, a need to belong.*

Ami tells: *My relationship with my voices changed when I learned to see them as a signal of my problems, when I learned to react positively to them. When they said to me 'Look at her, what a disaster', I looked in the mirror and thought 'They are right, I should dress properly'. From a negative influence they became a stimulus.*

Eleanor: *Over time I began to have more control of the times, and again it made me question how powerful is he really if he is willing to wait until after EastEnders to talk to me? Having realised these things made me think, well where is he coming from? He's not coming from outside, he can't be, it can only be from me. I was very intrigued by this idea and I began to slowly realise that yes, he is a demon but he was a personal demon.*

Flore: *Before I listened to the voice and just did what he said. I learned that I had my own opinion, my own mind. I did not have to follow the voice.*

Gina: *I have learned to ask them questions, and they appeared to be talking about the things I was thinking about. They told me things that were true. I could not afford such a high rent, I could not stay there.*

Hannelore: *I started to remember me before the time I heard voices, before I got into psychiatric care, and how I managed to cope with them.*

Stewart: *After I set myself up as self-employed, my relationship with my voices changed. I think because my self-esteem started to rise. Work gave me a purpose.*

Jeanette B: when she had challenged the power of her voices says: *This was a turning point. I realised they spoke nonsense and systematically closed them out, and started to concentrate on my own thoughts. Everything I did I thought about, like laying the table I thought 'this is a fork, this is a knife' etc. This gave me control. It took me five years before I had banned them for 100%, but I got rid of them.*

You can see here that the ways people change the relationship are very different, but this seems to be an essential prerequisite to recover from the distress with voices. Changing the relationship seems to become possible with the recognition that the person her/himself gives power to the voices, and by starting to take back power, it becomes possible to change the relationship with the voices. This can be by either becoming friendly and therefore less dependent on the voices (Antje), or by recognising that what the voices are saying has a value for the person (Ami, Sue). A third possibility seems to be taking back full power. We see the first two solutions of changing the relationship from a negative one into a positive less often with people with sexual abuse as the originating trauma. For these people, rather than a positive relationship, there is a growing independency. People become less of a victim and take back power by realising they have minds of their own to make decisions, finding solutions within themselves, and living their own life (Flore). In both situations there are preliminary needs, such as: the need to accept the voices as a reality; learning to talk about them with others; finding support; looking for their role in your life; testing the power of the voices; making choices in starting living one's own life; using voices as a helping hand, but not living their life.

9. Recognising one's own emotions and accepting them

Because traumatic experiences and emotional neglect distort one's emotions, it becomes more difficult not only to cope with them, but also to recognise emotions as one's own. In the case of hearing voices it seems as if there is a kind of 'placing outside' of emotions; and emotions are, in the beginning, felt to be provoked by the voices. Only in the process of recovery do emotions become recognised again as one's own. Some examples:

Eleanor: *Everyone has their private demons, and his [the voice's] demonic aspects were the unaccepted aspects of my self-image. The contempt and loathing that he expresses is actually to do with me in that it reflects how I feel about myself. He is like a very external form of my own insecurities, my own self-doubt.*

Debra: *I also began exploring other areas of my life and discovered what role the voices played in my life: the need to feel connected to someone, a need for a friend, a need to belong. The voices kept me so busy I had no time for any other relationship, and they also spared me the pain and hurt I had experienced by numerous rejections from people in the past. At least they didn't desert me. I decided I needed to take the risk of inviting real people into my world, and cautiously and clumsily this became my new quest.*

Jeannette W: *Because of the tolerance of my therapist I learned that emotions of anger and grief were my emotions, and they may be there. He said: 'I would also have been angry if what has happened to you had happened to me. How is it possible that you are angry and I don't see anything?'* Jeanette became conscious that she hardly knew who she was: *I am nobody, that's what has happened to me. Who I am is my voices. I didn't know who I was, I didn't know what my feelings were, what was from the voices and what was from others.* And later she discovered: *The girl that lay there, that was me. At last I had been able to feel the pain I felt at the time. The death agony I had was me. I felt my body again without missing a piece of it. I had to recognise myself and especially accept myself.*

Sasja: *You realise the consequences of hearing voices much later. You have to change yourself also, whether you like it or not. I don't like change. Now I am more philosophical but before I wanted to control everything.*

The more the process of recovery develops, the more the relationship with the voices becomes functional instead of pathological. They become the mirrors of the soul and well-being; a reflection of one's mental health and well-being.

CHAPTER 2

THE DISEASE CONCEPT OF HEARING VOICES AND ITS HARMFUL ASPECTS

MARIUS ROMME

Hearing voices has been reported throughout history, from the ancient civilisations of Egypt, Rome, Babylon, Tibet and Greece up to the modern day (Watkins, 1998). The earliest, well-known voice hearer was Socrates (469–399BC) and although he reported the voice of a demon, he valued the voice positively. Socrates' testimony of hearing voices was followed by the experience of religious figures, such as Mohammed, Jesus, George Fox (one of the founders of Quakerism), Saint Paul and Saint Teresa. Perhaps the best-known voice hearer was Joan of Arc. More recent names include politicians, Swedenborg and Ghandi; poets, Rilke and William Blake; the author Virginia Woolf, and the composer, Robert Schumann.

In some non-Western societies hearing voices is still interpreted as a relatively normal experience and often appreciated positively (Al-Issa, 1977; de Jong, 1987). However, in most parts of the Western world, a person who hears voices is immediately seen as someone with a psychiatric problem, typically suffering from schizophrenia. Confronted with different beliefs between past and present, and between non-Western and Western cultures, two questions surface: Did Socrates, Jesus, Mohammed, Joan of Arc and Ghandi suffer from an illness? And is this also true for voice hearers in modern Western societies? Or is it possible that voice hearers in our Western society are wrongly observed as being mentally ill and suffering from schizophrenia. The difference between the disease concept and modern epidemiological research will give us the answer.

THE DISEASE CONCEPT

Over the last thirty years, especially with so-called psychotic experiences like hearing voices, there has been a growing tendency to reduce mental health problems to symptoms of disease, rather than reactions to problems in the patient's life. The basic assumption of the 'clinical' psychiatric approach is the existence of a specific disease that leads to symptoms, including voice hearing, and experienced as an illness: illness being the subjective experience of the disease. This disease is called 'schizophrenia' and, with the development of psychiatric thinking, hearing voices has become linked to this disease. It is assumed that schizophrenia produces symptoms in a similar way to, say, diabetes. In diabetes, the symptoms of the disease are the result of a disturbance of sugar levels in the body; the disease is a process that affects the production of insulin, and the illness experience is how this makes us feel; we do not feel blood-sugar levels but their effect – for example, tiredness, dizziness, excessive thirst – and these are rightly interpreted as symptoms of the disease. It is argued that voices are, in the same way, an illness experience arising from the 'disease', schizophrenia. The difference is that with diabetes we know what causes the symptoms, for example, thirst is an understandable consequence of the disturbance of insulin production. In schizophrenia this is not the case since nobody really knows the cause of this disease, so symptoms such as hearing voices are neither logically nor understandably related to that disease. However, in the absence of other evidence about the origins of voice hearing, this idea of the experience being caused by the 'disease' schizophrenia has been kept alive.

WHAT DO WE NOW KNOW FROM EPIDEMIOLOGICAL RESEARCH?

We now know that we should not simply regard hearing voices as one of a collection of symptoms that, together, form evidence of disease. Instead, we should focus on the voice-hearing experience itself, because we now know, at least in most cases, that voices are reactions to problems in life and between people.

Studies in the 1990s have shown that hearing voices, meeting the psychiatric criteria of an auditory hallucination, are apparent in about 4% of the normal Western population, most of them without other signs or symptoms indicating a disease process (Tien, 1991; Eaton et al., 1991; Bijl et al., 1998; van Os et al., 2001; Johns & van Os, 2001). Evidence suggests that about one-third of this 4% are indeed in need of mental health care, but about two-thirds do not feel this need, i.e., they do not feel troubled or ill. Rather, this latter group mostly experiences their voices as helpful, for example, as a kind of advisor in the problems of daily life or with personal problems of an existential type. These epidemiological studies underpin the ideas that hearing voices is not in itself a sign of psychopathology but rather a signal of other problems, and that identifying hearing voices with a mental disease, especially schizophrenia, is not only scientifically wrong but also harmful, as the stories in this book show.

WHY A SIGNAL OF A PROBLEM?

We also now know that in 70% of 'patients' (meaning people who have difficulty in coping with this experience) the voices are related to trauma and/or powerless-making situations. Trauma includes: sexual abuse; physical abuse; emotional neglect; severe bullying; high levels of stress; and situations that have produced insecurity in the sensitive adolescent period. All these might lead to an intense feeling of powerlessness and can have a disrupting effect on coping with emotions. This has been studied on a personal level (Romme & Escher, 1989, 1996b, 2000, 2008a; Escher, 2005a; Ensink, 1992; and others) showing that trauma-related experiences are found in the characteristics, triggers and content of the voices. The relationship between hearing voices and experienced trauma has also been studied on an epidemiological level by Read et al (2005) who conclude from a literature review of 180 studies:

> Symptoms considered indicative of psychosis and schizophrenia, particularly hallucinations, are at least as strongly related to childhood abuse and neglect as many other mental health problems. Recent large-scale, general population studies indicate the relationship is a causal one, with a dose effect. (p. 1)

In the meantime, scientific criticism of the diagnosis 'schizophrenia' has been growing and argues that, scientifically speaking, the disease of schizophrenia does not really exist; rather, it is just a group of very different people labelled as such (Bentall, 1990, 2003; Boyle, 1990; Blom, 2003, and many others).

HARMFUL ASPECTS OF TRADITIONAL PSYCHIATRIC CARE AND TREATMENT

The stories in this book demonstrate quite literally how harmful it is to identify hearing voices with the 'disease' schizophrenia. This diagnosis alienates the voice hearer from their experience; it makes them a passive victim of disease; it inhibits an individual's existing capability and potential and so impedes recovery. The person is given a lot of negative and pessimistic information about the nature of the disease. Even now, the person is often made to believe that they will be ill for the rest of their lives with little or no possibility of recovery, and that they will need to adapt to lifelong disability. In short, the disease concept of hearing voices can destroy the potential for a helpful relationship between voice hearer and professional.

Research about recovery seems not to be believed by many mental health professionals. It seems that, because of their conviction that they are dealing with a real disease from which the symptoms stem, they have no reason to become interested in the cause of the individual symptoms, such as hearing voices. This sort of thinking ignores the problems that lie at the root of the hearing voices experience; they are not asked for, not analysed, but effectively denied and neglected. The problems of the voice hearer, who then becomes a patient, are not spoken about, and he/she is not helped to cope with them. On the contrary, the voices are seen as signs of madness, and this lowers the already challenged self-esteem of the voice hearer and diminishes the capacity to solve his/her problems. Voice hearers are not helped to detect the relationship between their voices and what has happened in their lives, nor are they helped with the distorted emotions as a consequence. People cannot, therefore, be helped to recover with this traditional way of thinking and practice in psychiatry. And it is not just psychiatry but society at large that persists in believing in this disease concept, creating a situation in which voices are something to be afraid of. Hearing voices in Western societies is wholly associated with the negative views and consequences of schizophrenia, distancing voice hearers from others, and preventing them from becoming part of society again, from getting a job, a mortgage, or even a driving licence.

THE STORIES IN THIS BOOK

The personal histories in this book tell a different story; they are stories of recovery, of using one's own capabilities and making one's own dreams come true. They show that it is entirely possible to learn to cope with one's voices, to take back power, and to live one's own life again. The necessary thing is not to get rid of the voices but, rather, to change one's relationship with them – a process in which medication sometimes plays an important but minor role. These stories also show that there are now mental health professionals who look differently at the voice-hearing experience and who can play an important role in starting the recovery process.

We are also shown the harmful outcomes of wrong treatment: total misunderstanding resulting from the missing link between the treatment and the patient's problem. This is well formulated by **Jacqui:**

> *I knew that what had happened to me as a child was the root cause of my distress. To my astonishment the psychiatrists that I tried to tell either denied my experience or told me that I would never, ever recover from what had happened. They told me that I had an illness. I was mentally ill. I was expected to be the passive recipient of treatment for a disorder I had; that medication was the only option open to me, and that, actually, I would never really get better anyway. No one ever asked me what I thought might help. The fact that I listened to my voices was evidence of my illness.*

To be able to more easily digest the information given in the stories we will give examples of the following harmful aspects of the traditional treatment and disease concept of hearing voices:

1. Equating hearing voices with the diagnosis of schizophrenia
2. The negative effects of psychiatric hospital admission
3. The 'no hope' and 'lifelong illness' message
4. The passive victim of a pathology approach; not encouraged to help oneself
5. The dominance of the diagnosis of schizophrenia, disregarding all other problems
6. 'Schizophrenia' as a lifelong label
7. Neither interest in the voices, nor in what underlies the experience
8. Inability to accept people's experience
9. When medication doesn't have the presumed effect, no alternatives suggested
10. Medication leading to social breakdown
11. The disease concept destroying the relationship between the voice hearer and the professional
12. Promoting a belief in society at large that hearing voices is a sign of madness
13. Difficulties of social acceptance arising from the diagnosis of schizophrenia

1. Equating hearing voices with the diagnosis of schizophrenia

This has a wide range of consequences, with psychiatrists seemingly convinced of the harmfulness of hearing voices.

Ronny: *My hearing voices increased when I moved away from home to start school. I struggled a lot with anxiety and confusion. After a while I was sent to an outpatient psychiatric clinic where my psychiatrist asked me if I heard voices. I answered 'No'. My psychiatrist was glad to hear that: 'Otherwise we would have to hospitalise you in a psychiatric institution,' he said.*

Eleanor: *The psychiatrist equated hearing voices with insanity. I got the diagnosis of 'schizophrenia'. What started off as experience became a symptom.*

Stewart: *I had been hacking into computers at school, somebody else got the blame. I felt guilty but unable to own up. I stopped going to school and just said I was not feeling well.*

After a while I was referred to a psychiatrist. I got medication. When I first took that medication I slept for a day, my tongue swelled and I couldn't stand up.

On that day, about eleven in the morning, I started hearing this really bad voice. I was given an injection and the side effects went away, but not for long. The voice also persisted. I was sent to a day centre. I was only fifteen and spending my day with older people. One day my mum, dad and me went to see a psychologist. I was told my diagnosis was schizophrenia and that my prospects for the future 'were not great'.

2. Being hospitalised, often only because of hearing voices, with the consequence of lowering already challenged self-esteem and self-confidence

Eleanor: *I made an appointment with my GP, who referred me to a psychiatrist. I presented myself as a confused, troubled eighteen-year-old who didn't have much self-esteem or confidence in herself and who was worried about her future. The psychiatrist disregarded all of this and honed in on what she perceived as this developing psychosis. She said: 'I would like you to come into hospital voluntarily, just for three days or so.' But I stayed much longer. It was a savage and terrifying experience. I was the youngest person there by about twenty years. It was hugely disempowering. It was all undermining my sense of self, exacerbating all my doubts about myself. The devastating impact just served to make the voices stronger and more aggressive.*

Many stories record that hospital care was not helpful regarding the hearing voices experience: Antje, Audrey, Caroline, Don, Frank, Gina, Hannelore, Jacqui, Jan, Jeannette W, Johnny, Jolanda, Mieke, Odi, Olga, Peggy, Peter B, Peter R, Ron, Ronny, Rufus, Sjon, Stewart and Sue. Others either don't talk about their hospital admissions or have not been admitted to a psychiatric hospital. Only two clearly positive psychiatric hospital treatment experiences are recorded: Elisabeth, on a traditional ward and only for a short time, and Mien, who received psychotherapy rather than traditional treatment because of being suicidal.

3. The 'no hope' and 'lifelong illness' message

Stewart: *I was only fifteen. I was given a diagnosis of schizophrenia, and different professionals – nurses, social workers, psychologists and psychiatrists – all gave the same sort of message, time and time again: my prospects for the future were 'not great'; I shouldn't have expectations about school, or work, or relationships.*

Olga: *I was a schizophrenic, they said 'please remember that, oh, and while you are at it, remember to stop thinking there is a cure, you are a chronic, a chronic schizophrenic, a biological defect with an incurable disease'.*

4. The passive victim of a pathology approach; not encouraged to help oneself

> **Audrey** tells of her psychiatric care experiences: *Going round in circles and not going anywhere. It was very frightening and I felt such hopelessness. No one in the psychiatric services gave me any hope. In fact, it was the opposite. In one week I had two appointments: on the Tuesday they told me that I had manic depression, and on the Thursday they told me it was schizophrenia. What do you do with that? They are completely bizarre words that don't mean anything.*

For **Eleanor,** having schizophrenia meant being seen as a passive victim and being given only drug therapy.

> *The psychiatrist equated hearing voices with insanity. I got the diagnosis of schizophrenia. With this I got the message that I was a passive victim of pathology. I wasn't encouraged to do anything to actively help myself. Therapy meant drug therapy.*

5. The dominance of the diagnosis of schizophrenia, disregarding all other problems

We have often observed this with people who started hearing voices after having problems in adolescence.

> **Johnny:** *I first heard the voices at the age of fifteen, during the school summer holidays. During that time and leading up to it I had been extensively bullied at school due to dyslexia and a slight speech impediment. I felt no control over the voices whatsoever. Over the next few years I became an alcoholic. If I became drunk enough, I had a little respite from the voices. I was eventually admitted to the local psychiatric hospital, but I still told no one of the voices. I was treated for my alcohol abuse and later for depression. During my third or fourth admission I finally told a student nurse I heard voices; the relief was immense. However, my diagnosis was quickly altered to that of schizophrenia and I was heavily medicated. The dose was increased each time I was asked if I still heard voices and said 'Yes'. The only result during ten years was more and more social isolation, inhibited by the voices, dulled by the medication and with no one ever talking about the original problems.*

> **Stewart** says: *I was generally feeling very insecure, and to cap it all I was being bullied by the head boy at school. I felt I had nowhere to turn. I stopped going to school and just said I was not feeling well. Eventually, my mum took me to the family doctor. I was referred to a specialist. I had no idea it was a psychiatrist. When I first had medication I slept for a day and when I woke up I just realised something was different, my tongue had swelled and I couldn't stand up. That day I started hearing this really bad voice. I recognised the voice as the bully from*

school: the head boy. I was sent to a day centre. I was then only fifteen and spent my day with people at least fifteen to twenty years older than me. One day my mum, dad and me went to see a psychologist and she asked if we had any idea about my psychosis. I mentioned schizophrenia because of what I'd learnt from talking to other patients. She said I was right. Stewart was not helped with his problems but sent in another direction and treated with medication only, which did not change his voices.

Rufus says: *At the age of eighteen I found myself in a boring job as an office junior. I was anxious about my future as I had failed in my education. On top of this, emotionally, I was struggling to adjust to the fact that my first girlfriend, who I had been with, been with for a year, had left me. This left a big hole in my life. Also, I found myself socially isolated: my best friend was in Germany and I was trying to avoid my former dope-smoking friends. I found psychiatric treatment very oppressive, the drugs I was being given slowed my thinking and made me weak and impotent. Nobody talked to me about my experiences and ideas. They thought this would encourage them and make them worse. Because my grandfather and aunt had been given diagnoses of schizophrenia, doctors were convinced I had this condition that they assumed was genetic.*

Not having an open-minded interest in what has happened to the voice hearer is not only related to diagnosis but also to the voice-hearing experience itself. It can lead to a change in what would have been the right treatment, as with Ami, or to ceasing to talk about what has happened, as with Mien and many others.

Ami tells us: *The second time in hospital I got Haldol and the doctor also gave me early retirement. It was well meant but came as a blow: 'I am worthless'. The voices did not react to Haldol so I stopped taking it. In an earlier period, when I had depressions in winter time, I got antidepressants which worked fine; it was only when they found out that I heard voices that I got neuroleptic medication. Why?*

Mien says: *The [sexual] abuse history still haunted me and therefore I became depressed. I was prescribed different kinds of medication which helped neither for the voices nor for my depression. However I was told to take my medication and not to talk about what had happened.*

6. 'Schizophrenia' as a lifelong label

The diagnosis of schizophrenia can have a stigmatising effect in the sense that, having been given this diagnosis, it becomes a convenient label – nobody looks further than the diagnosis and the patient continues to be treated the same way, even when they go to a different psychiatrist. There are exceptions however.

Dirk Corstens, one of the psychiatrists involved in this study, recalls of **Don**: *He was admitted to hospital because of a psychosis in 1984. He was given a diagnosis of schizophrenia. After that, he was admitted for some years to acute wards and follow-up departments and for the last seven years he had lived in a sheltered home. Most of his day was spent sitting in a chair and he hardly talked. When his wife brought him to me in 1999, he had already spent sixteen years in psychiatric care systems in this way. My conversation was mainly with his wife. He listened intently but was obviously tired. He told me that he was hardly hindered by his voices. After a few contacts I suggested his psychiatrist lower the dose of his medication, because his behaviour could possibly be explained by its negative effect. Slowly, he became more talkative. He read books again, spent more time at home with his wife and looked after himself better ... He also started to talk about the difficulties in his life before his psychosis. He changed to a low dose of medication and, four years later, was invited by me to reflect on his recovery.*

Don says: *I observed everything but I lost my identity. My feelings stood still. Slowly I regained my identity and returned to a state of harmony. I have made a decision to not go back to my native country because that has been always a reason for great stress.* **Dirk Corstens** says of this evaluation talk: *Don, compared with 1999, is a totally different man. He speaks clearly, makes jokes, has a vivid imagination and sees things in perspective. He has really outgrown the diagnosis of schizophrenia.*

7. **Neither interest in the voices, nor in what underlies the experience**
Helen, who was severely abused and criticised throughout her childhood by her father, says: *As a psychology undergraduate at Manchester University I sought help for my difficulties. I was referred to a clinical psychologist. After a few sessions she described herself as a Freudian therapist and informed me that my experiences of abuse were not real but the result of fantasy.* She goes on: *For the past sixteen years I have worked as a clinical psychologist in the mental health system. The prevailing psychiatric worldview offers no insight into the experience of psychological distress and voice hearing.*

This lack of interest in the voice-hearing experience becomes clear when people meet professionals who *are* interested.
Peggy: *Seven years ago I met Dr Phil Thomas and was relieved to meet someone who was really interested in voice hearing. Previously, no one had wanted to know, in spite of being admitted to hospital for ten weeks out of control of myself and others.*

Antje, who had spent many years in psychiatric hospitals, recalls: *At that time (after having met the Berlin Hearing Voices Network) I had a new doctor. She* *was different; she was the first one to ask if anything had happened to me at the start of my hearing voices experience.*

8. Inability to accept people's experiences

In all the stories we see psychiatry as being unable to accept people's hearing voices experiences. It also seems to be difficult for psychiatry to accept experience associated with cultural background. **Odi,** 37 years old and born in Nigeria, was tortured for three days in 2000 by an officially endorsed army group commonly known as the 'Bakassi Boys'.

Odi says: *I knew that I had to escape from Nigeria and, with the help of Amnesty International, I came to England. I was living in London, but the chaos of the city made my panic attacks worse and all I could hear was negative voices. I feared that people were following me and that they wanted to kill me. It was a very bad time. Because of the problems I was having, my GP arranged for a psychiatrist, and this doctor sent me to a psychiatric ward. They saw me as a mad person who was delusional, as I was still talking to my voices. They diagnosed me with schizophrenia. They told me that I needed medication and I said, 'But I am the doctor not you.' They asked to meet with some of my family and friends who said, 'Yes, this is our culture'. They began to understand me by reading my poems and looking at my paintings and sculptures. They began to see that I wasn't mad – I was a person. My voices helped me to combat the panic attacks and flashbacks.*

9. When medication doesn't have the presumed effect, and no alternatives are suggested

Eleanor: *Therapy meant drug therapy. It was hugely disempowering. It was all undermining my sense of self, exacerbating all my doubts about myself. The devastating impact just served to make the voices stronger and more aggressive. I went from hearing one mild rather banal voice, to three, then eight, then twelve voices, and then this dominant voice shows.*

Debra: *I had been under mental health services and, although I was heavily medicated, the voices persisted.*

Ron: *I received many different kinds of medication. The voices kept coming, and the response from the psychiatrist was to increase the dose or change the kind of medication. No matter what was done, the voices persisted.*

Ronny: *I tried to kill myself, but it only brought me into a psychiatric institution. During that period I was in and out of institutions several times. I was asked if I heard voices but no more than that. I received antipsychotic medication, but the voices were still there.*

Rufus: *I found psychiatric treatment very oppressive. The drugs slowed my thinking and made me weak and impotent. Nobody talked to me about my experiences and ideas. During my second hospital admission my close friend, Catherine, returned from abroad and started to visit me almost every day. She showed me an acceptance that was deeply healing. She believed I would get through this breakdown.*

10. Medication leading to social breakdown

Johnny: *The dosage was increased over a period of time because each time I was asked if I still heard voices, I said 'Yes'. During the next ten years I became more and more isolated, socially. I managed to continue living alone but with massive support from the social psychiatric home help. Inhibited by the voices and dulled by the medication, I slept sixteen to eighteen hours a day and ordered junk food so that I didn't have to go out or cook for myself. My only outside interest was chess, which I continued to pursue but found difficult due to interference by the voices.*

Ron: *I had been in and out psychiatric hospital for eight years. I received many different kinds of medication: Clozaril, Methotrimeprazine, Lithium, Procyclidine and Clomipramine. The voices kept coming and the response from the psychiatrist was to increase the dose or change the medication. No matter what was done, the voices persisted. My life was just a mess, a total mess. I had nothing anymore and neither was I interested in anything. I stayed in bed for about twenty hours a day. I did not want to talk to anybody. I was only interested in what was happening in my head.*

Antje: *When I think about all the years in psychiatry I have the impression that every time I was dismissed and went back to normal life, there was this reduction of possibilities in my life. Nearly ten years later, I was not interested in anything anymore. Now I think there is a relation between the voices and my life history but, then, I didn't think that.*

Don's story recalls: *He had been in a psychiatric hospital for sixteen years, treated nearly exclusively with neuroleptic medication. At the age of forty-six he was admitted with a psychosis in which he heard voices. The consequence of the medication, as was shown later, was that he could hardly speak and had isolated himself from the people around him.*

Debra: *I have been under mental health services and although I was heavily medicated, the voices persisted and my body was lethargic and agitated at the same time.*

Gina: *Medication never really helped me, but I muddled along with it for two years.*

11. The disease concept destroying the relationship between the voice hearer and the professional

In all the above-mentioned stories we see a negative relationship between voice hearer and professional (mainly psychiatrists) as a result of the disease concept, with a no-hope and lifelong illness message. The illness position promotes a passive victim role – not being listened to, being treated with medication only – helping neither with the voices nor addressing the person's problems. In the stories of Antje, Caroline, Debra, Don, Eleanor, Flore, Gavin, Gina, Jeannette W, Johnny, Jolanda, Karina, Mieke, Odi, Olga, Patsy, Peggy, Peter B, Ron, Ronny, Rufus, Sjon, Stewart and Sue, we see the negative influence counteracted by a professional who primarily takes up a relationship with them, shows them a way forward and offers another perspective. Positive influence comes from a variety of sources: a psychiatrist (Antje, Ami, Caroline, Don, Eleanor, Gina, Gavin, Jeannette W, Jolanda, Patsy and Peggy); a nurse (Audrey and Flore); a social worker (Hannelore, Johnny, Peter B, Ron and Ronny); a general practitioner (Stewart); a complementary therapist (Mieke and Antje); another voice hearer (Ron and Ami); a hearing voices group (Frank, Karina and Sue); a friend (Debra, Olga and Rufus); a family member (Antje and Odi) and our children's research (Sjon).

We have worked through these examples in Chapter 1 'Important Steps to Recovery with Voices', which illustrates that it is possible for mental health professionals, including psychiatrists, to take another perspective.

12. Promoting a belief in society at large that hearing voices is a sign of madness

The disease approach influences the reaction to hearing voices of both the voice hearers themselves and their families and friends. Identification with madness often starts for voice hearers with the fear they are going mad.

Hannelore says: *I was 16 when I first heard voices. I was so afraid of being seen as mad that I told nobody.*

Debra says: *I had not told my nurse of my beliefs as I was sworn to secrecy, therefore she was unaware and unable to assist me adequately.*

Friends are also frequently convinced of the illness concept; they then express their anxiety and advise people to seek psychiatric treatment.

Eleanor writes: *I made the fatal mistake of mentioning to one of my friends that I was hearing this voice and the impact that it had on me. She was absolutely horrified and said that hearing voices is not a good thing and that I should get some help.*

Not everybody listens to that kind of advice, for instance:

Sasja says: *I have a woman friend who told her psychiatrist about me hearing voices; she thought it was dangerous and that I needed medication, she tried to convince me to go to this psychiatrist. I thought about it briefly but decided not to go.*

13. Difficulties of social acceptance arising from the diagnosis of schizophrenia

There are drawbacks on different social levels, including blatant personal discrimination, as with **Eleanor**, who recalls:

I went into that hospital a troubled, confused, unhappy 18-year-old and came out a schizophrenic – and I was a good one. It all escalated. There was this terrible domino effect because the more people polarised and victimised me the more bizarre my behaviour became. I was spat at outside the Students Union and I became this really sad and lonely figure who would drift around campus on her own and sit on her own in lectures. I'd walk into a room and hear this flurry of laugher. People started calling me 'psycho'.

Less brutal on first sight, but also difficult to live with, are the prejudices in society about schizophrenia; a growing handicap for those who are given the diagnosis and yet like to live freely, without being discriminated against.

Frans was given the diagnosis of 'paranoid schizophrenia' having worked for many years in a large organisation as an IT specialist. He also has a Master's degree in physics.

Frans says: *Because of my diagnosis I am confronted with a number of consequences:*
- *No psychotherapy. There is no discussion about the experience of hearing voices, neither is there any discussion about the problems that lie at their roots.*
- *The advice not to have children because of the point of view that you have a genetic disease.*
- *When I report my health status to the occupational health doctor, that I perceive myself to be fully capable to work, it is interpreted as fraud.*
- *After telling the occupational health doctor that I hear voices, I am immediately treated like a child and information is requested from the psychiatrist or CPN about whether it is true that I am able to work.*
- *At my annual work assessment alarm bells ring – even after having worked for a year full time, a report is requested from the psychiatrist before my contract is renewed.*
- *With financial transactions I always have to make a written declaration that something is wrong with me, with the consequence that the cost of life insurance, for example, becomes higher.*

- *When I want to become self-employed I encounter the same problems with health insurance and unemployment insurance. This problem, twenty years later, still persists.*
- *As soon as the diagnosis of schizophrenia has been given, I am regarded as not able to speak for myself, I am measured according to an average norm and a medical doctor has to be consulted to approve what I have said.*

Not only do the negative influences of the traditional approach make recovery difficult, the lack of any positive input from the traditional approach makes it harder too, because, to recover, the voice hearer needs to be stimulated and supported in many ways. The eleven issues or steps that are important to helping recovery from distress with voices are outlined inc Chapter 1 'Important Steps to Recovery with Voices', with examples provided. They demonstrate that the road to recovery does not take the direction of suppressing the voices but moves toward changing the relationship with them. Most voice hearers who recover still hear voices.

WHAT MIGHT PSYCHIATRY HAVE BEEN DOING WITH PSYCHIATRIC PATIENTS HEARING VOICES?

It is hard to believe that there is no scientific basis for the way psychiatry has developed its blanket approach to psychotic experience. I have been a psychiatrist for some forty-five years and I, too, have experienced there being some truth in the categorisation of illness behaviour with psychiatric patients. For me it is true and I know from other psychiatrists that one can recognise people who are given a diagnosis of schizophrenia, dissociative disorder or borderline disorder – and with all three diagnoses it was mostly people who experienced hearing voices. But I was never able to answer the question: 'What is it that I recognise?' Now I think I know what it is. Most of my life as a psychiatrist I didn't recognise it because I didn't make comparisons between these three groups of people, nor did I have a clue what hearing voices was about. It has only been since studying these experiences intensively that I have come to understand what people are talking about when they speak of recognising a diagnostic label.

As we know, there are four categories of psychiatric illness in which hearing voices are often apparent: schizophrenia; dissociative disorder; borderline personality disorder; and depression with so-called 'psychotic traits'. When we compare these people, we can imagine what clinical psychiatry is more or less doing. They have tried to give labels on the basis of symptom combinations but, in reality, it looks as if they have given (strange) names to the emotional reaction patterns that people show after being traumatised.

Voice hearers as a group react, emotionally, quite differently to their trauma experiences. There are four main reactions to distinguish between. Some people become withdrawn; this is the reaction we usually see in those diagnosed with schizophrenia. Others express anger about what has happened to them but don't talk easily about it because of shame and anxiety, and because they find it to hard to live with the experience. They tend to fight for their interests and perceive themselves as not being heard; this reaction we see in the group often diagnosed with borderline personality disorder. We also see people who react by taking flight from the experience, literally escaping with their minds from the situation they are in; this we see with people diagnosed with dissociative disorder. The fourth reaction pattern is feeling guilty. Through powerlessness to change what has happened, they direct their anger towards themselves. They become depressed and are possibly diagnosed with depression. It is also possible to react by trying to control one's emotions by becoming obsessional. There are also descriptions of people not being able to accept their emotions and overruling them by becoming manic. This is not an attempt to restore a diagnostic system but just an (unscientific) attempt to understand what professionals perceive when they recognise diagnostic labels.

WHAT MIGHT BE CHANGED?

The most important change might be that the relationship between voice hearer and professional becomes the centre of the treatment. This means listening to each other, being interested in each other, believing each other, becoming unafraid of each other, trusting each other, supporting each other, exchanging and accepting experience, exchanging knowledge and thinking together.

The problems connected with the diagnosis of schizophrenia, however, provide sufficient reason to change aspects of this diagnosis. The evidence presented here begs for these changes:

1. It should be acknowledged that hearing voices is apparent in different categories of psychiatric illness, and is, therefore, not predominantly equated with schizophrenia; only one in six of all voice hearers meet the traditional psychiatric criteria for the diagnosis of schizophrenia.
2. It should also be acknowledged that hearing voices is related to traumatic experiences for many voice-hearers (70%) and that the voices are expressing emotions disturbed as a result of those traumas.

Therefore:

3. Psychiatrists should complete their diagnostic activities by exploring the background to the person's complaints – and this holds not only for voices but also for other 'symptoms'. This requires training to use instruments that are now available for hearing voices, delusions and self-harm. Instruments could also be developed for negative symptoms and obsessive-compulsive disorder (OCD) behaviour.

4. Psychiatrists should talk about illness on the basis of scientific knowledge rather than prejudice that cannot stand up to scientific standards, for example, the no-hope prognosis that is still regularly given in relation to the chronic course of psychiatric illness. And more consideration should be given to the effects of medication.

5. Psychiatrists should return to their original role of helping people, relating to patients in a supportive way, trying to find out (as in all other branches of medicine) the background to mental health problems, rather than ignoring possible causes of so-called 'psychosis'.

6. Psychiatry should change its practice of constructing diagnoses from symptom combinations only; it could instead categorise them according to the main complaint hindering the person. This would open the way to research on the basis of scientific, more valid and independent variables than the Diagnostic and Statistical Manual for Mental Disorders (DSM) categories.

7. Psychiatry and psychology should acknowledge that, on the basis of available epidemiological research, hearing voices and a number of other mental health problems are not, in themselves, signs of psychopathology, and that becoming ill can be the result of other circumstances, the consequences of experiencing trauma, which can be explored and understood.

8. Psychiatrists, psychologists, nurses and social workers, support workers and others involved in mental health care, should recognise that their profession is, above all, a profession dealing with people's disturbed emotions.

9. Prescribing neuroleptic medication for voice hearing should be neither an automatic, nor obvious solution. If used, the effects of the medication should at least be followed up in order to balance the positive and negative consequences.

CHAPTER 3

WHAT CAUSES HEARING VOICES?

MARIUS ROMME

The question, 'What causes people to hear voices?' can be answered at different levels, for instance, on the level of the voice hearer who recognises the voice. For example, when a voice hearer recognises the voice he/she hears as the voice of a deceased person, when asked about where the voice is coming from they will say, 'the voice is coming from so and so'; they *don't* say that this is the cause of their voice-hearing experience.

Another level of explanation, valuable to all voice hearers, is that of scientists who want to know what kind of brain problem or brain capacity or psychological process is responsible for the experience of hearing voices? This has led to many kinds of supposition, one example of which is, for people with a COMT gene disorder, the use of cannabis can lead to schizophrenia, because genetic variations might modify associations between schizophrenia and tobacco use – which, by the way, it doesn't (Zammit et al., 2007). Lately Aleman and Laroi (2008) have developed a complex model that shows how a hallucination can be the result of a complex interaction between psychological and biological factors. This is like explaining how the motor in a motor car works, but not how the car functions. This kind of research, whilst in itself interesting and providing quite a lot of information about the brain, has not yet given any plausible answer to the question of why someone hears voices.

Another level of evidence is about what happens in the brain when people hear voices. It is well known and moreover confirmed that when a person hears a voice there is at, the same time, activity in the speech centre of the brain (McGuire et al., 1995). However this is not a causal relationship, it merely shows that something is happening in the brain when hearing voices, more evidence of a reality base.

The level at which we prefer to answer the question, 'What causes the hearing of voices?' is through a combination of epidemiological and qualitative research into the experience of voice hearers themselves. On the epidemiological level, Read et al. (2005) have recently published a literature review of 180 studies and concluded:

> Symptoms considered indicative of psychosis and schizophrenia, particularly hallucinations, are at least as strongly related to childhood abuse and neglect as many other mental health problems. Recent large-scale general population studies indicate the relationship is a causal one, with a dose effect. (p. 330)

At the qualitative level of studying the experience of voice hearers, we have observed in our own research (in several studies adding up to around 350 voice hearers) that voices are expressing, by what they say and how they interact with the voice hearer, what has happened in the life of the voice hearer. From these two levels of research we think it becomes clear that traumatic experiences play an important causal part in people developing voice-hearing experiences. This qualitative type of study has also been undertaken by Ensink (1992), who looked at the relationship between sexual abuse and hearing voices or seeing images.

Hearing voices often starts as a helping influence. This can be the case with children during difficult times who are then helped by their voices telling them they are good and not guilty, and giving them hope for the future. They later become negative because others don't accept the voice hearing but, instead, identify it with illness. For example, as a child and throughout her adolescence, Caroline had accepted her voices and allowed them to protect her in an environment where she was neglected and misused. When she was about 21 she became a member of a religious sect. There, other members told her that the voices were instruments of the devil. From then on, Caroline wanted to get rid of the voices and they became ugly towards her. It is usually friends, family or family doctors who react negatively when told by the person that they hear voices, and who tell them to go to a psychiatrist (which does not tend to solve the problem; for more on this, see Chapter 2, 'The Disease Concept of Hearing Voices and Its Harmful Aspects'.

This chapter looks at the kinds of trauma that lie at the root of the hearing-voices experience. We answer the question: 'What has been experienced by voice hearers who have recovered from the distress caused by their voices?' This concerns voice hearers who have gained insight into the relationship between their voices and their traumatic background. The fifty stories in this book cover the following traumatic experiences (in order of frequency):

1. Sexual abuse (18, plus 3 combined with emotional and 3 combined with physical neglect)
2. Emotional neglect (11, plus 3 combined with sexual abuse)

3. Adolescent problems (6)
4. High levels of stress (4)
5. Being bullied (2)
6. Physical abuse (2, plus 3 combined with sexual abuse)
7. Not clear (7)

Giving numbers is always a tricky business because, as can be seen above, there are people whose stories include sexual abuse and who have also experienced emotional neglect. There are also quite a number of voice hearers who suffered emotional neglect as children and who later in their lives, when experiencing high levels of stress, started to hear voices. You could say that traumatic experience, such as emotional neglect during childhood, induces stress vulnerability. An emotionally neglected person has more difficulty coping with emotions, making him more vulnerable to stress, and this might trigger voice hearing. The stress is often quite specific, such as the stress of failure (Frank), or stress related to aggression (Frans). We see this vulnerability with other traumatic childhood experiences (for example, sexual abuse) because trauma leads to a distortion of emotions. Sexual abuse is usually a clearly remembered traumatic experience; this is less often the case with emotional neglect. In the following stories, emotional neglect is not always clearly an isolated experience. It is more often hidden, part of the traumatic background; a story within a story.

So the main objective of this study is not numbers but, rather, what voice hearers tell us about their traumatic experience and its relationship with their voices. To explore these links one could systematically interview the voice hearer about their experience; about the characteristics of each voice separately, because they might be similar to persons involved in the traumatic experience; about the beginning of the voice-hearing experience, because this can be the time traumatic experiences took place; about what the voices tell the person, because this can be about what has happened to the person or give an idea about the emotions involved; about what triggers the voices, because this can reflect the vulnerable emotions as a consequence of the traumatic experiences.

We will give examples of each kind of trauma we have differentiated:

1. Sexual abuse
Some people start hearing voices as soon as the abuse starts and experience the relationship between their voices and the sexual abuse from the beginning:

Jo: *I first started to hear a voice after an early traumatic episode of abuse. I remember my first voice so clearly because it took on the identity of the person who had abused me.*

Helen: *I suffered severe abuse throughout my childhood and have always known my voices to be related to this. I am very clear about the nature and origin of my voices. I see them as post-traumatic after-effects of the abuse; natural and normal in the circumstances.*

Others start to hear a voice later, and recognise it as that of the abuser. **Flore** started to hear a voice when she was 14. This was when she finally began the protest behaviour that ended the abuse she had suffered by a friend of her father, which had started when she was 6 years old.

She says: *With me, there was never any confusion about the voice. I recognised it; it was the abuser's.*

With others, voice hearing starts much later, with some trigger reminding the person more fiercely of the abuse; yet they don't automatically realise there is any connection with the abuse. They have to learn this – by talking about their voice in therapy, for example – from what the voice says, or from the characteristics of the voice and the abuser.

Lisette was sexually abused by her stepfather. She started to hear one voice when she was 15. She never related her voice to the abuse.

She says: *It was my therapist who showed me that there were similarities between my voice and my stepfather. For example, my voice sometimes forbade me to eat. My stepfather loved eating but had told me: 'Don't eat so much, you'll get fat'. Also, the name my voice had given himself was 'Stefan', a kind of sound metaphor for 'stepfather'. When my therapist told me about these resemblances I got a flashback of my stepfather.*

Most voice hearers in this book did not relate their voice-hearing experience spontaneously to the abuse they experienced. They have learned this relationship in hearing voices groups or therapies, even if the voice started right away, at the time of the abuse.

Mien started to hear voices when she was 7 years old, just after her Holy Communion. That was when the sexual abuse by the chaplain started.

She says: *As a child I was not confused about the voices, it was absolutely normal for me. I have never talked about them. I was not afraid of them.*

Many years later she went into psychotherapy because of being very depressed about the abuse she had always kept to herself.

She says of this therapy: *It has greatly helped me to accept the voices and the past, as well as the relationship between both.*

2. Emotional neglect

The term 'emotional neglect' is used for quite different experiences, but the consequences of these experiences are the same. People who suffer emotional neglect experience difficulty in coping with emotions, because expressing emotion has been forbidden, or frowned upon, or even dangerous. It could also be that the person has been criticised so often that they have become very insecure and constantly afraid of failure.

Ami: *In my family their was a message for living: 'Keep your emotions to yourself. Cry only in bed. Behave at all times, be restrained.' It hurt me more than my sisters because I could less easily escape it [because of her physical handicap]. I learnt to lie still and be as quiet as a mouse. Bullying came easily to my family.*

Ami has had two periods in her life in which she has heard voices: when she was 24 and, again, at 49. She says:

When I was 24, I was admitted to hospital, having tried to commit suicide. The birds started to talk to me and, some time later, a tree talked to me. This was a spiritual experience which stimulated me. My first suicide attempt was a reaction to the fact that I could not recognise my feelings. I was very much in love. It went to my head. I was so happy that I was afraid of going mad. Before I made my suicide attempt in this period I thought the world would be a better place without me. The first time I heard voices that I recognised as such I was 49. They were neighbours, two girls living next to me. I had been homeless for many years and I had just acquired an apartment. I was happy with it and wanted to lead a new life and make new friends. To get new friends I knew I had to lie about myself. This kept me busy. And I became psychotic after two months, for about six weeks. I did not know how to get new friends, how to explain myself. I isolated myself with a concept of the future in which I was alone in my flat. I was paranoid; I was hiding myself in the flat and crouching down below the windows when anybody passed by, in order not to be seen. This was when the voices came.'

Because Ami had not been taught to cope with emotions she was not able to express them. This became highly troublesome when the expression of emotion was necessary, as in love and friendship.

Frank started to hear voices after he failed at university where he studied biology and psychology and failed them both just before the end of the course; having always been told he was no good, he expressed a need to fail.

Frank: *My mother died at the age of 25, when I was 2 years old. My mother was very important to me. I needed a good mother and I was hoping that I might be able to get one. My father remarried after one year but my second mother was very aggressive towards me. She demanded that I listened to what she said and I was expected to be obedient. She often chose not to communicate with me and I* *was made to feel guilty for everything. She used me as a way of dealing with her own aggression – this was a psychologically destructive relationship for me. The children from the second marriage were better off. My voice is quite young, 10 to 12 years old, but I know it's my mother. I have asked her and, about three years ago, she answered: 'I am your mother and I can become any voice I want.'*

Frans has a different story:
Frans: *I believe that incidents in my past have also made me vulnerable for a breakdown. I think that my mother's psychosis when I was very young and of which I was very scared played a role. After that it was not allowed to show emotions at home. From the age of 8 onwards my parents did not touch me anymore. I was too old for that.*

Frans hears two voices: one is very emotional and the other very rational. They first came after an emotionally overwhelming row when he was 27, a situation in which he could not express his anger.

3. Adolescent problems

In this category we have included voice hearers who began to hear voices in their adolescence when they had severe problems in their lives.

Antje: *I was 17 when I started to hear three voices. I will explain my situation. I had just started living on my own because I had got a flat. I had also just changed schools. I went to a special science school where we concentrated on mathematics and physics. I started to hear voices when I was in the third week of this new school. I had real difficulties with mathematics. I had never had that before. I had already been sitting at my desk for three hours, not knowing where to start, getting very agitated, when I heard a very clear voice saying: 'Are you stupid?'*

Eleanor: *I went to university when I was 18 to do a degree in English. I'd never been away from home before and I was quite naïve. I was accruing a massive debt. The group I got into at university were very different people to the kind I had known prior to going. They were very outgoing; they didn't take their work very seriously. I felt torn between wanting to follow that path and feeling that I ought to be working hard, taking it seriously and being a conscientious and diligent student. I felt that I didn't really know who I was anymore. It was around that time that this voice turned up. It was banal, mundane; it just commented on what I was doing.*

Rufus: *At the age of 18 I found myself in a boring job as an office junior. I was anxious about my future. I had failed in my education and I had failed to get* into the advertising business. On top of this, emotionally I was struggling to adjust to the fact that my first girlfriend, who I had been with for a year, had left me. This left a big hole in my life. (In hindsight this emotional loss echoed an earlier experience of abandonment that I'd had when I was 11.) Also, I found myself socially isolated. I felt socially left out in the cold. Instead of getting depressed, I gradually entered an alternative reality that had spiritual undertones. My experience also included the television and radio talking to me.

At the first contact Sasja had heard voices for three months. The first voice started at the funeral of a classmate who had lived opposite her and died in a motor accident. She didn't know what to say to his parents. Sasja thinks the voices have to do with a certain sensitivity. She experiences them as a loss of control. The first contact was in her final school examination. She lives in a small village with a lot of her family around her and there is a high level of social control. She is going to a university seventy-five miles from home. Much later, when she has adapted, is happy with student life and has lost the voices, **Sasja** says:

The consequences of hearing a voice you come to understand much later. You have to change, whether you like it or not. I don't like changing, but I have become more philosophical. Before I began to hear voices I wanted to control everything.

Stewart: *My journey as a voice hearer started around the age of 14, a very difficult time for me. My parents were in the process of splitting up and at the same time two grandparents passed away. I had also been told my brother had roughly twenty-four hours to live, which really shook me. Separation and loss had become a big part of my life. At the same time, a lot was going on at school. I had been hacking into computers and messing about and, when it was discovered, somebody else got the blame and was expelled for what I had done. I felt very guilty but unable to own up. And to cap it all I was being bullied by the head boy. But things really came to a head one day when a kid from another school tried to rob me, pulling some kind of knife in the park. I stopped going to school and just said I was not feeling well. I started hearing this real bad voice. It told me I was a really bad person. I recognised the voice as the bully from school, the head boy. I also started to hear my teacher's voice asking me why I wasn't going to school and saying she knew I was 'wagging' it.*

The sadness of the first three of these stories is that, in psychiatry, their problems were equated with schizophrenia and they were not helped in any way. The story of Sasja makes clear that this is avoidable.

4. High levels of stress

One could also say that the adolescents above were suffering from a high level of stress. We have categorised them under 'adolescent problems' because of their age. We will give two examples of adult voice hearers who also began to hear voices during periods in which they experienced a high level of stress.

Gina began to hear voices when she was 28. In psychotherapy she started to explore what had happened to her before the voices came, and she recognised that what had happened had disempowered her; she had lost the boyfriend she had been living with, she had lost her job, and she was living in a neighbourhood with a high level of crime.

Mieke, who began to hear voices when she was 40: *I start to hear voices when I am in a situation that threatens my existence, like my divorce and, six years later, buying a house on my own with all the financial risks. The voices express my emotional struggle with wanting to face my problem as well as wanting to fly away.*

5. Being bullied

For some people, being bullied at school continues over a long period. This induces feelings of helplessness and insecurity. We observed two voice hearers for whom being bullied seems to be the main cause of their hearing voices. They also experience that the bullying is sustained by the voices.

Karina: *The strongest and most negative voices came from the people I used to go to school with. These were a mixed group. I was bullied at school a lot and the content of the voices came from this time, like I was carrying past voices around with me in the present.*

Johnny: *I had been extensively bullied at school due to dyslexia and a slight speech impediment. The typical themes for the voices are that I am stupid, ugly and worthless. The bullying seemed to be carried on by the voices, although I didn't connect the two things at first.*

6. Physical abuse

Physical abuse might be the only trauma or it might occur in combination with sexual abuse, a combination that might also result in emotional neglect. For people with these experiences coping with emotions becomes more difficult.

When quite young, **Daan** was physically abused by his mother and stepfather and, later, he was sent to a foster family.

I thought I was bad because the voices called me all sorts of names. Later, I realised that the voices were related to the physical abuse, because they have the characteristics of those who abused me.

Helen: *Throughout my childhood my father made me feel more like an object than a human being. He never provided any sort of love, kindness or support. My brother and I seemed to be useful only as outlets for his abusive behaviour, as punch bags, or as objects to be used, abused and then thrown away.*

Jacqui: *My early years were filled with many terrifying and disturbing experiences that literally shattered me into pieces. My family were involved with a group of organised, sadistic paedophiles who abused children and took part in extreme sado-masochistic practices. To be betrayed and exploited by those who are meant to protect you leaves a profound sense of terror, isolation and shame. To survive, I developed a number of self-sufficient strategies. As well as hearing voices, I began to self-harm at an early age. I also developed a complex relationship with food which created an illusion of control over the arbitrary and cruel world I existed in. I hear many kinds of voices, voices born from my experience.*

CONCLUSION

Most voice hearers who have recovered are quite clear about the causal relationship between their voices and their traumatic experiences. However, the voices express what has happened to the voice hearer in different ways: by their characteristics; by what they say; in metaphors, or directly; by the triggers that sets them off, and so on (see also Chapter 5 'Making Sense of Voices' and Chapter 6 'Metaphors and Emotions').

It is very important to explore the links between the voices, the trauma and the involved emotions that lie at the roots of the voice-hearing experience. To learn to cope with these emotions is more relevant for the recovery process then learning to cope with the voices alone. To get more control over the voices, however, opens the gateway to getting at the social-emotional problems that are at the roots. Voices serve as a defence mechanism, avoiding confrontation with those problems and the emotions involved. Voice hearers often transfer their anxiety and shame for what has happened onto the people around them. Mental health professionals and others should not avoid these issues. Coping with these problems and emotions is needed to lead a full life of one's own.

CHAPTER 4

ACCEPTING VOICES AND FINDING A WAY OUT

SANDRA ESCHER

In this book all the voice hearers describe that accepting their voices is an essential step in the process of learning to cope with them. However, all the voices hearers in this book have recovered, which means they can cope with this experience. Stories of people who could not accept their voices have not been included; for them, coping has continued to be problematic. Reflecting on the stories in this book one can see that acceptance has become so obvious that for the most part it is not specifically mentioned, so instead it needs to be looked for between the lines. Acceptance is not usually an isolated element, it is also related to the acceptance of the voices by others, or to information from others.

Self-help groups are often mentioned as important:

Flore: *The positive effect of the self-help was that when hearing voices was accepted by others and myself, I could control it more.*

Karina: *I used to go to the group in Manchester every month; it was my only lifeline to sanity then. I talked to the group ... Helen Heap was running it and Terence McLaughlin was attending then ... I used to share my voice-hearing experience with the group and it felt great to be able to talk about it to people who understood what I was going through, and even to have a laugh about the strange things the voices sometimes said.*

For some people, it was going to a lecture:

Jan: *When I heard Marius and Sandra speaking back in 1992 saying voices made sense, I instinctively knew that was right. I had wanted to work that way for eleven years and it was trained out of me.*

Ami: *I came across advertising on a billboard that somebody would be giving a lecture about hearing voices. This lecture was given by Liz Bodil [one of the first voice hearers to promote accepting voices in Sweden]. This was the turning point.*

For others, reading about acceptance of the voices by others was important:

Antje: *It was nearly ten years later that I changed that idea. It was around the year 2000. I myself was at a point in my life where I really said to myself: 'This cannot be life'. My conclusion was to bring it to an end definitively. At this time I was not interested in anything anymore. My mother was very worried. She then saw Hannelore, the coordinator of the German Hearing Voices Network, on TV. My mother got the address. She went there, participated in a group, and after that told me about it. But I really didn't want to know. She left a paper on my desk beside my bed. It was a short flyer about the book 'Accepting Voices'. I said: 'You can take it with you, I am not interested in it.' However, she left it there. After she left I became interested and I read it. I was very surprised to read that a psychiatrist was writing in a different way about voices. As far as I recall, no one had ever asked me about the voices, even though it was the voices that made life impossible for me. All the talking I had in hospital was about a lot of things, but somehow not connected to me. It was always about things around me and around different things connected to me, but not really about me.*

Gina: *Someone at her work advised my mother, who was very worried about me, to read the book 'Accepting Voices'. My mother and I read the book; we found the address of Prof Romme, and I went to see him. He took my voice-hearing experience seriously.*

Karina: *I came into contact with the accepting voices approach in the early 90s, joining the Hearing Voices Network when it was in its infancy. I started to read all the literature by Romme and Escher and Paul Baker and Nigel Rose, etc.*

Eleanor: *My psychiatrist, Pat Bracken, told me about the importance of conceptualising it in my own way. There is a context to it and a meaning in it. I started reading about this and thought 'Whoa! Maybe I can profit from it.'*

Ami: *Liz Bodil also sold books. At that time I was neither able to read books, nor anything else, but that book ['Accepting Voices'] I read in one night. I just felt 'This is for me. This is it.' I understood the concept of hearing voices. This described my experience and it also told me there is a reason for voices.*

Some voice hearers describe how their therapist set them on the road to accepting their voices:

Johnny: *On the way home from Maastricht to Denmark, Trevor (my therapist) encouraged me to make, for the first time, a deal with the voices, suggesting that I would talk to them when we got home if they left me in peace to sleep throughout the night. To my amazement it worked! This too was a turning point for me as I* *realised that I had some form of control over the voices. It became a strategy that I used on a daily basis.*

Mien: *Up to then I had never told anyone about my voices. At the institute I had been in, there was no special therapy for voice hearing. Now, I got psychotherapy. Because of this I got more inside in myself. I could understand the phenomenon of voice hearing better.*

Mieke: *I then contacted Pieter Langendijk, a psychologist and alternative therapist who is married to a voice hearer. He put me at rest by telling me that hearing voices was not so special. It was not madness, and that one can cope with the voices through a dialogue, and to talk to them and try to make them positive.*

One element that was specifically mentioned was normalising the experience:
Eleanor: *There was one big barrier between me and the future and that was the voices. Pat Bracken told me about the philosophy of Marius Romme and Sandra Escher, and about the Hearing Voices Network and that it was just a normal human experience.*

Mien also describes what happened during therapy: *It helped me enormously to realise that hearing voices is quite a normal experience, that one can talk about it, and that the voices express what is happening to me.* And the consequence for **Mien:** *I no longer feel ashamed about the voices, and I can even talk with my family about it. I can do it because I have changed my mind about it being my fault. I had to say to myself over and over again the opposite: I was not to blame.*

FINDING A WAY OUT

Accepting voices is often described as finding a way out of a negative and overpowering relationship with the voices. However, in order to accept the voices, one has to change one's mindset by finding a way out of the belief that the voices are in charge of one's life, both by their presence and by their cause. If the voices are perceived as symptoms of an illness, as a powerless-making dominant force that has nothing to do with oneself other than as a result of having a brain disease, then one cannot become open to and interested in them, nor to accepting them.

Looking at the stories, it is possible to distinguish five elements to acceptance, and each element has different consequences:
- accepting that the voices are real
- accepting that the voices belong to the hearer (and are a part of that person)

- accepting that the voices are related to the life history
- accepting that the voices originate with the hearer
- self-acceptance

ACCEPTING THAT THE VOICES ARE REAL

Ron says: *Anne Walton, a fellow voice hearer, at my first hearing voices group asked me if I heard voices. When I replied that I did, she told me that they were real. It does not sound like much but that one sentence has been a compass for me, showing me the direction I needed to travel, underpinning my belief in the recovery process.*

Sue got in touch with the Hearing Voices Network in Manchester. She obtained information about membership, conferences, self-help group meetings and other events within the network. She became an active member and found the support she needed. Sue describes the road she then took:

At first I had denied the voices were real. This brought utter conflict within me and fear, extreme fear. They completely took over. Once I accepted the voices were real, the relationship changed. I stopped trying to get rid of them, but accepted them as personal.

ACCEPTING THAT THE VOICES BELONG TO YOU

Accepting the voices as real is one thing, but that does not mean that the hearer feels the voices belong to them. As the stories in this book show, voice hearing mostly begins after some kind of trauma (in our research, and the research of others, a high percentage of trauma was found: Romme & Escher, 1989, 2006a; Read et al., 2005). Voices are personal experiences, and they talk about trauma and about emotions related to these traumas, such as shame and guilt. As voices evoke often intense anxiety, they are perceived as bad news, not something to relate to.

It is probably most clearly described by **Lisette**:

When I first heard about the book 'Accepting Voices' it took some time before I wanted to order it. And when I received it, it took another few weeks before I could read it. The title 'Accepting Voices' did not appeal to me. I had the idea that I could not accept something like that. I have accepted it now, but though I still do not like the voices, I have accepted that they belong to me.

Mien: *I accepted that the voices are there and found a way to cope with them. They belong to me.*

Accepting the voices is a step in developing a (more) positive relationship with them:

> **Hannelore:** *In the beginning I had big problems in making it clear to the voices that they should not interfere too much with my life. They belong to me, and they can guide me, and give me advice and tips.*

ACCEPTING THAT THE VOICES ARE RELATED TO THE LIFE HISTORY

Acceptance by the voice hearer that the voices belong to them is not the same as connecting their voices to their life history. It is also not a step that everyone is able to take. For some people making the connection might be too threatening as the voices are often related to a troubled past, for example, with parents who the person wants to keep a good relationship with. Interestingly, some people are able to see a connection between their voices and their life history from the start, and are able to accept the voices as a reaction to a problem and not as an illness.

> **Stewart:** *I know I started hearing voices because of what was happening to me at that time, although I still don't know why those things came to me as voices. I just accept that it is me and all in all things have turned out OK.*

> **Jo:** *All the voices are part of me due to my life events.*

> **Helen:** *I suffered severe abuse throughout my childhood and have always known my voices to be related to this. I am very clear about the nature and origin of my voices. I see them as post-traumatic aftereffects of the abuse, natural and normal in the circumstances.*

> **Johnny:** *Trevor (my therapist) and I decided to complete the Maastricht Interview and go to the Netherlands together and partake in a voice-dialogue course in Maastricht. Marius, Sandra and Dirk Corstens worked with groups from Denmark and Sweden. I recall this as the toughest few days of my life. This was also a turning point for me as I began to relate my past life experiences to the voices, and could see how they had affected me.*

ACCEPTING THAT THE VOICES ORIGINATE WITH THE HEARER

In therapy, the aim is for voice hearers to understand that their voices are created by themselves, and accepting this fact is seen as being cured. However, this aim is not often mentioned by voice hearers themselves, as only a few come to that conclusion; most aim to change their relationship with their voices. It even angers voice hearers if this is specifically brought into the therapeutic discussion as it is seen as the aim of the therapist. However, it is mentioned by some people in this book:

John E: *I recently realised that I created my voices, that they come from my mind; my unconscious, as my dreams do.*

Mien: *I have had the most benefit, and I still have, by assuming that in one way or another, I create the voices myself.*

SELF-ACCEPTANCE

Jeannette W: *My first choice was to stay alive. That was an important decision as I stopped myself not wanting to live. The next step was to see if I felt OK about myself. The psychiatrist thought I was OK, more than OK even, and said: 'I do not understand why you think so negatively about yourself, because if there is someone with capacities it is you.' I reasoned that if this is true, why don't I believe I am someone? After this I started to think slowly about what I was doing to myself. Why did I make such high demands on myself? What was so bad about me? Why didn't I have any rights? One day that psychiatrist asked: 'Who are you really?' I totally freaked out. I panicked. Later I started to think about it, why I had become so terribly afraid of the remark. Then I thought: 'I am nothing at all. That is what has happened to me. Who I am is my voices, that is who I am and nothing more.' I did not know what I was feeling, what came from the voices and what came from others. Because of the tolerance of the psychiatrist I learnt to feel emotions like anger and sadness as belonging to me, and that I just could have them.*

Mien: *It has everything to do with how I perceive myself. For years I had lived with the idea that it was totally my fault, that I was a child of the devil and doomed from birth. This conviction I had to turn around.*

SUMMARY

Accepting the voices is the first step in the process of changing the relationship with the voices, and might lead to changing the relationship with oneself. Accepting is a personal process, and a difficult one, as it involves accepting something that is negative and frightening, and implies learning to cope with emotions that are triggered by the voices. Accepting is seldom an isolated process. Others must accept that the voice hearer will be able to accept their voices; something that is denied to voice hearers by the disease model.

CHAPTER 5

MAKING SENSE OF VOICES:
THE RELATIONSHIP BETWEEN THE VOICES AND THE LIFE HISTORY

SANDRA ESCHER

Most people find it difficult to believe that it is possible to make sense out of hearing voices. Making sense of voices is like putting together a jigsaw puzzle. In the beginning, when a voice hearer talks about his or her experience, it is like having a heap of puzzle pieces without having a picture next to it that shows what the puzzle will look like when finally put together. In such a situation it is necessary to have a strategy for organising the pieces so that the puzzle will be completed. We have, therefore, developed such a strategy to organise the information about what the voice hearer tells about their voices, in such a way that it is possible to lay out the puzzle and, by doing so, construct a relationship between the voices and the life experiences. The tools that can be used to piece the puzzle together are the Maastricht Hearing Voices Interview; a report of this interview, and the construct scheme (Romme & Escher, 2000a). What we call a construct is called a formulation by some psychologists (see Dallos & Johnstone, 2006) but seldom done with hearing voices.

    The stories in this book provide sufficient evidence of a relationship between trauma and hearing voices to beg the question: is there a relationship between the voices and the person's life history? Can we make sense of voices? In the voice hearers' stories there are sufficient links between different aspects of the voices and the traumatic experience of the involved emotions to come to the conclusion that voices make sense and tell us many things about the life of the voice hearer. In the first part of this chapter, quotations are selected to indicate these links. In the second part of this chapter, the elements that link voices to people's life histories are put together to make a 'construct' that systemises the information.

    What do voice hearers say about the relationship between the voices and their lives? These links are:

1. What happened at the onset of the voices: feeling threatened, enduring high levels of stress, traumatising experience of abuse, emotional neglect, being bullied, etc.

2. What the voices say: their possible reference to trauma experiences and to difficult emotions, feeling worthless or guilty, or in need of support
3. Emotions triggering voices: for example, feelings of insecurity or aggression
4. The characteristics of the voices, indicating one or more people involved in the trauma, or troubling emotions
5. The age of the different voices, indicating the time when different traumas happened
6. The use of the voices: voices can be a survival strategy or, in psychotherapeutic language, a defence mechanism against overwhelming or specific negative emotions
7. Voices can also be indirectly related to trauma through intermediating paranoia and/or social isolation

1. **What happened at the onset of hearing voices**
   Mieke: *I start to hear voices when I am in a threatening situation, like my divorce and six years later when buying a house of my own, with all the financial risks involved. On both occasions my voices presented the choices of flight (which would have made me none the wiser) and help in analysing my problems. The voices express my emotional struggle with wanting to face my problems and wanting to fly away.*

Mieke is a clear example of the relationship between the problem and the onset of voice hearing. When she feels threatened in her daily life she begins to hear voices.

2. **What the voices say**
The relationship between what the voices say and traumatic experience is well described by Karina and Johnny, whose voices repeat the terrible things that were said to them during bullying at school.

   Karina: *The strongest and most negative voices came from the people I used to go to school with. These were a mixed group. I was bullied at school and a lot of the content of the voices came from this time, like I was carrying past voices around with me in the present.*

   Johnny: *During that time and leading up to it, I had been extensively bullied at school due to dyslexia and a slight speech impediment. Typical themes for the voices are that I am stupid, ugly and worthless. I have always felt sad and very hurt by the things the voices have said, but began to believe them more and more as time went by. I went to a self-help group and this made me extremely motivated to work with Trevor (my therapist) and explore the voices. This was also a turning* *point for me as I began to relate my past life experiences to the voices and to see how they had affected me. The bullying seemed to be carried on by the voices, although I didn't connect the two things at first.*

The content of the voices might also relate to what the voice hearer is actually feeling.

Gina: *I began to understand that what the voices said was my own thoughts. The voice talked about things relating to the situation. They talked about money because I really couldn't afford to live in such a beautiful apartment on social welfare. In the sessions with Romme I discovered that a lot had happened before the voices came and I had mostly thought it was my own fault. I think I hear voices because of low self-esteem and they confirm this by telling me I'm not good enough.*

Gina's voices express her own worries and feelings of insecurity. These emotions are the result of her highly stressful personal situation: losing her boyfriend and her job, and her financially insecurity.

3. Emotions triggering voices

The voices might express emotions that the voice hearer feels, or they might come at times when it would be natural to feel emotion but the person is not able to do so. The emotions or their lack are often the trigger.

Sue: *The relationship with my voices has always been related to suppressed emotions and the identity of my human spirit. I believe my voices are emotions that I denied myself. They talk about abuse, self-doubt, insecurity and inadequacy.*

Patsy, when asked in the interview if certain emotions triggered the voices, answered: *I'm never angry. When I should be angry, the voices get angry.*

Antje: *It took me a while to see a relationship between the voices and my life. One of the relationships was the relationship between my emotions and the way the voices spoke. When I was angry and didn't express my anger they became angry with me.*

4. The characteristics of the voices

This is most often the case with sexual abuse, but we meet it in all kinds of trauma.

Lisette: *My therapist made me aware that there was a resemblance between my voices and my stepfather. When she told me this I got a flashback and I saw my stepfather. I understood that they are not the same but that the voice sounds like him and asks me to do the same things. When I became aware of the resemblance* between my voice called Stefan and my stepfather, I could complete the jigsaw. It all fitted together.*

Flore: *With me, there never was any confusion. I recognised the voice. It was my abuser. I was afraid of the voice and felt powerless against it.*

We might also see this with physical abuse:
Daan hears the voices of family members scolding him and during his recovery his interpretation becomes more discerning when he says: *They are related to my physical abuse by my mother and her man friend. The voices are coming from when I was still at home, they have crept into me.*

To recognise and accept the reality of being physically abused by his mother is very difficult for him.

5. The age of the different voices, indicating the time when different traumas happened

Jolanda: *I hear three voices and they all have names: Nina, Eva and Hannah. I hear them through my ears. All three are female. Nina is about 7 years of age. She is still a child. Nina originates from a long time ago and she is connected to the sexual abuse. I think Eva is 18 or 20 years old … Eva came when I was 18 and my family withdrew the formal complaint to the police about the person who had sexually abused me.*

6. The use of voices

Voices are functional, they are used to keep certain memories and emotions at a distance. It can be a survival strategy or, in psychotherapeutic language, a defence mechanism against overwhelming or specific negative emotions. For example:

Jolanda: *Nina cries a lot but is also immediately present when other people, or I myself, want to have bodily contact. At that moment Nina sets the rules. She does not get angry but she takes control over me and behaves like a 7-year-old child. I might even say things that come from Nina. If something happens that I do not want, I hear Nina crying. It might also be that Nina starts singing, as she did during the abuse … Eva has done me a favour by making me more defended from others. Eva wanted me to act sturdier. That wasn't such a bad idea, as managing to live at that moment it was the best attitude.*

7. Voices can also be indirectly related to trauma

Ami for example, had grown up in a family where expressing emotions was strongly discouraged. This made her vulnerable to overwhelming emotion, but she reacted differently to emotion in different periods of her life and after different emotional experiences.

Ami: *When I was born I initially stayed in hospital with my mother who had cancer. As a child my body did not function well. My teeth were discoloured and I had difficulty walking because of twisted legs. As a small child I had a lot of therapy which planted the idea that I was not good enough. My sisters didn't like me. I was a nuisance to them as they had to take me to therapy. I was very unhappy. In my family the message was always 'keep your emotions to yourself'. Cry only in bed. Behave at all times and always be restrained. It hurt me more than my sisters because I could less easily escape from it. I learned to lie. I kept as silent as a mouse. Bullying came easily to my family. My older sister was an A-student in everything. If she got a hundred and I got ninety-eight, I was criticised. One summer they sent my sister away to let me develop, but this was not much compensation.*

Ami talks about two periods of overwhelming emotions: *My first suicide attempt (at 24) was a reaction to the fact that I could not recognise my feelings. I was very much in love and it went to my head. I was so happy that I was afraid of going mad. I could not cope. I thought the world would be a better place without me. The first time I heard voices that I recognised as such I was 49. They were neighbours, two girls living next to me. I had been homeless for many years and I had just acquired an apartment. I was happy with it and wanted to lead a new life and make new friends. To get new friends I knew I had to lie about myself. This kept me busy. And, after two months of this I became psychotic for about six weeks. I did not know how to make new friends or how to explain myself. I isolated myself with a concept of the future in which I would be alone in my flat. I was paranoid. I would hide myself in the flat, crouching down behind the windows when somebody passed so as not to be seen. This was when the voices came.*

CONSTRUCTS

Making sense of voices acknowledges the relationship between the voices and traumatic experiences. It needs an open and empathic attitude combined with a systematic approach in observing and gathering significant information. In order to retrieve information about the relationship between the voices and life events the 'code' of defence must be broken. This code in patients hearing voices is often a destructive way of communication and an exaggerated and often negative way of expressing individual emotional problems.

This systematic but open search for meaning leads to a dynamic psychosocial formulation that Romme and Escher (2000a) call a 'construct'. The construct is the result of information gathered by the Maastricht interview. From the interview a report is made. The report is a short summary of the thirteen items of the Maastricht Interview Schedule and is used, in discussion with the voice hearer, to ensure that the most important information has been gathered. The report helps to achieve an overview that the voice hearer can memorise and is a way of avoiding a chaotic collection of information. From the interview report, six areas of information are used to form the construct; we have observed that these six items give most information about the relationship between the voices and the life history. They are:

- Identity
- Characteristics
- History of the voices
- Content of the voices
- Triggers
- Childhood history

With the construct two questions are asked:
1. Who are the people the voices represent?
2. What problems do the voices represent?

1. Who are the people the voices represent?

Experience has taught us that traumatic events are represented in the voice-hearing experience by the other people involved, as well as connected emotions that the person finds difficult to cope with. In the interview, identity is derived from the identity and characteristics of the voices; many people give their voices names or have voices who give themselves a name. Identity can also be derived from other characteristics of each voice, for example, age, sex, metaphorical forms of expression. Other connecting characteristics might be the way the voice speaks to the person: commanding, critical, helpful. The idea behind establishing this information is to get a picture of people who might have been involved in the trauma or time of stress, or who have been helpful in difficult times.

As in the story of Lisette, whose voice resembled her stepfather, the identity and characteristics of the voices can be very important in identifying the person involved in the trauma. They might also illustrate the emotions involved in the traumatic situation (as with Jolanda, whose voices represent defferent emotional problems resulting from her traumatic experiences).

2. What problems do the voices represent?

This question is directed to the circumstances or events at the root of the voice-hearing experience.

It is important to identify the time of onset as part of the history of the voice-hearing experience. A chronology needs to be established: when the person first started to hear voices; when more voices came; if and when voices changed character. This chronology links the circumstances surrounding the voice-hearing experience and should make it possible to identify the root cause. We have shown the relationship between voices and stress (Mieke and Ami); the relationship between voices and certain kinds of trauma (Karina, Johnny and Gina); and disturbed emotions that trigger voices (Antje, Patsy and Sue). These three issues – history, content, triggers – are important for analysing the problems that the person has experienced in their life and for indicating which of these problems the voices represent.

Finally, 'childhood history' is important in detecting the traumatic experiences that have made the person vulnerable to hearing voices (or to other mental health problems, such as paranoia or delusions); the person may have found it difficult to cope with emotions arising from experienced trauma. Of course, there is not a clear relationship in one hundred per cent of cases. There are voice hearers whose problems have occurred in later life rather than childhood: these might include severe conflict at work; a difficult home situation; confusion about sexual identity; loyalty conflicts; etc., and the voices talk about these problems. Identifying these issues will help in providing a suitable treatment plan.

There are also voice hearers who do not describe a clear relationship between voices and life history, although these account for only seven of the stories in this book. There might be a reason for this: for example, it could feel too threatening, or the person might see the issue as too private to discuss or it might not have become clear to them, a situation we often see with emotional neglect. Greater awareness helps the voice hearer to understand the experience in relation to what has happened in his or her life rather than hanging on to the idea of a debilitating biological illness. In seventy to eighty per cent of cases voice hearing is undoubtedly a reaction to actual social problems, based on the traumatic vulnerability of the individual. The identity, content, characteristics of the voices and their history of origin might indicate whom they represent, whilst the history, content and triggers might show what problems they represent. Sometimes collaborative imagination is needed in order to find the 'who' behind the voices.

We will now give an example of a construct using the information Jolanda has given in her interview. Jolanda is 30 years old at the time of the interview and hears three voices.

The identity of the voices
They all have a name: Nina, Eva and Hannah.

The characteristics of the voice
Nina is 7 years old, cries a lot or shouts if Jolanda doesn't listen to her. Eva is 19, thinks Jolanda worthless, and is aggressive towards her most of the time. Hannah is the same age as Jolanda and is a positive and helpful voice.

The history of the voices
Nina came when Jolanda was 7 years old. This was when the sexual abuse by an uncle started. It lasted until she was 12. Eva showed up when Jolanda was 19. At that age Jolanda wanted her parents to help her to officially accuse the uncle and bring him to trial. Just before the formal court hearing, the parents withdrew the charge and then the voice of Eva came. Hannah entered the scene when Jolanda had therapy; this voice helps Jolanda to cope with the other voices.

The content of the voices
Nina wants to tell Jolanda what happened when she was abused and will cry or shout if Jolanda doesn't listen to her. Eva accuses Jolanda of being weak and of not being assertive enough in defending herself against others. Eva bullies Jolanda and tells her to kill herself for being 'such a wimp'. Hannah gives advice, for example, not to listen to the other voices and to look for something that distracts her.

Triggers
For Nina, triggers are visits to the Jolanda's parents, when talk turns to family matters and there are confrontations about sexuality in her life. Triggers for Eva are when Jolanda should make a stand but is afraid of doing so, and often when Jolanda visits her family or comes into contact with men, because Eva doesn't want her to relate to men. Hannah comes when the other voices, especially Eva, are aggressive and when Jolanda is afraid of them or contemplates doing what Eva tells her to do.

Childhood history
Jolanda had a much protected upbringing where she didn't learn how to stand up for herself and her anger was rejected.

The construct
Who do the voices represent? The voices Nina and Eva don't represent real people but Jolanda's emotions in relation to the sexual abuse. Hannah represents Jolanda herself.

What problems do the voices represent?

Jolanda agrees that all the information points to her difficulties with coping with the sexual abuse in her past. She agrees with the construct. The voice of Nina represents her emotional reactions to the abuse and, later, her anger with her family who seemed to prefer her as a patient, rather than the victim of her uncle's sexual appetite. The relationship with the life history allowed her to change her relationship with her voices, but this was not an easy process. Jolanda started to develop herself. She embarked on a course of education and has become the proud mother of a son. She has found her way to recover.

Breaking the code

Breaking the code is not the individual activity of the professional but a collaboration between the voice hearer and the professional, or even between the voice hearer and a group when the construct is conducted in a group. In such a group, other voice hearers and professionals generate associations that can be very relevant for the individual in understanding the meaning of their voices. Experienced voice hearers can be of great support in this process and can act as professional helpers.

SUMMARY

There is a relationship between the voice and the life history and the way people are able to cope with their voices. In the stories, the voice hearers describe several elements that are indicative of this relationship: identity, characteristics, history, triggers, content and childhood. Together, these elements make sense of the voices for the voice hearer and for others involved with the voice hearer, such as family, partner and therapist.

CHAPTER 6

METAPHORS AND EMOTIONS

MARIUS ROMME

Metaphors are described as figures of speech in which a term or phrase is applied to something to which it is not literally applicable in order to suggest a resemblance. A connection between the two subjects is not direct or immediately obvious but, rather, the term or phrase is used because it contains symbolic or certain qualities found in the other.

With hearing voices these seemingly unrelated subjects are the voices and the voice hearer. When we say the voices speak in metaphors we indicate that 'what a voice says to the voice hearer' tells something about 'a problem of the voice hearer'. For example: when Ami looks in the mirror and sees the homeless woman she once was, her voice says: 'what a disaster', Ami first thought she was being scolded, but now she knows that the voice gives her realistic advice because, as she looks in the mirror 'Ami looks not well cared for', and realises herself 'I have to dress more properly'.

So when the voice says 'what a disaster', for Ami it seems to be a metaphorical way of expressing: 'Ami looks not well cared for'. It took Ami quite some time, as with most voice hearers, to learn to understand these metaphors. In the beginning she thought that she was being scolded by the voices, but now understands it as advice, and this has led to a quite different feeling about her voice. Her voice has not changed, but Ami has changed her relationship with it in that she now listens for the purpose behind what the voice is saying, in order to understand what the voice wants to say to her.

In general, we have observed that what voices say can be related to a characteristic of the various difficulties in life of the voice hearer, and mostly this is an emotional problem. The voice that is being critical in its way of speaking to Ami reflects the fact that Ami is highly critical of herself and, in turn, this can be explained by a lack of self-esteem. A low self-esteem can be a result of being scolded and unappreciated as a child. So 'what a disaster' is also Ami's emotion about herself, and might refer back to what was said to her. We have observed regularly that scolding voices have a metaphorical link for voice hearers with low self-esteem.

There is nothing mystifying in what voices say, but the metaphorical meaning has to be translated in order to understand the problem. It is not so strange that voices are metaphorical, because what they say points directly to problems that are difficult to accept for the voice hearer. In this way the metaphor protects the voice hearer from direct confrontation with their emotions. When voice hearers or professionals want to understand what voices are saying, they have to discuss the metaphors the voices are using by asking questions about them. Because of the protective function of the metaphor and the potential for many interpretations, a translation should not be imposed upon the voice hearer. The metaphor should be discussed, reflected upon, and can only be helpful if the voice hearer is up to it – in his/her time schedule.

The metaphors the voices employ have multiple connections to the voice hearer's problems. For example, the age of the voice might tell the hearer's age when the trauma happened; often the voice stays at that age and does not grow any older. It might also be that the age of the voice tells us the age of the main person involved in the trauma, and these voices mostly grow older with the voice hearer. This fact might also indicate that the abuser is still around and the problem is still not resolved. Here we also see the need to reflect, as one might make a mistake and look at the wrong person, as in the case of a voice hearer who heard a voice who was 45 years old, and the father had abused her as a child when he was 45: Was it the father? Discussing the metaphor, the voice hearer told the therapist that the voice had grown older, and she then realised that the voice represented her brother who had abused her for years and, by coincidence, was at the time of the interview also 45 years old, living in the same village, and she still felt threatened by him.

Furthermore, what the voice tells the voice hearer can indicate metaphorically the kind of trauma. For instance 'you are a whore' could refer to being abused, or could refer to the abuser suggesting that the voice hearer seduced the abuser; turning around the facts and making the voice hearer more insecure. It could also be that what the voices say refers to the actual insecurities of the voice hearer, as with Ami's experience above. What the voices say might also refer metaphorically to the emotions of the voice hearer, emotions that are involved with different traumatic experiences. The different voices of one person can metaphorically express different emotions connected with different problems; an example of this metaphorical complexity can be seen in the story of Jolanda.

Jolanda hears three voices, named Nina, Eva and Hannah. Jolanda started to hear her first voice 'Nina' at 7 years of age when the sexual abuse began. Nina has not grown older, so is still a child of around the age of 7. Nina takes over when Jolanda starts an intimate relationship by protesting and starting to cry as a reminder of the situation of the sexual abuse. So Nina has, metaphorically, two functions: she indicates by her age, Jolanda's age when the sexual abuse started; and by starting to cry when someone is becoming intimate, she indicates what the trauma is, reminding Jolanda of what happened when she was 7. The voice is, in a way, protectively warning her of the emotional consequences of intimacy.

Eva, Jolanda's second voice, started when she was 18, the time when Jolanda had a good reason to be very angry but was also powerless, because the family had promised to go to the police with a complaint against the person who abused her. The family subsequently retreated from their promise, and Eva is the voice that represents Jolanda's aggressiveness, stimulating her to promote her own interests more aggressively. Eva represents metaphorically, Jolanda's aggression and sense of self-worth. Eva has remained 18 years old; like Nina she also has not grown older. In discovering the metaphorical meaning of Eva's interfering, Jolanda has learnt to stand up for herself, as she still meets situations in which she finds this difficult. In this sense the voice has also been functional.

Hannah, the last of her three voices, represents Jolanda herself by being the wise voice, trying to come to peace with the other voices and with her problems.

Metaphorically voices can express very different things:

1. They each refer to an emotional problem based on a real problem, as in Jolanda's situation. In this chapter we will give examples of different problems that voices refer to metaphorically, including: sexual abuse; physical abuse; emotional neglect; being bullied; and threatening situations.
2. The characteristics of the voices can metaphorically refer to people involved in the traumatic experiences, those who were the aggressors, and those who were helpful.
3. They can metaphorically imitate the circumstances of the trauma.
4. They can metaphorically represent what other people have told the voice hearer.
5. The triggers that bring voices forward or make them worse can metaphorically refer to different time aspects related to the trauma, like the time of year, or memorable days such as a death or confrontations with the abuser or aggressor.
6. They can metaphorically refer to problematic emotions, such as aggression, shame or guilt feelings.
7. The age of the voice can metaphorically refer to the time in life that the trauma took place (as with Jolanda and the voices Nina and Eva)

8. They can metaphorically indicate intellectual problems, either (a) not being able to follow the level of education, or (b) the anxiety about failure.
9. They can metaphorically express that the voice hearer is not safe and in this way protects the voice hearer.

1. Metaphoric relationship with different kind of problems
Sexual abuse
Sexual abuse quite often lies at the root of the voice-hearing experience. The metaphor can indicate the emotions involved, such as guilt feelings. Mien was sexually abused by the village priest, and so she hears a voice telling her she is the devil's child – a metaphor for being bad because of the sexual abuse explained by the priest as punishment.

Physical abuse
With physical abuse, being beaten up and being in no position to fight back provokes a lot of aggression. Later on, this aggression might make the person afraid of him/herself, as the aggression might bring all manner of fantasies to mind, fantasies that the person may then want to act out on others. When this happens for the voice hearer, it brings about conflict. The person finds it difficult to experience the aggression as his own, does not agree with the acts of aggression, nor being like the abuser, someone who beats others.

Daan was 7 years old when he started to hear voices, a time when he was seriously physically abused, and later placed in a foster home. Daan is afraid of his voices who tell him to 'go after your brother with a knife'. Although he's not sure he can resist the commands of the voices, he doesn't want to do it because he does not agree with aggression. The aggressive commands metaphorically point both to the aggression he suffered in his youth, and to aggression being a problem with him, thus provoking a conflict of mind.

Emotional neglect
This describes formative experiences where the child is very much criticised and has learnt to avoid emotion, creating a sense of safety and protection against the situation where expressing emotions is dangerous. This might also happen when carers themselves cannot tolerate emotion, and literally disallow emotions by belittling the child when expressing them. We see that belittling over a long period is really harmful for self-esteem. Voices give words to such situations and emotions, as with Frank who says: 'My voices are three small boys. The three together sing like they are in a choir: 'Drown yourself, you have no chance.' This is probably a metaphor for Frank's situation as a youngster. Frank tells that his mother died when he was 2 years old and his father remarried a year later. 'My second mother was very aggressive, and

she used me to get rid of her aggression. I was simply guilty of everything.' The age of the voices suggest they are both a metaphor for the age that Frank as a youngster lived in very difficult circumstances, and the time when he was the target of his stepmother's aggression. He was not able to defend himself against her, just as the voices said: 'You have no chance.'

Being bullied

When being bullied lies at the roots of voice hearing, the characteristics of the voices and what they say may metaphorically point to what has happened. For example, Karina tells about the characteristics of her voices: 'I heard many different voices. The strongest and most negative came from the people I used to go to school with.'

Another story in which bullying plays a role is the story of Johnny, who does not show us a metaphorical relationship, but experiences this relationship more directly during his recovery process when he says: 'The bullying seemed to be carried on by the voices.'

A threatening situation; not feeling safe; intensive stress

Gina started to hear voices after a year of intensive stress with her job, being made redundant unfairly, and living in a flat in a high crime-rate area that she shared with a friend, who then left because she couldn't cope with her troubles in dealing with the stress. She did not want to live in the flat any longer, and unexpectedly got offered a very nice but rather expensive flat. Relieved, she wanted to move to this new flat as soon as possible. She worked long hours painting all rooms, felt extremely tired and started to hear a voice saying: 'I will destroy you, I will get you, and I will ruin you mentally.' She panicked and did not understand what was happening. She got very paranoid and her mother persuaded her to see a psychiatrist. She was admitted to a hospital, given medication and got stuck in the psychiatric system that intended to cure her of the voices. Two years later her mother found her a psychiatrist who looked differently at Gina's experience, one that accepted her voices. In therapy they looked together at the meaning of the voices and then discovered that, after all, the voices were right because she couldn't afford such an expensive flat. The metaphor is that the word 'I' meant '*It*', i.e., the flat, '*it* will ruin you, because you can't afford *it*.'

The voice gave word to an anxiety about moving into a financially dangerous situation, because the reality was that Gina would be unable to afford the rent. The message of the voices wasn't a welcome reality check at that time. Originally the voice was functional in the sense of being protective, but it wasn't interpreted that way. Only later when the voice was understood did it then become a step toward changing her relationship with the voice.

2. Characteristics of voices

The voice hearer can be afraid of their voices as they might represent the person or persons involved in the traumatic experience. It is also possible that the voices are helpful when they represent, for example, the therapist who really helped. In both cases the voice might mimic some characteristics of the person involved in the traumatic experience. Characteristics we have observed include identity, age, sex, personality, way of speaking, and often what the voice says may remind the voice hearer of the trauma. For example: Lisette was sexually abuse by her stepfather. She started to hear one voice when she was 17. She never connected her voice to the abuse.

> She says: *The voice is male and called Stefan. My therapist made it clear that there was a similarity between my voice and my stepfather. As soon as she told me that I got a flashback and saw my stepfather. I also understood that they are not really similar but that the voice resembles him and asks me to do the same things. For example, the ban on eating: my stepfather loved good meals but would say to me: 'Don't eat too much because it will make you fat.' The voice forbids me to eat too. When I became aware of the similarity between Stefan and my stepfather I could start to complete the puzzle.*

The metaphoric meaning can also change from negative to positive, depending on the voice hearer's development.

> As **Ami** says: *My relationship with my voices changed when I learnt to see them as a signal for my problems, and learnt to react to them positively. For example, when they said to me; 'Look at her, what a disaster', I saw it as a negative critical remark, breaking me down. Now I know that they relate to my low self-esteem. Nowadays I am able to look in the mirror and think that they are right, I should 'dress more properly', 'go to a dentist'. Or I would look around in my room and think 'it is time to clean up'. A negative influence has become a stimulus.*

An example of a helping voice is given by **Mien**:

> *I got a therapist who supported me and helped me to get more insight into myself, making a connection with my traumatic childhood and, as a result, I understand my voice better than before. After my therapy I sometimes heard the voice of my therapist, especially when I tended to think about myself in a negative way again.*

3. Voices can metaphorically imitate the circumstances of the trauma

This can be clearly seen with bullying. Bullying was the main problem for Karina, and she describes many metaphors referring to bullying in the description of her voices. For example, with her triggers she says: 'The most important trigger for the voices is when I go out into crowded places like pubs, in a busy street or on a bus'. As with being bullied, the voice also happens when in a crowd and feeling overwhelmed. Another metaphor involves the influence of the voices, as Karina says: 'Voices made me afraid and tearful, and had the ability to strip my dignity and self-respect'. This sounds very much like the influence of bullying, where bullies make people tearful and strip away their dignity. She also describes the lack of influence she has on her voices, which is much the same as the lack of influence experienced when being bullied. She says: 'I could not make them go away', as with being bullied and being unable to make them go away.

4. The voices can metaphorically refer to what has been said to the voice hearer

Below (see No. 6) is an example with the voice of Mien, calling her 'a devil's child'.

5. Situations that trigger the voices or intensify them can be a metaphor for problems

Daan was physically abused by his stepfather and mother in a family where fighting was routine, so he was placed in a foster family. He says that the voices become worse when there are serious conflicts at the foster family home, provoking anxiety within Daan, who is reminded of his own family home situation.

Voices might also be triggered at times that bring up memories of past dangers, something we came across with Patsy. Her voices became more frequent and intrusive twice a year, in November and May. In the month of November she burnt her face, after which she thought she was going to die and she started to hear voices. In the month of May her father, who was strongly interwoven with her problems with aggression, died.

6. Voices refer in a metaphorical way to troublesome emotions

The story of Mien tells about guilt feelings following sexual abuse, being called 'a devil's child' by the voices, a metaphor for the conviction that it was entirely her fault. Mien heard voices from the age of 7 years, the time when her abuse by the village priest started.

> She says: *I had two ugly voices and one nice one. One of the ugly voices said I was a devil's child and was good for nothing; he told me that the abuse was a punishment because I was stupid and lazy. The other voice talked about the same things, like 'you are good for nothing', 'you may be glad with what crumbs are left over after eating'*. In therapy she changed her ideas: *From the moment I understood that the roots of my voice-hearing experience lay in my youth, I started working on my self-esteem, because the voices had to do with the way I perceived myself. What the voices told me was said to me by the priest and by my mother.*

For many years I have lived with the conviction that it was my entire fault. I was a devil's child already from birth. This conviction I had to turn around.

7. Age of voices

The age of a voice can refer to the time in life when a trauma happened. We have already given an example with Jolanda in the introduction to this chapter. One of her voices was 7 years old, the age at which Jolanda's trauma started. (See also Frank's story where he hears the voices of three small boys, commenting on his behaviour, just as his second mother did when he was young.) The age of the voice can also be a characteristic of a person involved in the trauma, as with the age of the abusing brother of the voice hearer, also discussed earlier in this chapter.

8. Intellectual problems

(a) The metaphor indicates the inability to follow the level of education

In the child research carried out by Escher (2005a), children told about the influence of their voices, for example, when the voices mixed up numbers in their heads so they became confused. The relationship between the voices and the problem in this example was that the level of education was too high in relation the child's capacities. Tim (not a story from this book, but a child who participated in the children's research, Escher, 2005a) heard voices especially at school. When he had to do mathematics his voices mixed up the numbers in his head. He became confused at that moment and failed to give the right answer. When an IQ test was completed it showed he had an IQ of 85, indicating that the level of the school was too high for his intelligence. The metaphor is that voices mixing up numbers might refer to the voice hearer being unable to perform well at mathematics at this level of education.

(b) The metaphor indicates an anxiety about failing

> **Antje** explains: *I started to hear voices when I was in the third week of this new school. I had real difficulties with mathematics. I never had that before. I was already sitting at my desk for 3 hours not knowing where to start, getting very agitated, when I heard a very clear voice saying: 'Are you stupid?' After that he laughed very unpleasantly.*

The metaphor is rather clear: the voice gives words to what Antje fears – failure. She is a very intelligent child but now, suddenly, she is confronted with something she doesn't understand. The voice turns her fear of being stupid into words. Although the voices stayed, Antje finished school and sat the final exam.

9. A protective function of voice expressed metaphorically

Patsy did not dare to speak about her voices, because they forbade her to talk about them during her therapy sessions with me. So we came to a compromise; she would write about them at home, and then let me read what she had written. This was in the first year of our contact, and at this time she still had to convince me that her voices were real. When I had accepted the reality of her voices they no longer forbade her to talk about them. The metaphor is: voices forbid talking about them while it isn't safe to talk about them, and it is not safe as long as the other person does not accept them. We see in a lot of stories that the voice hearer actively avoids talking about their voices. This is rather wise when taking into consideration the potentially awful consequences this has had for many voice hearers. This is particularly true when starting to talk about voices to people, especially psychiatrists, who do not accept their voices, as can be seen in the stories of Antje, Eleanor, Hannelore, Johnny and Stewart.

CONCLUSION

Strangely, it seems a rather new idea to mental health care that we should work with the content of what the voices literally say to the voice hearer. Voices have not been recognised as a source of information to work with, yet the metaphors expressed by voices reflect a wealth of different aspects of life, as represented by the voice-hearing experience. In this chapter we have tried to demonstrate that voices might metaphorically express the relationship that exists between what the voices tell the voice hearer, and the voice hearers emotions connected to various situations; memories, experience of trauma, and so on. These metaphors are very instructive in learning about the problems that lie at the roots of the voice-hearing experience. These problems are hard to live with and give rise to overwhelming emotions, as they are problems and emotions mostly rooted in serious traumatic experiences; problems and emotions that the voice-hearer often tries to put out of mind, out of consciousness.

Through metaphors, the voices provide a key to opening the door to the problems that lie at their roots. To analyse the relationship between voices and the life story of the voice hearer, metaphors can be helpful in thinking about the meaning voices might have for the voice hearer. Working with metaphors means working from the point of view that the experience can be accepted, and the voice hearer's knowledge is as important as the theoretical framework of the therapist. The metaphors represent issues to be discussed with the voice hearer. It needs training to become sensitised to recognising metaphors. It needs wisdom to show there are similarities, but not to impose these connections on the voice hearer. After all, it is only helpful when it becomes part of the thinking of the voice hearer. The examples given in this chapter might well set you, the reader, on a journey of discovery. However, metaphors can also be problematic because they can be interpreted in many ways, and not everything that voices say is a metaphorical expression of the problems of the voice hearer. With this in mind, in 'Making Sense of Voices' (Chapter 7, Romme & Escher, 2000a), we described a method that we have called 'making a construct', a more systematic way to explore and analyse the relationship between aspects of the voice-hearing experience and the life story.

CHAPTER 7

HEARING VOICES GROUPS

MARIUS ROMME

Because many voice hearers who have recovered from their distress with their voices did this with the help of a hearing voices group, we will report in what ways they found these groups helpful. Before that, we will give some information about the history of these groups and about the research done with them.

HISTORY

Julie Downs (2001), the coordinator of the English Hearing Voices Network writes, 'The Hearing Voices Network has developed from a handful of groups to become part of a national and international network. It was based on the research of Prof Marius Romme and Dr Sandra Escher. Their research proposed that the way to cope with hearing voices was to talk about them, to get people who heard voices to get together to talk to each other about their experiences. Whilst this may not sound very revolutionary it nevertheless was. At the time of the research (1987), classical psychiatry regarded hearing voices as a delusion, a psychotic symptom, a symptom of schizophrenia. To talk to the person hearing voices was to collude with their delusion. The treatment was to ignore the voices and give the person medication to get rid of them; if this did not work the dosage was increased. Sadly some people still do not get the help they feel they want and this is where hearing voices groups fill a need.'

The first hearing voices group was formed in Holland in 1987. This led to the foundation of Resonance. One of the conferences organised by Sandra Escher in those years was visited by Paul Baker (2003) who wrote, 'fundamental to the approach adopted by Romme and Escher and Resonance has been its emphasis on partnership between voice hearers themselves and professionals who followed this lead; this was a refreshing change from most of the approaches I had come across before, which rarely – if ever, gave such importance to the views to those who had actually experienced the mental health difficulties under consideration.'

The first hearing voices group in the UK was formed by Paul Baker in 1988. Members were Anne Walton, John Williams, Helen Heap and Ron Coleman. In the time since 1987 there has been a development of hearing voices groups in 20 countries, in which England has developed the most with about 180 groups, second is Finland with 24 groups, which is in fact many because of the much smaller population of 5 million people.

RESEARCH

The first study was done in Holland by Pennings and Romme (1997). It was an experiment by forming four groups who came together, each for 10 times; two groups of voice hearers who were living at home and in contact with the ambulatory mental health care system; and two groups of people staying at the psychiatric hospital in Maastricht. The purpose was to learn about how voice hearers appreciate talking with other voice hearers about their experience. The evaluation concerned the following sub-goals:

1. To overcome diffidence to talk about one's voices: Participants found it easier to speak about their voices with other voice hearers than with non-voice hearers
2. To recognise one's experience with others: Nearly everyone recognised their experiences in what others said mostly concerning the negative sides of their voices
3. To accept their voices more after participating than before: 58% of the voice hearers in the clinic and 78% of the voice hearers living at home did become more accepting
4. To change the way of coping with their voices: Reported changes concerned: accepting one's voices more; not doing what the voices ask one to do; being less impressed by what the voices say; a different attitude like realising: 'I don't have to be afraid because voices can't really do anything'; 'things came up I have never talked about and I will discuss them with my support worker'; 'I discovered when I am bothered a lot by my voices, I also have many problems in my daily life.'

Another question was whether the voices increased by participating in the hearing voices group. It showed that only in the beginning the voices might be more frequent. Forty per cent reported that just after the meeting they weren't more hindered, but they were more busy with their voices. It did not lead to decompensate with any of the voice hearers. More then 80% said that they would advise other voice hearers to take part in a voice-hearing group.

A second study was done by the English Hearing Voices Network and published by Julie Downs (2001). It was a joint venture between groups in Leicester, Manchester, Sheffield and Portsmouth. It describes the experience of setting up a group; the planning procedure; how it should be run; the benefits; the facilitator's role; important communication aspects; and responsibility. As far as responsibility is concerned, I like to quote Chris Stowers from this publication (Downs, 2001: 29):

> The issue of responsibility is complicated. If the group is to be given a chance to outgrow the needs of its facilitators, it is important that the staff members do not direct things within the group all the time. As NHS (National Health Service) staff we are trained to assume responsibility for people at times of need. To some extent we have to back off from this stance and learn a different way of supporting people. We need to get a balance between providing structured help and allowing group members to take responsibility for the work they need to do.

A third study was also done by the English Hearing Voices Network (Downs, 2005). They held an inventory among voice hearers participating in groups and describe why people go to a hearing voices group (p. 8). The results were: an opportunity to talk freely about voices and other sensations; to have their experience accepted as real and not necessarily as negative; to share ideas and coping strategies; to become less isolated; to no longer have to deny or keep quiet about their experience; to feel supported; to be in a non-judgemental atmosphere; and to gain positive reinforcement.

There are also a number of studies by professionals who set up a group and evaluated certain outcomes:

Til Wykes et al., (1999) evaluated a hearing voices group, which they called group treatment, but which looked more like an exchange of experiences and psycho-education combined. There was quite some drop-out; 8 out of 21. The participants were middle-aged (average age, 40) had a long duration of illness, heard voices for 14 years on average, and half were living in psychiatric residences. After the twelve sessions there were changes in the perceived power and distress of the voices, as well as increases in the number and effectiveness of the coping strategies. These changes were maintained at the follow-up session after three months. The 'reduction of pathology' score on the Brief Psychiatric Rating Scale (BPRS) after the treatment phase were not maintained at follow-up.

Sara Meddings et al. (2006) evaluated a hearing voices group with twelve participants involved in the full evaluation after six months, with pre- and post-measurements. They report as social benefits: reduced isolation; relating better; increased social opportunities; feeling more confident socially; increased self-esteem and confidence; less hospitalisation. They found that average hospital admission rates decreased following participation in the group from a mean 39 days each per year over the three years prior to joining the group to 8 days each in the year after joining. This was statistically significant.

Terry Conway (2006) describes a model of a twelve-week hearing voices group in a medium secure psychiatric hospital. He says 'the participants contributed well when prompted but the group left both facilitators drained afterwards. This pattern continued for most of the twelve weeks, with the facilitators often doubting whether the group was of any value to the participants.' After some years they changed the format with more focus on what participants benefited from in the previous years. The facilitators adopted a more democratic style and became a more exploratory type of group. Conway writes: 'It was far easier to facilitate when patients were encouraged to take responsibility for the direction of the group and define its purpose. Based on the feedback of the members the group was such a success, we decided to run it on a regular rolling basis every week rather then just the usual twelve-week period before Christmas.'

Rebecca Morland (2003) looked at the benefits and difficulties members had experienced attending a hearing voices group after four months. She comes to the conclusion 'by giving people a safe place to go to, they may start to share their experiences and give and receive support which is of benefit to them'. This cycle of a safe place, sharing, being there for each other and other benefits can continue and lead to closer relationships being formed which then leads to increased trust and disclosure. In this book we see that in the stories of Sue and Peter R.

Terry McLeod et al. (2007) evaluated the effect of a hearing voices group with ten participant voice hearers, in which they discussed eight different themes in eight sessions. They compared the effect of the group with a so-called control group of the same number of voice hearers who underwent psychiatric 'treatment as usual' (not specified). They called the voices group a 'cognitive behavioral therapy group'. They did pre- and post-measurements and found as results that the discussions led to a reduction in the frequency of voices; a reduction in the perceived power of the voices and a trend towards reduction in the level of stress in the voices group as compared with those who received treatment as usual. Because the results of this more structured group with a programme are not different from other results with hearing voices groups who are less structured and not called therapy groups, it would be nice to know if a structured group speeds up the results in coping and feeling less overpowered, so that possibly a time benefit is to be gained. We don't know yet. The themes used in the McLeod group were not exceptional but nice to use and are regularly used in groups. They involve discussion about: sharing common features of voices; the effects of the voices upon their lives; sharing real life experiences and ways to cope with them; examining the beliefs about the voices' power; possibilities to increase coping strategies; practising coping strategies in the group; development of coping strategies and consolidation.

Elisabeth Newton et al. (2007) give an extensive report on interviews with eight voice hearers who had followed a hearing voices group which was also called a CBT group. The members found the group a safe place to talk; normalising and destigmatising; learning from and helping others by providing role models and suggestions for coping. The role of the facilitators was appreciated as they encouraged turn-taking and allowed quieter members to be heard. They thought it also had a positive impact on the participants' self-esteem. It was also observed by the reporters that 'however, the way in which the voices were described by each voice hearer revealed striking commonalities.' Each individual clearly described a pattern of interactions between a number of elements:

1. The content of the voices
2. The person's preferred explanations and beliefs about the source of the voices
3. The person's perception of the power of their voices
4. Their emotional responses to these experiences
5. Their coping repertoire for managing these experiences

They then discuss these relationships from a point of view of coping, not from a point of making sense of these experiences. All these research projects stopped at a coping level.

HELPFULNESS OF HEARING VOICES GROUPS AS TOLD IN THE STORIES IN THIS BOOK

Sixteen voice hearers tell about their experience with a group and found it helpful. Nineteen out of the fifty were helped by a voice-hearing group. There were relatively more people helped within a voice hearing group in England than, for instance, in Holland. This is mainly because there are quite a few more groups in England than there are in Holland. We will give examples of how voice hearers were being helped by a hearing voices group:

1. To kick-start their recovery process
2. Being helped along the whole path of their recovery
3. With parts of their recovery or with certain issues
4. At the end of their recovery

1. **Helped to kick-start their recovery process**
   Ron tells us: *Anne Walton, a fellow voice hearer, at my first hearing voices group, asked me if I heard voices. When I replied that I did she told me that they were real. It does not sound much but that one sentence has been a compass for me showing me the direction I needed to travel and underpinning my belief in the recovering process.*

He participated for about two years and was further helped by new friends who supported him to use his capacities again. He was encouraged to contact people who had nothing to do with psychiatry. He read a lot and developed with Julie Downs and Terry McLaughlin their ideas about training and mental health. He became an outstanding promoter of the hearing voices movement, within a recovery perspective.

> **Antje** describes: *I went to the self-help group for some weeks. I only listened. I did not really say anything. I think I became more awake during this time. I had been asleep. Still my decision to commit suicide was clear to me. Only it was not the right time. When I went back to the network I met some interesting people. So I woke up. I started to talk and I was very surprised to have a voice, to be able to speak.*

Later on she became active in the German network and followed different psychotherapies which together worked positively on her recovery. She is now the coordinator of the German Network.

> **Johnny** thinks: *The importance of joining a group and speaking with other voice hearers can't be emphasised enough. After the first meeting I felt almost elated at having spoken openly about the voices to people whom I'd not met before.*

Other courses, therapy and developing the Danish network together with other voice hearers and professionals worked favourably at achieving his recovery.

> **Karina** says: *I came into contact with the accepting voices approach in the early 1990s. I used to go to the group in Manchester every month. It was my only lifeline to sanity then. It was great to talk about it to people who understood what I was going through. I also started to go to a psychotherapy centre.*

2. **Being helped along the whole path of their recovery**

Sue: *No one other than I could help me to recover from the problems I had with my voices. But there were people who helped to support me. These were other voice hearers, who shared their experiences with me during self-help group meetings, where I was the leader of the group. I was just providing and allowing voice hearers to explore experiences along with myself included. We made an atmosphere of well-being and healing. We could relate to each other through our experiences. Working together with other voice hearers I learnt a lot about my voice-hearing experiences. Out of that I compiled focusing/self-help techniques to help other voice hearers to explore their voices and find their own individual experience and meaning. There was no set background theory, only our own experiences. As part of the process of looking within oneself and our voices we naturally develop an understanding of the relationship between our voices and our life history. And so it starts to make sense, the more we explore our voices, the more we discover and start to understand. With this I used my own strength, priorities and positive capacities to recover from my problems with my voices.*

Fernand reports about the issues he found important in the hearing voices group: *My experiences were seen as normal and not as only negative; I learned to know different point of views and ways of coping; For me it was the first step of being able to cope with my problem; I became less isolated, because I could talk more openly about my voices; I didn't have to keep them secret; I felt supported; I experienced an open atmosphere without prejudices; I was supported with the small steps I took; I recognised the relationship with my earlier life; I could cope better with the average normal life issues. I started to work again.*

Peter R: *When I first went to the hearing voices group I was very depressed, very down and I didn't speak for about three months, I didn't know if I was safe. I discovered that most people had similar problems to me. Everyone seemed to be suffering alone until they came to the group. Just being part of the group helped me a lot. We exchanged coping strategies ideas, and advice. In the group I spent time talking about my guilt in relation to what had happened between me and my sister in law. In the group I was made to feel that it was okay to enjoy a part of it but that it was wrong to feel guilty about all of it. It's 32 years now that I have been hearing voices. I've learned a lot about myself and about other people. I haven't been back in hospital for nearly six years. I now have insight into the voices, gained through the voices group. I cope very well with my voices now. I challenge them more than I used to because I have gained confidence and self-esteem. I've got a network of friends now, they are all voice hearers and we ring each other up when we've got problems and help each other out. I got more involved in the group in facilitation and I really grew from that.*

Flore says that she has heard a voice from the time she was 14 and had taken medication for thirty years. She then met a woman who also heard voices and with whom she fell in love. This woman facilitated a self-help group for voice hearers and guided Flore in the seven very difficult weeks after she stopped her medication. No doubt that falling in love is an effective base for identification and learning. Flore's recovery from the distress with her voices however was a learning process she developed by participating in the hearing voices group and later on by facilitating a hearing voices group herself. In the interview with her she confirmed all the important elements a voices group has to offer, which you will find in the summary of this chapter.

3. **Being helped with parts of their recovery or with certain issues**
   Frank: *I have participated in the hearing voices group in Berlin. Beforehand I hadn't been theorising, I just started because I knew: 'You need friends because otherwise you might fall in a hole of loneliness again', but I also knew that psychotherapy was more important for me. I knew that my voices are a reaction to experiences. My first suicide attempt was a reaction to loneliness and estrangement. I wanted psychotherapy because of my guilt feelings and anxieties in social groups. I wanted to become more self-confident.*

   Hannelore: *I have developed myself from victim to expert of my own experience. Thank God I have freed myself from the victim role; here Ron Coleman was a great example. Without my involvement in the German network 'NeSt', I would not be where I am today. I always say: when I try to help others, I also help myself.*

   John E: *A hearing voices group started at my local Mind, which I attended. It was extremely liberating, being able to talk about my voices openly and freely. Before this the very mention that I was hearing voices, even to warm and understanding counsellors brought the reaction, 'You'd better see your psychiatrist'. One other reaction to the voices group was for me to think very deeply about what my voices were. Talking to other voice hearers, swapping stories and experiences was highly stimulating and positive. The idea that voices were our own creation was talked about. I couldn't accept this at the time. After a while the group folded, but it had left a very positive mark on me.*

Then more or less on his own he changes the relationship with his voices, discovers that he also creates them himself, but at the same time they can be advisors who give practical advice.

   Andreas had changed his relationship with his voices long time before he became a member of a hearing voices group. He says: *It was refreshing how honest and involved people worked with their voice-hearing experience. For me it* *was the first time to talk about my experiences without being laughed at. Because of that I learned to look at my voices from different angles and this helped me to get control over my voices in my daily life.*

Riny heard only one voice and that voice was a positive voice. She had experienced herself as deviant, because other people around her found it crazy. She was helped in community mental health care with her problems with her sexual abuse, but they never accepted the fact of her hearing a voice.

She says: *In the hearing voices group I experienced the importance that others accept your hearing voices. The hearing voices group made me more self-confident. Others see that you have grown, before I kept myself very much to myself, now I am a blossoming flower.*

Ruth: *The hearing voices group:*
- *Gave me the vocabulary to talk about what I experience*
- *I could listen to others talking about things I could relate to*
- *It has to do with feeling accepted, normalising the experience (it is not that weird anymore as it is experienced by all the others)*
- *It is also about being honest about yourself (like having a stressful week, how that is experienced emotionally and understand the relation between the stress and what the voices say)*
- *It is like talking about the whole of my life, the whole of me because others understand you*
- *It stimulated me to get more insight. My main voice is the voice of someone who treated me badly when I was young. I don't feel myself anymore to be so much a victim since I became conscious that I was not in the wrong*

Mien was helped and became more self-confident by a hearing voices group in the last phase of her recovery. She had had quite extensive psychotherapy and learned to cope with her past of sexual abuse and emotional neglect.

She tells: *With two other women we have started the foundation 'willpower' and organised groups for women with the same kind of problem we had experienced. In these groups I really felt understood because you have to have the experience yourself.* About the self-help group for voice hearers she says: *I started to really talk about my voices in and after the hearing voices group. Before I tended to isolate myself in myself and I was very lonely. In the group I learned to talk also about voices outside the group and that reduced my isolation. I also didn't become afraid anymore, and when I didn't become afraid anymore I also didn't see shades and devils anymore. The voluntary work made me more self-confident. I didn't have dips anymore.*

Elisabeth first started individual therapy with a physiotherapist: *I felt able again to be in my body and to feel emotions.* After that she had individual therapy with Trevor (social worker). *I could work through my deep fear of loss and feeling of abandonment connected to the absence of my father.* It was only in a later phase that she participated in a voices group. *As it turned out the group became a natural part of my life, something I would not want to be without. The possibility of sharing, listening and expressing – to see how the group and every individual in the group moved, changed and developed. To learn to give and to receive support – and just being together about something that is so essential to each of the group members. Creating a 'fellowship' around voice hearing gives the experience, the recognition, the weight of reality, the value that it truly has to every voice hearer.*

Feeling connected again is an important later phase in the recovery process. Besides Mien and Elisabeth, this is also described very nicely in literature by Judith Herman (1992).

4. Setting up a self-help group and becoming helpful at the end of their recovery

A few voice hearers, at the end of their recovery, start a hearing voices group themselves. They then develop ways of working themselves, like selecting key points to be covered in hearing voices groups. We saw this with Debra, Flore, Hannelore, Jacqui, John R, Peter B, Mien and Riny.

Debra, who lives in New Zealand, describes this development towards the end of her recovery process when she had found a way to deal with her voices and saw her own needs. She reports:

Instead of having a life totally consumed by voices now I began to devour my ordinary life. I thought of the role the voices played in my life and discovered they fulfilled a need in me, a need to belong. Developing relationships and being exposed to people who showed they could be kind, caring and flawed just like me, freed me from the need for voices.

I was approached by a clinician who wanted to start up therapy groups for voice hearers. We discussed the key points I learnt from my own process of dealing with voices. On reflection these key points were as follows:

- *The voices have something important to say but they communicate in a clunky way*
- *To make sense of the voices I needed to interpret what they are trying to tell me*
- *I realised that what they have to say is important, so they won't let you ignore them*
- *There is a strong relationship between voices and stress*

- *Arguing with them doesn't help; they always win*
- *They can't always be trusted to tell the truth so I need to evaluate what they are saying*
- *The only power they have is the power I give them. I'm in charge here*
- *I will decide what I do as it is only I who must face the consequences, not the voices*
- *They react like they are approached. I greeted them with kindness and respect*
- *As a consequence my fear reduced*
- *They might fulfill a need in one's life. For me a need to feel connected, to belong*
- *They might fill a void of feelings of loss and grief*
- *They might represent the demons in one's life. I took back the power of my demons*

SUMMARY

It becomes clear that quite a number of people can be helped by a hearing voices group. It especially seems to be a good start overcoming shyness and opening up for talking about the experience and to being accepted with it, so it is beneficial in the first phase when people don't have any idea about what to do with their voices. Also along the lines of an otherwise initiated recovery process, hearing voices groups can be helpful in discovering more about possible backgrounds of the hearing voices experience and how it might be connected to one's life history. However, we often see that there is more needed than just the hearing voices group to complete the recovery process. Other people, especially devoted friends, but in many cases also psychotherapy are necessary to complete the job. Psychotherapy is especially helpful in coping with the original traumatic experiences and emotional neglect and the emotions involved. A helpful psychotherapy teaches the person to recognise their emotions as their own and learn to cope with them. We will report on psychotherapy with the recovered people in this book in a separate chapter. Also, in a later stage of the recovery process it must be said that the hearing voices networks in different countries and the hearing voices groups can do a great job in giving the voice hearer a purpose in life again, a fulfillment of their ambitions to help others; the need to belong. Many have found a job in this work as coordinators of the network; setting up groups; being facilitators of groups; organising training and conferences; bringing out newsletters or periodicals; organising websites etc. These tasks can also lead to becoming self-employed in the care and training field, or finding a job in mental health care. All these elements can be quite essential in building up self-esteem, self-awareness, self-worth and a more stable self-confidence, and make people less vulnerable than they were at the start of their hearing voices experience.

We now summarise all the very important reasons why a self-help group can be helpful. We learned these elements from a study by the English Hearing Voices Network (Downs et al., 2005). These were confirmed and also extended by studying the fifty stories in this book. The profitable elements of a hearing voices group are:

1. The possibility to talk about the experience and about other experiences in an open, free and respectful atmosphere
2. The acceptance of the experience as real and not only as a negative experience
3. To be confronted with other voice hearers and realising your are not the only one
4. To experience not having to hide the experience or defend yourself because of hearing voices
5. To feel supported because of being accepted, and learn to talk about the voices without being laughed at or belittled. To feel good because the voices are not being rejected or denied
6. To become less isolated because of being able to talk about the experience
7. To exchange experiences about coping, and to improve your coping
8. To realise that you can work with your voices and not only have to suppress them
9. To recognise that there are different phases in learning to cope with voices
10. To recognise when to expect the voices, because of certain situations or emotions
11. To get positive feedback about the small progressions one makes.
12. To realise more and more that the voices have to do with you as a person
13. To realise that you just don't have to do what the voices say, but that you do have your own opinion and your own power
14. To realise that the only power they have is the power you give them
15. To learn to listen to your voices better and try to understand what they really want to tell you and learn to really talk with them
16. Because of talking with your voices you can start discussing topics that you kept to yourself up to then
17. To become more active again, also in your daily life: shopping, sport, going to the cinema, socialising
18. To become a member of a club again or begin to follow courses in order to start work again

19. Feeling better in your daily life which also helps in coping better with one's voices
20. Changing the relationship with one's voices, becoming friendly with them, which has as a consequence – they become friendly with you

The first eleven are shared with several studies about hearing voices groups; the main inventory by the English Hearing Voices Network and the studies of Pennings and Romme (1997); Wykes, Parr & Landau (1999); Downs (2001, 2005); Morland (2003); Medding et al. (2006); Conway (2006); McLeod et al. (2007).

CHAPTER 8

PSYCHOTHERAPY WITH HEARING VOICES

MARIUS ROMME

Talking in self-help groups is for many voice hearers not enough to overcome their emotional and behavioural difficulties as a consequence of their experienced trauma. It is not enough for them to recognise their emotions as their own, and not only provoked by their voices. Besides, hearing voices groups were not available for a number of voice hearers in this book, so they needed another way to recognise the relationship between their voices and what has happened in their lives; they both need psychotherapy.

Simply explained, psychotherapy is talking therapy. This involves learning to express oneself and being supported with one's problems: problems with the voices; problems in the life of the voice hearer; problems with coping with emotions; recognising reaction patterns like dissociation, repression etc.; recognising triggers; understanding the relation between anxiety, shame, aggression and sadness; insecurities and powerlessness as a consequence of experienced trauma; realising and understanding the consequences of emotional neglect; trying to understand that carers could behave in such distorted ways, and making choices; learning to recognise one's needs and emotions, accepting them, and learning to feel them and express them. Psychotherapy is also talking about the background of all these problems; talking about the way the person might change his/her ideas about these problems; how to stop being a prisoner of these problems and the emotions involved; freeing oneself from controlling care systems, and becoming able to make choices and live one's life in a more free way; and being less disturbed by all these problems. It isn't as easy as it sounds because the therapist has to know a lot about how people's emotions and behaviour get distorted, about the many ways people react to problems, and how to approach such a person so that he/she becomes open to change.

We will differentiate the five psychotherapeutic orientations that we've met in this book:

1. *Making sense of voices psychotherapy.* Oriented on the experience of hearing voices, following the phase of development of the voice hearer in relation to their voices. Starting with accepting their voices and helping them to get more control over their voices and become less anxious about them. Creating a safe and supporting relationship. Then in the organisation phase, searching with the voice hearer for the relationship of the voices to what has happened in their life, and their distorted emotions and behaviour as a consequence. Doing the voices interview and making a construct or problem formulation. Then working through the feelings of shame, guilt and aggression related to the traumatic experiences, and learning to understand the metaphors. Then in the third phase, supporting the person to take back power from the voices and make choices to realise goals in real life. Recognising their emotions and changing the relationship with their voices. This process is more or less a combination of the next three below but also, like the next, more led by the experience and development of the voice hearer.

2. *The workbook of Ron Coleman and Mike Smith.* It is a kind of protocol that the voice hearer works through on his own or supported and stimulated by anyone else who the voice hearer chooses him/herself.

3. *Psychodynamic psychotherapy.* Oriented primarily on the emotional make-up of the person and working through the social emotional consequences of the trauma.

4. *Cognitive behavioural psychotherapy (CBT).* Oriented on the way people think about what is happening in their lives, what feelings and behaviour results from the way they think; directed primarily on reduction of anxiety and getting more control, more oriented on the coping with voices, thoughts and emotions than on the causal problem.

5. *Complementary psychotherapies and recovery-directed psychotherapy.* Oriented on the experience of hearing voices itself and changing the relationship with that experience, and using the person's own strengths and capacities to direct their life. Complementary therapists give more attention to spirituality and spiritual forces, recovery-oriented is more directed to making choices.

Some of this is also done in hearing voices groups, but in psychotherapy one goes more deeply into the various consequences and backgrounds of the voice-hearing experience. To do this requires more knowledge, which might be available in psychotherapy because of the psychotherapist's training in helping people to cope with their difficulty with accepting emotions. It is therefore seldom done in hearing voices groups although in principle it is possible and the story of Sue shows that possibility. We also see this done by voice hearers themselves without a therapist, but only infrequently, although in the stories of Rufus, Ron and Debra we see these voice hearers being their own psychotherapist. We also observe that sometimes only a simple direction given by a therapist can promote this self-help process, for example, Peter B, when he is advised to go after his demons in his past.

The content of the psychotherapy in the stories does not always become very clear because of the difference in the way they are described (see Frank, Karina, Fernand, Johnny S, Ronny). We did not ask for a specific description of this as the interview schedule was mainly oriented on the process of recovery, so this is very understandable. The therapies, however, were experienced by them as important parts in their recovery.

There are many voice hearers who did psychotherapy with themselves in order to work through their feelings of shame and guilt etc., and worked on their personal problems either in groups of voice hearers (see Sue) or with the help of another voices hearer or a friend (see Debra).

We will now describe different kinds of professional psychotherapy and illustrated with examples.

CATEGORY ONE:
MAKING SENSE OF VOICES PSYCHOTHERAPY

This category combines voices oriented with relating them to what has happened in the person's life, their involved emotions and their recovery.

Peggy: *Seven years ago I met Dr Phil Thomas, and was relieved to meet someone who was really interested in voice hearing. No one before had wanted to know, in spite of being admitted to hospital for ten weeks out of control of myself and others. Phil had me admitted to Dyll y Cas for two weeks and with intensive therapy I found I could be open and discuss my voices, and in fact a new one appeared and took over, thus enabling me to cope with the destructive ones. He encouraged me to be more open and to talk to him and to Sheila, my friend, of things I had repressed for many years, e.g., my adoption, my schizophrenia. As a result of Phil's work and Sheila's support I coped very well, handling the voices and enjoying a more positive and free way of life. Previously I was suppressing and introverted, preferring to stay indoors if I could.*

Caroline: Her therapist, Dr Dirk Corstens, says: *The Maastricht Hearing Voices interview told me that she heard four male voices. In the first session of talking directly to each of the voices separately, all four told us their names, which Caroline* didn't know. They said that they urged Caroline to kill herself. Asked for the reason, they talked about the moment Caroline had become a member of a religious sect. There the other members had told her that the voices were instruments of the devil. Before that Caroline had accepted the voices and they had been allowed to protect her in her environment where she had been emotionally neglected and misused.

Each of the voices told Dirk that they were angry with Caroline because they had lost their influence. From the moment Caroline had rejected them, they had started to fight her. They wanted to have a meaning in her life once again. At that point Caroline began to negotiate with them again. From thereon two voices disappeared and Caroline came to an agreement with the other two (see her story for more details).

Gina heard voices and after a highly stressful period. She says: *After two years sitting at home and taking medication that did not help me with my voices, I read the book 'Accepting Voices' and because Prof Romme lived not far away I asked my GP to refer me to him. He took my voices seriously and talked with me about how they disturbed me and made me afraid. He was also interested in all that had happened in my life before I started to hear these voices. I wanted to get rid of them but he said that was not possible. I should first try to find out how to cope with them better to get more control, like listen to what they say and see if that is right or not. So together we started to look for what I could do. I discovered that I could ask questions of the voices, so I perceived that what they said could not be true. I also first thought that they were critical but then I discovered that I was more or less thinking the same things as the voices. So slowly it became more clear that what they were saying was rather realistic but in a way it sounds overdone. Then it became clear they were talking about the problem that lay at the root of my hearing voices. I found it difficult to accept that, but I had to, because it was just reality and had nothing to do with feeling guilty.*

I went back to my mother and gave up the flat I couldn't afford. We then began to discuss what my plans were for my life and I decided to start a course, although I still heard voices. I overcame my insecurity by just starting. I did the course, I got a certificate and I started my own business as a hairdresser. Slowly I discovered that the voices just were my worries fed by my insecurity. In a voice-dialogue session, I realised who the most awful voice represented, but the time of difficulties with that man I realised was in the past. When I discovered all that and succeeded with my business they vanished.

Lisette has been sexually abused by her stepfather. She started to hear one voice when she was 17. She never related her voice to the abuse. *It was my* *therapist who showed me that there were similarities between my voice and my stepfather, for example, my voice forbade me from time to time to eat. My stepfather loved eating, but to me he said, 'Don't eat so much, or you'll get too fat'. Also the name my voice had given himself, 'Stefan', was a kind of sound metaphor for 'stepfather'. When my therapist told me about these resemblances I got a flashback seeing my stepfather. This made me afraid and I am glad that anxiety for my therapist was not a sign to stop. I understood that the voice and my stepfather were not the same, but that there is a resemblance as he asked me to do the same things as my stepfather did. It was only when I became conscious of the relationship between my voice and my stepfather, that I could put the missing pieces of the puzzle together. However there was still some chaos in my head, the voice, the flashbacks, my incest past, all were mixed up. My therapist taught me that certain pictures I saw belonged to a certain age period. I could not place them. I learned to become conscious of what had happened in the past and that was not easy. Another helpful skill of my therapist was that she sometimes said things the voice also said to me. That recognition was helpful. We have worked through the incest. I have learned from her how I react why I react and how I also could react differently.*

CATEGORY TWO:
THE WORKBOOK OF RON COLEMAN AND MIKE SMITH

As already described it is a kind of protocol that the voice hearer works through, and is best understood by looking through the workbook (Coleman & Smith, 1997). It is difficult to define this way of working and best explained with an example here:

Audrey: *Blue voice is the voice of a guy who abused me when I was 8. One of the things I did was to support Aud Junior* [child's voice]. *It took quite a lot supporting her to stand up to him and to tell him what he did was wrong. He did back off and she became stronger, more confident and felt less like she was wrong. Abuse raises a lot of issues in your head. One of the big ones is guilt. I was able to say, 'Well I did nothing wrong.' What seemed more important was not that I'd done nothing wrong but that the 8-year-old girl knew that she'd done nothing wrong.*

CATEGORY THREE:
PSYCHODYNAMIC PSYCHOTHERAPY

Psychodynamic psychotherapies are mainly oriented on working through the emotional problems that lie at the roots of the voice-hearing experience. We will give two examples in which the therapy part is well described. First is Jeannette W. You can best read the story itself. Here we only give some essentials, showing the positive support as a main helping issue in this therapy from someone acquainted with the emotional make-up. The second example is that of Mien. Both learned to recognise their distorted emotions as the consequence of the trauma of sexual abuse and having not been able to express themselves afterwards.

> **Jeannette W:** After years of psychiatric treatment that did not help she was referred to a psychiatrist psychotherapist. *We then started the therapy, which was horrible! This was one of the most difficult periods in my life (but she took the strain). Rather soon he said, 'Your voices are saying things that become true.' By putting it in this way he confirmed that part of me was not psychotic, but rather well knew what could happen in the future. The voices predicted but also were there because I coped strangely with my emotions. I had made a split between what were good and bad emotions. The main thing in therapy I learned was that I am all right. For example he often asked, 'Don't you see how clever you are?' and then I said, 'No because I don't understand people.' He then said. 'Don't you understand people or do people not understand you. If you think that quick you, you might well jump further away and people do not understand you.' Because of the tolerance of my therapist I also learned that emotions of anger and grief were my emotions and they may be there. For example he said: 'I would be angry about what has happened to you, so why am I not seeing your anger? How is it possible that you are angry and I don't see your anger?'*

He then organised a therapy in which she once could act out her aggression while experiencing that she not really harmed anybody. **Jeannette** became conscious that she hardly knew who she was, telling:

> *I didn't know who I was any more. I didn't know what my feelings were and, what belonged to the voices and what belonged to others.* And later she discovered: *The girl that lay there, that was me. That was me. I could finally feel the pain that I felt at that time. The extreme fear and anxiety of dying was my anxiety. That was the first time that I was in my body, feeling my whole body without missing a part of it. I had to rediscover myself and, above all, accept myself.*

> **Mien:** *Around my 50th birthday my energy was gone, I was exhausted and asked my support worker to help me to end my life. Only then they woke up and mediated treatment in a psychotherapeutic clinic. There I was greatly helped because my therapist was not afraid of hearing voices and helped me work through my abuse and explained the relationship between the two. I didn't get a special therapy for my voices but I learned to know myself better. For years I had lived with the conviction*

that it was all my fault. I was a child of the devil already doomed from birth. I have learned to turn this conviction around, by using my brain and consequently telling myself the truth was the contrary, I have been able to turn that conviction around. It sounds simple but it is hard work and it goes step by step.

CATEGORY FOUR:
COGNITIVE BEHAVIOURAL THERAPY

In this series of stories we find only one person who's had cognitive behavioural therapy, but not over a longer period and not extensively described (Frans). The lack of more people being helped by cognitive behavioural therapy might well be a consequence of the period when people who are telling their stories recovered. This was in nineties, the same time-span when the cognitive therapy with voice hearers was slowly developing, and in this period mainly in England. It might also be that there is a somewhat negative view in the voice-hearing networks about cognitive therapy, because in cognitive therapy hearing voices is still possibly too much seen as a sign of mental illness. It might also be that cognitive therapy emphasises the thoughts that give rise to emotions, while with hearing voices it might be more important to centralise the emotions that give rise to thoughts? Paul Chadwick (2006) in his book on cognitive therapy, acknowledges 'that the greatest threat to relationship building is the therapist's beliefs and assumptions'. When he talks about accepting voices and the person he says: 'Establishing radical collaboration is a process of allowing clients to find their own goals.'

Frans: *In the second period of my recovery I started to work on the perception of my emotions. I used for that emotional body therapy in which you become conscious of the emotions you feel in your body. I also participated in a Zen meditation group, where you try to perceive your emotions consciously. I also followed a cognitive behaviour therapy in which I learned to give a name to my emotions and to describe them. I still do the latter, but nowadays at home on my laptop.*

CATEGORY FIVE:
COMPLEMENTARY PSYCHOTHERAPY

We only see a clear complementary therapy in one of the stories in this book. This is a pity because in the research with children (Escher, 2005a) we met a lot of children who heard voices and were helped by complementary therapists often in combination with psychodynamic therapies, as is the case in the story of Antje. This combination worked well because complementary therapists have more experience and are not afraid of going into the voice-hearing experience itself and change the relationship with the voice, while the psychodynamic therapist knows more about people's emotional make-up, and go deeper into that part of life. The complementary therapists also often attend to spiritual aspects which are unusual for the other therapists.

> **Antje:** *I then met a shaman, a woman with whom I discussed my voices and she gave me very concrete hints about how to talk to a voice. I had no idea myself. I started in an aggressive way and the voices reacted with aggression. The shaman taught me to talk to the voices in a friendly way. And when I tried, my voices reacted in a friendly way, which was strange to me. She also taught me to speak to the voices very slowly. After three or four weeks talking three or four times a day in this friendly, slow way to the voices, they slowed down and became quieter. She also gave reasons why people hear spiritual entities. Voices, she told me, were lost souls and you have to encourage them to find their way back. From our discussions I think the most important result was that I found my self again. A topic I was keen to be busy with. I discovered that only when I was young had I been myself, but thereafter, for many years, I had lost myself. Making peace with my voices had not been possible without preparatory work with the shaman, as well as with a psychologist with whom I worked through Ron Coleman and Mike Smith's book 'Working with Voices', which made it possible for me to see the relationship between my voices and my life.*

CONCLUSION

We think that psychotherapy is often necessary to become able to work through the distorted emotions which are a consequence of traumatic experiences. In the stories in this book we observed this was most frequently the case with the trauma of sexual abuse. Psychotherapy is also helpful with the traumatic experience of highly stressful circumstances as well as with voice hearers who have been bullied. We less often saw stories of those with a history of emotional neglect making use of psychotherapy. Those voice hearers mostly managed to recover on their own, when they succeeded in making contacts in the outside world and did not isolate themselves any longer. To accept severe traumatisation as having really happened is a difficult process because it seems so difficult to accept the unfairness of life. Isolating themselves seems a rather dangerous reaction for people with a history of traumatisation. It also seems to take a long time to acknowledge and accept emotional neglect because it is such a hidden form of traumatisation. It takes some time to accept the reality of this situation and acknowledge the consequences in the person's difficulties with coping with emotions. In this book most voice hearers with a history of emotional neglect received a diagnosis of schizophrenia. Statistics are not very reliable as too many voice hearers receive that diagnosis as hearing voices is too easily equated with schizophrenia.

This chapter about psychotherapy with psychosis or with trauma at the base of psychosis is far from complete. This a developing field and rather controversial. I think that psychotherapies which start from people's experience are preferable to therapies which begin with theories. The only description that was mentioned by recovered voice hearers as very helpful was Judith Herman's book *Trauma and Recovery* (1992, and translated into many languages). This clearly works from experience not from theory. Jacqui Dillon refers to this book as follows:

So often people are impeded because of the feelings that they experienced at the time of the trauma and this stops them from talking about the painful things in order to be liberated from them. That is why Judith Herman's work was so important to me many years ago when I was embarking on my journey. I learned and understood this natural reluctance to shy away from frightening and painful experiences but also that we will continue to be haunted by them if we do not choose to face them. To this end psychotherapy has been vital to me in making sense of my experiences. I think that this knowledge needs to become more widely known because then people might feel more motivated to look at the painful things and have the chance to be free of them.

CHAPTER 9

MEDICATION

MARIUS ROMME

In psychiatry there seems to be an automatic response of prescribing neuroleptic medication as soon as a person talks about hearing voices. The dominant argument is that hearing voices is in itself pathological and labelled as a psychotic symptom, if not diagnosed as schizophrenia. From the stories in this book it is apparent that medication is prescribed far too often and usually in too high a dosage. On top of this, the effect of medication in relation to the effect of the complaints is not evaluated.

It is important to recognise that there are voice hearers who describe a positive outcome from medication; the most beneficial effect being that it diminishes emotional sensitivity. However, this positive effect is only experienced with low doses. A high dose of medication is rarely, if ever, experienced as helpful; on the contrary, it diminishes the possibility of using one's own capacities. The effect is typically described as making people feel 'like a zombie'. So a low dose can be effective when it diminishes overwhelming emotions and opens a road to developing the capabilities to recover. In this book, there are only four voice hearers who clearly describe how medication helped them. Most voice hearers explicitly state that neuroleptic medication did not help and so they stopped taking them. Others reduced the medication dose and found a better balance between dose and effect. As a broad conclusion we can state that if a low dose does not work then neither will a high dose.

There is a further issue related to whether the right kind of medication is given. Too often neuroleptic medication is given to people whose strategy for coping with their emotions is to dissociate. With these people neuroleptics hardly have any effect, or can even have the opposite effect. It often has a damaging influence on self-esteem and self-confidence and/or has a negative influence on their potential for coping with their voices. It's a pity that there is such a lack of attention given to dissociative experience in the diagnostic procedures of most psychiatric services. This is even more true for people who hear voices as most people who hear voices have traumatic experiences lying at the root of their experience. Dissociation is often used as a way of coping with trauma, but of course this is not recognised if there is an assumption that hearing voices is explained by the disease of schizophrenia.

If we look at the kind of trauma, and the effect of medication in relation to the trauma experience, we can observe differences. Voice hearers who have suffered emotional neglect are clearly afraid of emotions, either because feelings were forbidden, or came to be regarded as dangerous. Neuroleptic medication for these people can create a sense of distance from their voices because medication diminishes emotionality. Neuroleptic medication also helps to diminish confusion because emotional neglect easily leads to confusion when confronted with emotions. We can observe this in the stories; of the ten voice hearers who describe emotional neglect, six continue to use medication. By contrast, of the nineteen who suffered sexual abuse only three still take medication and four have never taken medication.

With physical abuse, and to a lesser extent with sexual abuse, the powerlessness over the traumatic event and the associated aggression can in turn lead to powerful aggressive emotions that the voice hearer may well be afraid of. If the person isn't able to express their anger, medication may help to feel it less and suffer less confusion. However, in the long run, it is more helpful when the aggression is recognised as very understandable and the person is helped to express their anger (Jeannette W). Some have to learn to feel their anger and accept it as very reasonable in relation to the traumatic experiences (Frank, Frans). If the person is able to express their anger but does it in a rather unbalanced way, medication is not helpful. It is often taken because 'we don't know better' (Flore). These people are fighters, and it is better finding something to fight for rather than being restricted in the traditional way with medication and hospital restraints. They can be better helped by working through their emotional problem and finding a purpose in life.

There are voice hearers who have been seriously traumatised but not emotionally neglected, who have reacted to the trauma by trying to put aside all their emotions. However, they didn't close up within themselves, and the voices gave words to their emotions. For them too, neuroleptics were not effective. They needed to face the demons in their lives and find something to fight for (Ron, Peter B). Traumatisation might also result in having serious problems with social contact. Those voice hearers might be easily discouraged and are afraid to fail. Voices can fill in for this lack of social relationships and loneliness. However it is more helpful to build up one's self-esteem through social contact with real people and having something to fight for (Debra).

Voice hearers whose experiences are related to depression are better helped with antidepressants, as well as exploring their problems, than with neuroleptics (Ami).

Our fifty interviews generated the following statistics:
- 44 out of 50 voice hearers were prescribed neuroleptic medication
- 4 out of 50 have never taken medication; one has taken homeopathic medication and one has given no information on medication
- 30 out of these 44 explicitly state that medication did not help them and stopped taking it
- 14 out of these 44 said that medication helped in part; medication alone did not help
- 12 out of 44 still use some, or sometimes use, medication
- 6 out of these 12 explain how medication helped them

Recovery is always described in combination with changing the relationship with the voices. Medication alone never helped people to recover.

Six people explain how medication helps them

Don: The psychiatrist in charge prescribed him Olanzapine 5mg. Then began what Don called his 'stable period': *More stable than ever before.*

Frans: *I still work full-time in the IT sector, but I am also taking a small amount of Risperdal. Without Risperdal I am earlier finished with working and can only go on until three in the afternoon. With Risperdal I just work on for the whole day. I am less excitable.*

Karina: *What helped me was the support I got from the Hearing Voices Network. Feeling a part of something and being accepted for who I was. I don't hear voices now, but I did up till a year ago. I heard voices for more than ten years without taking medication. Now I take medication that suits me and at a low dose and I hardly hear voices at all now.*

Peggy: *As a result of Phil's [psychiatrist] work and Sheila's [friend] support, I coped very well, handling the voices and enjoying a more positive and free way of life. Previously I was suppressed and introverted, preferring to stay indoors if I could. It was suggested I no longer needed Depricol injections and I was weaned off them. Sadly it did not work for me and I now have a small daily dose of Olanzapine. The voices are now back under my control and I scarcely hear them.*

Peter R: *One of my six voices is the man that my mother had an affair with. He talks to me about my mother sometimes. What he says is very crude and horrible. That is the time when I will take medication because he is so destructive and he hurts me.*

Ruth: *I have more recently been taking Citalopram and it has helped me through some depressive episodes. I think the reason that medication is helpful to me now is because I have an understanding of how it can help me and a realisation that it will not solve my problems so that I can supplement it with other efforts to help me.*

Lowering the dose brought a better balance

It is rather important to look at the minimum effective dose.

After sixteen years of treatment with a high dose of neuroleptic medication **Don** had become totally silent. He just sat in a chair most of the time. After his wife consulted a psychiatrist familiar with the accepting voices approach the dose was lowered and Don became his old active self again. On a dose of 5 mg Olanzapine he entered a stable period 'more stable then ever before', as he said. After that he was able to live at home with his wife again, and he has done so for several years.

I became clearer in my mind as my medication was reduced. I didn't feel that haze around me anymore. My identity became connected again with the rest of my being.

Andreas: *In the clinic I got a high dose which lamed me totally. Now my new psychiatrist lowered the dose of the same medication, discussed the effect with me and gave me the lowest effective dose. This made it possible for me to enjoy life again. This psychiatrist thinks it is important to have pleasure in life and be able to work according your capacities.*

Stewart: *He (my GP) started reducing the medication and that was really a big thing for me because I started to feel things again, you know, feeling emotions and that sort of stuff. It was from then that I started to feel more like a normal person. I am now discharged from psychiatric services and if I need anything I go and see my family doctor. I still take a small amount of antipsychotics and antidepressants.*

Audrey: *When I came off the medication the positive voices became stronger and got louder and I got a lot of support and a lot of good ideas from them.*

High doses can have a damaging effect

Eleanor: *Therapy meant drug therapy. It was hugely disempowering. It was all undermining my sense of self, exacerbating all my doubts about myself. The devastating impact just served to make the voices stronger and more aggressive because I became so frightened of them. What started off as experience became symptoms. When I heard the voice I would get very agitated. I went from hearing one, mild rather banal voice, which then became three, became eight became twelve voices.*

For six people the medication is taken as a kind of safety net after becoming used to them

Stewart: *I still take a small amount of antipsychotics and antidepressants, partly because I feel OK on them, partly because they are like a psychological crutch, I don't know what I'd be without them, but equally I have no idea what they do for me.*

This holds also for the other five who still are taking medication and are not given an explicit example of a clear reason why they take medication.

Hearing voices might well be related to depression and neuroleptics might be of no use

Ami: *In this period I had still spells of depression, especially in the winter, but I started in September to take antidepressant medication. During these ten years I worked as an account keeper in a business. I had a well-paid job.* In another period, years later: *After six weeks somebody came to my door and helped me to go to hospital just to visit a doctor. I got Haldol. The voices did not react to the Haldol, so I stopped after a week, because I had to be on guard.*

Why voice hearers do not take medication

Just a few examples:

Ami: *The voices did not react to the Haldol so I stopped.*

Debra: *I had been under mental health services for several years and although I was heavily medicated the voices persisted and my body was lethargic and yet agitated all at the same time.*

Eleanor: *I then asked Pat [psychiatrist] if I could come off medication and he agreed to support me in that process.*

Elisabeth: *They diagnosed me with schizophrenia and immediately took me off the antidepressant and put me on Zyprexa. The medicine helped me to gradually restore my normal sleep pattern. After six months I stopped taking medication and have not taken any since.*

Flore: *I was given medication from the time I was 14 years old, for thirty years. I then fell in love with a woman who involved me in a hearing voices group and helped me to kick the medication. It took seven weeks and was a hell of a time, each time a tablet less.*

Hannelore: *I landed one last time in psychiatry. This time I was so shocked by the treatment that I went away after a few days. Since then I have not been in psychiatry and have never taken psychopharmaca any more.*

CONCLUSION

Neuroleptic medication can be helpful in a low dose to help with coping with emotions, especially in people with whom expressing emotions was not learnt or even forbidden from when they were young and over a long period. It is much less helpful with a trauma like sexual abuse, which can be better worked through emotionally in psychotherapy or hearing voices groups. High doses never work favourably toward recovery, and medication alone isn't any help either.

In psychiatry the professional should be more attentive to dissociative experiences, because that way of dealing with emotions is either not much or not at all helped by medication. The traumatic experience should be worked through in special groups or therapy, or with the help of friends.

Mental health professionals, family, friends and voice hearers should change their therapeutic agenda:

1. Instead of treatment to get rid of voices, help the voice hearer to change their relationship with their voices
2. Organise hearing voices support groups, or find a network of voice hearers
3. Organise psychotherapy to work through shame, guilt feelings and aggression
4. Find a complementary therapist (Antje)
5. Be a good helpful friend, or try to find a buddy who supports when the voice hearer seems able to do the recovery work mostly on their own (Debra)
6. Support their own chosen coping strategy (Helen)
7. Use medication wisely and in low doses
8. Find out what lies at the root of the hearing voices experience

INTRODUCTION TO THE FIFTY STORIES

MERVYN MORRIS

In the introduction to this book we outlined the way in which the fifty stories were brought together. Here we want to explain both a little more about this process and, in particular, outline what editing has taken place.

Retaining the authentic voice of the storyteller has been a central concern for the editors. We have tried to keep the original words and phrases that people have used, even over-ruling grammatical rules of written English because, when people talk or write about their personal experience, their use of language is very different. Where we have made changes, it is only as a last resort to make sure that each story is readable. This means that some of the stories read quite differently because, as well as personal differences, they cross languages and cultures. Our publishers have also made suggestions to which we have responded following the above 'rule' about minimal interference.

For those stories that are self-authored, we have made few changes. Some of the stories are not directly told by the voice hearer, but by their interviewer. In these stories we have still retained the words and phrases of the original interview, even though they are not told in the first person. Where stories have required translation into English, in most cases this has also been undertaken by their interviewer. However some stories have been translated by Mrs Betty Gold, a professional translator, familiar with previous work of this kind. We also want to reiterate that because of the complexities of this, and the process of translation, some sections of text used as exemplars in the first part of the book vary slightly from the text in the stories themselves.

In terms of ordering the stories, we have chosen to put them in alphabetical order so that they are easy to find when following up quotes from the first part of the book. Each story breathes life and meaning into the experience of voice hearing. We hope you find them both inspiring and helpful.

ALPHABETICAL NAME LIST

Story	Written in	Country	Written by/with*	Edited by
Ami Rohnitz	English	Sweden	Marius	Jacqui
Andreas Gehrke	German	Germany	Marius	Jacqui
Antje Müller	English	Germany	Sandra	Jacqui
Audrey Reid	English	Scotland	Jacqui	Jacqui
Caroline	Dutch	Holland	Dirk	Mervyn
Daan Marsman	Dutch	Holland	Marius	Mrs Gold
Debra Lampshire	English	New Zealand	self	self
Denise Bosman	Dutch	Holland	Sandra/Dirk	Mervyn
Don Dugger	Dutch	Holland	Dirk	Mervyn
Eleanor Longden	English	England	Jacqui	Jacqui
Elisabeth Svanholmer	English	Denmark	Trevor	Jacqui
Fernand Chappin	Dutch	Holland	Dirk	Mervyn
Flore Brummans	Dutch	Holland	Marius	Mrs Gold
Frank Dahmen	German	Germany	Marius	Jacqui
Frans de Graaf	Dutch	Holland	Marius	Mrs Gold
Gavin Young	English	America	self	self
Gina Rohmit	Dutch	Holland	Marius	Mervyn
Hannelore Klafki	German	Germany	Marius	Jacqui
Helen	English	England	Jacqui	Jacqui
Mrs Hutten	Dutch	Holland	Dirk	Mervyn
Jacqui Dillon	English	England	self	self
Jan Holloway	English	England	Jacqui	Jacqui
Jeanette Brink	Dutch	Holland	Marius	Mrs Gold
Jeannette Woolthuis	Dutch	Holland	Sandra	Jacqui
Jo	English	England	self	self
John Exell	English	England	self	self/Marius
John Robinson	English	England	Jacqui	Jacqui
Johnny Sparvang	English	Denmark	Trevor	Jacqui
Jolanda van Hoeij	Dutch	Holland	Sandra	Mervyn
Karina Carlyn	English	England	self	self
Lisette de Klerk	Dutch	Holland	Sandra	Dirk/Mervyn
Marion Aslan	English	England	self	self
Mieke Simons	Dutch	Holland	Sandra	Mrs Gold
Mien Sonnemans	Dutch	Holland	Marius	Dirk/Mervyn
Odi Oquosa	English	England	Jacqui	Jacqui
Olga Runciman	English	Denmark	self	self

Patsy Hage	Dutch	Holland	Marius	Mrs. Gold
Peggy Davies	English	Wales	self/Phil	self/Phil
Peter Bullimore	English	England	Sandra/Marius	Mervyn
Peter Reynolds	English	England	Jacqui	Jacqui
Riny Selder	Dutch	Holland	Marius	Mrs. Gold
Robert Huisman	Dutch	Holland	Sandra	Mrs. Gold
Ron Coleman	English	Scotland	Marius/Sandra	Mervyn
Ronny Nilson	English	Norway	Geir	Jacqui
Rufus May	English	England	self	self
Ruth Forrest	English	England	self	self
Sasja Slotenmakers	Dutch	Holland	Marius/Sandra	Mrs Gold
Sjon Gijsen	Dutch	Holland	Sandra	Mrs Gold
Stewart Hendry	English	England	self/Mervyn	Mervyn/self
Sue Clarkson	English	England	self	self

*In addition to the editors, stories were written with the following colleagues:
Geir: Geir Fredrikson, a Norwegian social worker and dramatherapist
Phil: Phil Thomas, an English psychiatrist
Trevor: Trevor Eyles, an English psychiatric nurse living in Denmark

AMI ROHNITZ

WITH MARIUS ROMME

Ami Rohnitz is a 57-year-old divorced Swedish woman. After her Gymnasium she studied economics at a merchant school. She is now doing voluntary work at RMSH, the Swedish user organisation. She is working with voice hearer groups and trains mental health professionals in hospitals as well as in community mental health centres. There have been two periods in her life during which she has heard voices: a period of about seven years from the age of 24 and a period of about six years from the age of 49.

CHILDHOOD HISTORY

I was one of three children, the middle one. My mother had cancer when I was born and stayed in hospital after my birth. My body didn't function well. My teeth were grey and I had difficulty walking because of twisted legs. As a small child I got a great deal of therapy to be changed, which already planted the idea that I am not good enough. My two sisters didn't like me because I was a bit of a burden on them as they had to take me to the therapies. When I was 8 years old I fell from a tree and was really badly hurt, and afterwards had to learn to walk again because I'd been in bed for a long time. 'This is why I am built like a question mark.' Up to age 16 I always had restriction in my freedom of movement. After that time I became stronger in my spine because I trained myself. This was also a reason for exclusion and difficulty getting friends because when there was any action I had to stay aside in a corner in order not to be hurt. I became very introverted and had no self-esteem. I felt not good about myself. I was difficult for my parents. 'I was a problem.'

In my family there was a message for living: 'We should keep our emotions to ourselves'. Cry only in bed. 'We should behave all the time', and there were many restraints (the Martin Luther way). It hurt me more than my sisters, because I could less easily escape from it. I learnt to lie still, to keep as silent as a mouse. They were also easily hitting out in my family. My older sister was an 'A' student in everything. If she got 100 and I got 98, I was criticised. One summer they sent my sister away to let me grow, but this wasn't enough compensation.

THE FIRST PERIOD

When I was 24, I was admitted to hospital after having tried to commit suicide. The birds started to talk to me and sometime later a tree talked to me. This was a spiritual experience, which stimulated me. It gave me some insight, a big feeling of being connected with the universe. The birds told me that I was their friend, that I was part of the universe. This experience was positive and I didn't think of it as hearing voices. During this period I was not able to talk, I was in a mental state of isolation. Shut off from the world around me, shut up in myself. For myself I was in a creative state of mind, involved in triangles and numbers, but I could not express myself. However it felt good like I was in a higher state of mind. I also had other experiences, like only being able to talk in colours. When I was asked something I answered Red or Brown. This also isolated me from others in the hospital. I didn't understand this experience; that something was happening within me, a kind of power.

My first suicide attempt was a reaction to the fact that I could not recognise my feelings. I was very much in love. It went to my head. I was so happy that I was afraid of going mad. In the hospital they tried to treat me without medication, but with talk and support. I felt safe with this treatment and with this doctor. Life was such a mystery to me during that time, I did things I didn't want to, like the suicide attempt. There was a power within me that made me do these things. Before I made the suicide attempt at this time I thought the world would be a better place without me. I had to make a sacrifice, but I couldn't understand this power in myself. I had the idea the doctor understood and therefore I felt safe.

Then, after a year, this kind of supportive treatment stopped. I was given medication. This was a kind of black to white shift from one kind of treatment to a totally different one. Medication was a frightening experience for me, because I lost control over my body, and I needed my thoughts, but I could not keep them anymore. I went in and out hospital for seven years, always being admitted after a suicide attempt, and always with the diagnosis of depression. I usually stayed at home for only a short time, two or three months, and then hospital again.

After this seven-year period I stayed fully OK for ten years (from 33 to 43 years of age). In this period I had still spells of depression, especially in the winter, but I started, in the September, to take antidepressant medication. During these ten years I worked as an account keeper for a business. I had a well-paid job. I cared for my son who was around 13, and who had been with my parents during the time I went in and out hospital. After two years I also got a boyfriend and we lived like a family for eight years. I then married this boyfriend, but he changed dramatically. He went on honeymoon with another girl and he began to beat me up. At that time my son had already left home, he was 23 by then, and I was 43. I tried to get some crisis help but didn't succeed. As a reaction to the change I sort of gave up. I just left home with my toothbrush, went into town and started to live on the street. I just went away not to kill myself but to vanish, to slowly die. I went to town and looked for drugs. In the beginning I had some money. Later on drug people liked me because I was calm and looking normal and healthy, so they thought they could use me and send me to the post office to cash some stolen cheques. I sounded civilised; I didn't speak street language. I also looked civilised so was used as a courier, and didn't have to prostitute myself. I kept my apartment for 9 months but didn't use it, and did not pay rent so then they closed it. Everything I owned was in the apartment but I left it there.

THE SECOND PERIOD

The first time I heard voices, that I recognised as such, was when I was 49. They were the neighbours, two girls living next to me. I had been homeless for many years (about six years) and had just acquired an apartment. I was happy with it and wanted to lead a new life and make new friends. To get new friends, I knew I had to lie about myself. This kept me busy all the time, and after two months I became psychotic for about six weeks. I didn't know how to get new friends, how to explain myself. I isolated myself with a concept of my future being alone in the flat. I was paranoid, I was hiding myself in the flat, and went down behind the windows whenever somebody passed by in order not to bee seen. This was when the voices came.

After six weeks somebody came to my door and helped me to go to hospital just to visit a doctor. I got Haldol and the doctor also gave me early retirement. It was meant well, but it came like a blow; 'I am worthless'. (In an earlier period when I had depressions in winter time, I got antidepressants which worked fine; only when they heard that I heard voices I got neuroleptic medication. Why?) The voices did not react to Haldol, so I stopped taking it after a week, because I had to be on my guard. The voices were there all the time, except when sleeping. I thought I would go crazy because the doctor had not given any hope of recovery. I became even more isolated for another two years. [In that time Ami didn't realise the relationship between isolation and her voices and her paranoia.] I went shopping as little as possible, about once a month. If I go crazy in my apartment the murderers will come, I thought. I bought a dog in order to be able to go into the woods, to be with my madness in a nice surrounding. It was then that I came across an advertisement on a billboard that someone was giving a lecture about hearing voices; a lecture given by Liz Bodil [one of the first voice hearers to promote accepting voices in Sweden]. This was the turning point. Liz Bodil also sold books. At that time I was neither able to read books, nor anything else, but that book [about accepting voices] I read in one night. I just felt this is for me. This is it. I understood the concept of hearing voices, it described my experience and it also told me that there is a reason for the voices. While at the time I didn't know the reason why I heard voices, that there was a reason made it concrete, not abstract. Here a process of building-up was described, with logical reasoning, whilst the doctor mystified voices in craziness without hope.

I then went twice to the self-help group Liz had started. After that during a night with thunder and lightening, I just sat up and looked at this spectacle, and then another powerful voice, quite different from the voices I was used to hearing, said in a low tone 'You have heard enough', and the voices I was used to, stopped. It was silent for half a year, and during those six months I was involved with the voice-hearer group and got engaged in their activities.

The voices came back but not with the same frequency. They weren't there all the time. I could handle them. I pulled myself together and reacted positively to them. When they said 'look at her what a disaster', I then looked at myself in the mirror and agreed and took a shower, and dressed myself properly or cleaned the house. From a negative influence it became now a signal and a stimulus. I am not isolated any more. I have no time to fall apart.

ANDREAS GEHRKE

WITH MARIUS ROMME

I am 55 years of age, a father of two adult children and I live in Berlin. I have been married since 1968 and I am still extraordinarily thankful to my wife as she has stood by me during the incredibly difficult times when I was hearing voices. I am an archivist by trade and finished a course of study in history in 1989. When I was younger, I was involved with theoretical nuclear physics, however, I am now involved in teaching people in this country about voice hearing.

It was in 1986, at the age of 40, that I started hearing voices. I had somehow become the chosen, the one to intervene in the fight between heaven and hell. I believed I was Jesus Christ himself, lord of the world or God's substitute, and similar megalomaniac ideas. The voices only ever came from the outside. I was able to distinguish their direction, their sound, their characters and even their dialect without any difficulties. I had my neighbour on my side, or at least that is how she introduced herself when I heard her voice stating that she was a living angel. In addition, there were two witches, who had already perished, who were staying in our flat and who were controlling what I was doing minute by minute. There were different devils that functioned as their counterparts. They would switch in accordance with how successful or not they were in blackmailing a signature out of me.

All in all I was hearing voices for about eleven years at different periods, especially the evil voices. This was interspersed with various stays in psychiatric hospital following fifteen severe psychotic episodes where I was prescribed large doses of neuroleptic medication. However, I did not really use the periods in between to work through what I was experiencing, but pushed it away instead. Angels and witches, sometimes even St Peter himself came to me, in principle, to help me. However, I was petrified when I found out that the angels and witches had been taken away. This was a complete disaster for me, since I was being accused of their disappearance and I was blamed for their alleged deaths. I was also scrutinising the neighbour, for if anything bad was to happen to her in real life, then I would certainly not have survived. This was evident in the gruesome and harsh way in which the evil voices, mainly several devils speaking at the same time, had been acting. Their greatest means of pressurising me were the constant death threats, which first and foremost were made against me. Even at night-time when I was in bed, they appeared to have me 'die' step by step. When this also failed they surprised me one night with the message that my whole family was going to be extinguished within the next few months. This was at a point when I had already been hearing voices for ten years and I would still believe whatever they told me.

I was going crazy with fear, when a feeling – or was it a voice – told me: 'The voices do not master life and death'. This was a real turning point for me.

What in all honesty were the voices really capable of doing other than sounding hard, being verbally abusive, threatening, ridiculing me, etc? Was it not I who was ultimately able to actively change my actions and thus my environment? Eventually I started to get a sense of superiority, even towards the most evil of voices. All of a sudden an interesting question arose for me: how come the voices were coming to me and not to others? It was only later that I started to understand that all of this malaise had started off with me striving to become a rock-hard man, having been a rather soft youngster prior to that. It was not only a response to the fear of failure that I felt but also how I had lost myself in the process – I had gotten lost on the path of life that I had chosen for myself. Nothing in life appeared to be working properly any more. It was only on reflection later that I found that the voices had in fact been right. Yes, I did actually have problems with the way I was looking at the world and nature. Yes, I did have problems in relating to other people. Yes, I did have problems with my self-confidence. Yes, I did have problems with sexuality. Yes, I did have problems with how I was looking at life and death. Yes, I did have a lot of anxieties. Yes …

In an awfully mean manner, by using real catastrophes, the voices had in fact uncovered all of these things that I had consciously been trying to avoid feeling or thinking. As part of this process I became a believer, with strong, individual traits. The uncovered problem areas now actually helped me to redefine my role in life. Today, four years on, I usually only hear the voices when I start to meditate or when there is absolute silence. The following fact also shows how my own attitude towards the voices has changed. Today, the voices are allowed to tell me anything, even how things are with my soul and which problems are there to be resolved. The voices have now become good friends of mine. Just recently I experienced a return to old times. Voices were powerfully telling me how I was to conduct myself in relation to the gross and nasty behaviour of people, as this was something that I had not yet learned to become immune to. I was told to trust in myself, in other people and especially in God. As I understand it now, along with other statements, this was the core message of the voices. Interestingly enough, this was an area where I was still having the greatest difficulties in relation to my thinking and feeling.

I personally think that the voices are transported from the subconscious into the conscious mind. This hypothesis is supported by my experience of finding that every voice-hearing person has individual experiences. It may also be the case that a collective super-conscious helps us to balance out certain deficits. I think that all attempts to explain this are important, since an explanation is always better than none at all. Of course some ideas make more sense to me than others. Long before I became involved with the German Hearing Voices Network and was familiar with the methods described in *Accepting Voices*, I had come to see that the chain of continual hatred in the relationship to my voices had to be transformed. It was only when I recognised that a lot of what the voices were stating was actually right, that I was able to forgive them. However, this wasn't enough to create the necessary changes, so with a heavy heart, I made myself ask the evil voices for forgiveness and then slowly, my depression started to lift. I was even a little frightened when I found myself smiling spontaneously. This was an astounding matter, since I recognised that I had done just as much damage to the voices as they had done to me, by responding with such hatred. This was certainly no way to treat friends and I have since been able to carry out many acts of kindness in our relationships. If you dear reader believe that the chain of practising forgiveness is far off from being completed then you are certainly right.

Anyway, let's get back to the method as described in *Accepting Voices*. I learned about this method in a Berlin-based 'closed' group. It was really refreshing to see the sincerity and commitment with which the different group members embarked upon this task. For me, it was one of the first steps in a process of dealing with the voices from a more complex point of view. It was the first time that I was allowed to talk about my experiences without being condescendingly smiled at. Through this, I was able to learn to assess my voices from different points of view and eventually managed to get my daily life with my voices under control. By this I mean that it is no longer awful at all.

May I also take this opportunity to point out that my psychiatrist has enabled me to have the maximum enjoyment out of life by giving me the minimum amount of medication. His attitude to all of this has been, 'let the man experience joy, let him work within the network according to his abilities, let him become happy'. In complete contrast to this, when I was in a psychiatric hospital recently, I was given a high amount of the same kind of medication which meant I was completely out of action. I wish it was possible for courageous psychiatrists like mine to play a leading role in discussions, and for his point of view to be listened to and followed.

As I have already mentioned, I have been involved in the hearing voices movement since the spring of 2000. I enjoy being involved and it makes good use of my free time. At home, as my wife still works as a sales assistant, I am largely responsible for keeping the house. My living situation is very good and financially I am secure, thanks to a modest pension.

I often encounter scepticism when I recount my experiences with the voices. The most common objection is: 'Is it at all possible to have a good and friendly relationship with evil voices?' To this I tend to say that we have to live with all creatures, whether we want to or not. I think that all of them have a right to be and as a human being, I must love all people especially those that only talk, do no harm and are frequently right. I must love them with an earnest heart; so that I will ultimately learn to love all of my own parts in just the same way.

ANTJE MÜLLER

INTERVIEW WITH SANDRA ESCHER

I am 32 years old and I was born in Berlin, Germany. After leaving secondary school I did not complete any professional qualifications but I do have lots of hobbies. I like to write, paint, sing, make music and read and I like plants and animals. My parents divorced when I was 9 and I went to live on my own when I was 17.

I was 17 when I started to hear three voices. I had just started living on my own. By chance I had been lucky enough to find a flat, which was rare in East Berlin. I had also just changed schools. The East Berlin school provided special education for talented children. At the first school, we concentrated on languages, then in year 11, I went to a special science school where we concentrated on mathematics and physics. I started to hear voices when I was in the third week of this new school. I had real difficulties with the mathematics which I'd never had before. I'd been sitting at my desk for three hours not knowing where to start, getting very agitated, when I heard a very clear voice saying: 'are you stupid?' After that he laughed very unpleasantly. I did not know what was happening so I looked around me but there was no one there. I then searched my flat, looking for someone who might be there, but I was alone. Then I looked outside to see if there could be something else that had produced the noise. I lived in a very quiet area and I saw nothing special so after half an hour, I thought I must have imagined it.

A day later, he came again. It was during a math's lesson and I was sitting, staring at my desk. The same voice said to me, 'There is no need to have a close look. You will never be able to understand this.' After that he started to scold me and belittle me. He told me I was not able to do anything. After a few minutes, two other voices joined him and they said the same things. It was like a choir. After that they were always there, not always talking but sometimes just making noises. When they spoke they always said the same things. The voices stayed with me for the next thirteen years. I continued with my education but the voices became a handicap.

I heard these voices through my ears. They sounded very normal to me, in the same way that I perceive other external people speaking. The voices are not me – the way they talk to me is as if they perceive things differently and they talk about other topics. All three voices were male voices. I estimate their age at around 40 years old, so when I was 17, I thought the voices were old. They never went away and they never changed. However, they had different ways of influencing me, always in negative ways. They sometimes drove me crazy because they would comment on everything I was doing. They'd discuss topics I was occupied with and then confuse me rather than help me. For instance, I can remember that I had to do an exam in physics. I needed a formula and they started to change the formula so that I became uncertain about what I knew or didn't know. It was so difficult to concentrate. The consequence was that I had to compensate and learn a lot to be really, really sure of what I knew. Although the voices were there, I managed to complete my studies in mathematics. I made the final exam but I was completely burned out and I felt that I could not continue with this kind of study. I considered studying medicine but I was unsure if I could do that so I began studying nursing to get some experience within the medical field.

It was still in the time of the DDR [the former East Germany] so I could not choose which hospital I studied at so I had to attend a school and the school would select the hospital that you would work in. It sounds funny now but at the time it was not funny. They made me a nurse in a psychiatric hospital. I studied for one year and then I became a psychiatric patient myself.

I found my work as a psychiatric nurse very hard as I met a lot of ill people and I was afraid that I was similar to them. I then developed real sleep problems. I could not sleep for days and then my pet got very ill. It was only a mouse but I was fond of it. I decided to go to the vet and to let her die. This decision was too difficult for me and I had a breakdown. I started crying. Normally I did not cry but now I cried and cried. And then suddenly, I could not breathe anymore and my hands and nose turned blue. My boyfriend at the time called a doctor, and he came and gave me an injection, which I now know was Valium. He also told me that I should look for psychotherapeutic help. Not far from my home was a psychiatric hospital and I decided to go there. They gave me an appointment with a psychologist that same day. She talked to me for a while asking me what had happened. I told her about the death of my pet and she then said she wanted to admit me to the hospital for psychotherapy. I did not tell her that I heard voices – we were only talking about this nervous breakdown. I did not perceive myself as ill.

So I was admitted to psychiatric hospital for the first time, three years after the voices started. I had no experience with the system as a patient so I was not suspicious in any way. I stayed there for eight weeks and nothing happened. I did not really talk to the psychologist properly. I felt no need and when we were talking we were always beating about the bush, avoiding all problematic issues.

Then something happened. I had a nightmare, which was not unusual and I woke up feeling really anxious. The other patients in the room went to look for a doctor. A medical doctor, not a psychologist came and he asked what had happened. I answered: 'These voices are driving me crazy.' I told him I heard voices. I had never told anyone about the voices before because I had always felt it was like a deficit, something negative that was private.

The doctor took me downstairs to a locked psychiatric ward. The next morning they brought me back to the psychotherapeutic ward, but they had put me on medication. They gave me Haldol [haloperidol]. Within three days I was hardly able to speak anymore. I felt really terrible. It did not make sense; why they had given me medication? Although I was terrified of the locked psychiatric ward, they took me from the psychotherapeutic ward and brought me back to the locked ward. I stayed there for one year.

When I left the hospital, I tried to forget the whole business and start a new life. I wanted to become an architect. Whilst in hospital, I had taken the telephone directory and written down the addresses of architecture businesses, and with the help of my boyfriend, I wrote letters to them applying for a job. I got a response from an architect's company so I asked for a day off from the ward and went to see this architect company. Of course I did not tell them that I was in a psychiatric hospital. They told me that they would take me on. I was discharged from the psychiatric ward on Friday and I started work on Monday where I would learn to become a draughtsperson. I taught myself something that the others could not do. In the evening, after work had finished, I sat down behind the computer and studied an architectural program that no one was able to handle. After some weeks, I could use it, which gave me the freedom to work at different offices. I was well paid for this. I had a good a life, in some ways. I was able to buy myself a horse when I was only 22 years old.

I left the architecture company and began studying architecture at university. In my first year there were about a hundred people, so there were always a lot of people around me, but I found it difficult to have contact with people. It was more difficult for me because of the voices. The voices were problematic when I was going to meet other people so I became even more afraid. The voices blackmailed me and threatened me – they often said that they would kill someone I liked. It seemed like the voices did not want me to have emotions. At that time, I never tried to have any influence over the voices. For example, I never thought of talking to them. I was never sure if they could do something or not. The voices always told me that I was worthless and I came to agree with them. I wanted to commit suicide which resulted in me going back into hospital again.

I have forgotten a lot of things from that time. I had ECT and because of that I have lost some of my memory. The second time I was in hospital for two years. I have been in psychiatric hospital twelve or thirteen times. When

I think about all the years in psychiatry I have the sense that every time I was discharged and went back to normal life, there was this reduction of possibilities in my life. I did not think about problems. I did not have the idea that there were problems. I only had the idea that I did not function in a normal way. Now I think there is a relationship between the voices and my life history but at that time, in my mind, I did not think so.

RECOVERY

It was nearly ten years later that I changed that way of thinking. It was around the year 2000 and I was at a point in my life when I finally said to myself: 'This cannot be life'. My conclusion was to finally bring it to an end. At the same time I was not interested in anything anymore. My mother was very worried. She then saw Hannelore, the coordinator of the German Hearing Voices Network, on the TV. My mother got the address of the German Hearing Voices Network. She went there and participated in a group and after that she told me about it but I wasn't really interested. She left a paper on the desk beside my bed. It was a short flyer about the book *Accepting Voices*. She put it down and I said: 'You can take it with you. I am not interested in it.' However she left it there. When she left, I became interested and read it. I was very surprised to read that a psychiatrist was writing in a different way about voices. As far as I recalled no one had ever asked me anything about the voices even though it was the voices that made life impossible for me. So all the talking I had done in hospital was about a lot of things, but somehow they were not connected to me. It was always about things around me and around different things connected to me, but not really about me.

At first I was only surprised by what I read but I did not really react. Later I started to ask my mama about what they talked about in this group she went to. I had only read the flyer, and then I saw another patient reading the book. He was sitting in a kind of living room and reading it. I asked: 'What are you reading? Is it interesting?' I did not know he had voices. He said it was very interesting. I did not ask any more but I kept it in mind. Because he was a person I liked very much, we discussed the book and he told me he was going to this group of people hearing voices. He was talking about it a lot. He suddenly said where it was located and then I realised that it was the same group my mama was going to. Then I asked: 'Do you think I could come with you?'

At that time I also had a new doctor. She was different, different from the others I had seen before. She was the first who asked if anything had happened to me when I began hearing voices. I asked her if I could go to the self-help group. She said: 'Yes, please do it.' The man from the hospital and I got permission to go there together, late one evening. This is how I first came to the Network. The first times, I only sat there and listened to what people were talking about in relation to their voices. I had never considered the idea of having contact with my voices or somehow acknowledging them as complete beings. That one could do this was a surprise for me. It felt strange that people were talking about their voices as if they were neighbours.

I went to the self-help group for some weeks. I only listened and I did not really speak. I became more awake during this time. I had been asleep before. Still, my decision to commit suicide was clear to me. Only it was not the right time to do it as I did not have enough medication.

When I became more awake I had the feeling that I was living between two worlds. During this time I had contact with a social worker, who helped me with my daily needs, to go shopping, keep my flat in order and pay my rent. This made me connect with normal human life. When I went back to the Network I met some interesting people. The people in the group had changed a little bit. There were now people I was interested in and I still have a very close relationship with them to this day. So I woke up. I started to talk and I was very surprised to find I have a voice. I can speak. It took a while for me to see a relationship between the voices and my life. I started to listen to what people were talking about and how they coped with their voices. The first thing I tried was to make an appointment with my voices but it was really hard work and it did not work.

I then met a shaman, a woman with whom I had discussed my voices and she gave me very concrete tips about how to talk to a voice as I had no idea myself. I started in an aggressive way and the voices reacted with aggression. The shaman taught me to talk to the voices in a friendly way and when I tried my voices reacted in a friendly way, which was strange to me. She also taught me to speak to the voices very slowly. After three or four weeks talking three or four times a day in this friendly, slow way to the voices, they slowed down and became quieter. She also gave reasons why people hear spiritual entities. Voices, she told me, were lost souls and you have to encourage them to find their way back. From these discussions, I think the most important result was that I found myself again. I discovered that when I was younger I had been myself but thereafter, for many years, I had lost myself. This realisation made it possible to let the three voices that I had heard for so many years vanish.

I succeeded after I had talked for about a year with the shaman. The most important part of the voices vanishing was to change my attitude towards my voices. I approached them with love and asked them to go to the place they belonged to and originally came from. Making peace with my voices would not have been possible without preparatory work with the shaman as well as with a psychologist with whom I worked through the *Working with Voices* a workbook by Ron Coleman and Mike Smith. This made it possible for me to see the relationship between my voices and my life. Very soon we came to the content of the voices and the relationship between my emotions and the way the voices spoke. When I was angry and did not express my anger they became angry at me.

I also got a lot of literature tips from the voices; they gave me the title of a book that I should read. In the book, there were themes which I discussed with my therapist, like the book by Alice Miller *The Drama of the Gifted Child*. A theme about my parents, especially about my father, came into focus. After the divorce he did not want to have any contact with me anymore. I started to think about myself and to realise that experiences in my life connect with the voices.

Antje Müller is now the coordinator of the German Hearing Voices Network situated in Berlin. The network organises hearing voices groups and hold a congress every two years. They also teach professionals about coping with voices and have formed a support network for other voice hearers.

AUDREY REID

WITH JACQUI DILLON

Audrey is a 34-year-old woman. She lives in Dundee with her partner Maria where she lives a relaxed and contented life. She does voluntary work for the Hearing Voices Network in Dundee. She enjoys playing computer games, losing herself in a good book, taking her dog for walks, walking in open spaces, travelling and meeting new people. She is a former chef and enjoys cooking.

I don't remember a time when I didn't hear voices. They have been there since I was really small. As a small child you just accept what happens with your mind because you don't know any different. I didn't really think about myself hearing voices until I first went into hospital, when I was 24. I then was very paranoid and didn't tell about my voices.

Ten years ago I was at university and I was also working to try and support myself. I think I was doing too much. I was living on my own for the first time and trying to keep on top of a degree and working as well, as a professional chef. I first left home when I was 17. Before living on my own I had lived in shared accommodation for seven or eight years – staff accommodation when I was working, then a shared student flat for the first two years of university. At 24, this was the first time I was totally living alone. I became depressed and then I started drinking too much which didn't help the depression. At the same time I started seeing crows in the house that I was living in. I was really frightened to be seeing things that no one else could see.

My GP told me to stop drinking and he gave me Prozac. The effect it had on me was that I felt very detached so I didn't have any feelings, but I still had the same thoughts racing through my head. I became really intensely paranoid and very frightened. The crows started coming a lot; they came when I was falling asleep. They turned up when I was working. My natural reaction was to throw something at them and because I was a chef I was holding this big knife which I threw across the kitchen, which freaked out my colleagues. I had to give up university as I wasn't able to concentrate and, after the knife across the kitchen incident, I gave up work as well. Then I started living in my own little paranoid world. Eventually they took me off Prozac and put me on Chlorpromazine, so I slept with a few hours of being really, really paranoid in between.

I was first admitted to hospital when I went to see my GP and told him to take me in. I believed that I had an implant in my head. I was having a lot of migraines so I had a lot of pain in my head, and it felt like there was something just above my brow which was the root of the pain; and I was dopey with the drugs so it made sense to me. I did feel very controlled, and like a lot of people were out to get me. I had a real go at my GP saying, 'You are part of a conspiracy and take this fucking implant out of my head.' This was a sure way of ending up in hospital!

I was back in hospital after about three months. It all seemed so pointless. Nothing changed, nothing got better. It was just a place to go when things got out of control. The second time I was admitted I was so angry. I went in voluntary because otherwise they would have sectioned me. Again I was feeling very angry and fearful. I had been sleeping with knives under the bed. They sent me on an anger management course which just made me intensely angry! Why wasn't I allowed to be angry?

The drugs made me sleep so much, and the short times when I was awake I was cracking up and it was a really despairing time. I was 26 years old and I was asking, 'What am I doing with my life?' Going round in circles and not going anywhere. It was very frightening and I felt such hopelessness. No one in the psychiatric services gave me any hope, in fact, it was the opposite. In one week I had two appointments and on the Tuesday they told me that I had manic depression, and on the Thursday they told me it was schizophrenia. What do you do with that? They are completely bizarre words that don't mean anything. How do you know how to combat that or what to do with that? I can't even spell schizophrenia so what are you supposed to do with these bizarre diagnoses? And all they are actually doing is giving you drugs. You think they'll help. They've trained for a long time so you put your faith in them and put yourself into the hands of psychiatric services because you don't know what else to do. I was at the end of my tether and very suicidal. If I hadn't been sleeping so much because of the antipsychotics I would probably have tried to kill myself. I didn't because I was too tired. I still hadn't told anyone about hearing voices because from what I'd seen, the people in hospital who admitted to hearing voices had been in there a long time, so I wasn't going to admit it.

I heard seven voices, and four of them were present most of the time. The first was the voice of a guy who abused me when I was 8. His voice started when I was about 13 or 14, when I was moving from being a wee girl into a woman. His voice started because I was growing up and because I became a bit more aware of what had happened and what that meant. He is just a horrible, critical, dark voice that at one time would tell me that I was filthy and shit. The language this voice uses is quite graphically sexual. I don't think I would even have had the language to explain the abuse when I was younger – the impact of what it meant only really made sense after I became more sexually aware in my early teens. I never told anyone about the abuse. I think I had pushed it quite deep down inside; at the time I started seeing the crows I didn't remember it had happened.

Aud Junior is the voice of me as an 8-year-old child. She felt bad and she wasn't at all strong at first. She was a small, frightened voice. I'm not very sure when Aud Jnr arrived. I remember her being there at the time of the crows, but I can't consciously say she was there before. She came in very quietly. She says she has been there since then, but before that she was there but didn't really speak. As things are now I hear Aud Jnr, who is a fairly happy voice now, occasionally, like maybe once a month or less – if I'm really low he can turn up – but it's not often I hear the abuser's voice. The critical woman's (red) voice turns up when I'm feeling insecure, or when I'm trying to work something out, not every day, probably once or twice in a week.

There was also the voice of a woman that I worked for who was probably quite mentally unstable. She started when I was 24 or so – when things were getting out of control. Some days she was really friendly, and on others she was really foul-tempered and lashed out at everyone. She was really very difficult to cope with. She seems to jump on things and just tell me that everything that I'm doing is wrong. She is really critical. She pulls apart things that I have said or done and tells me what I have done wrong. She turns up sometimes now, but I'm much better able to deal with her.

Then there was the voice of another woman. She ages with me. I don't remember when she started; I think she is one of the voices I have always heard. She got quieter and harder to find when I was on antipsychotics. She can be jealous but she can also be supportive and fun, and she will occasionally have an argument with the other woman to defend me. She's great at knowing where I'm at and what I can do for myself. She's a very pragmatic voice. This voice is still around now.

RECOVERY

It was a CPN (community psychiatric nurse) who read between the lines – I kept going to services and saying, 'this medication is not working' – and she seemed to hear that. So she started looking outside of the box for what else there was. I told her about my voices and put me in touch with the Hearing Voices Network in Dundee. I think the CPN was trying to find anything that might have been helpful. She knew Pat Webster who had set up a voices group in Dundee and this seemed like something different, like something that people could move through and become more well, and the medication didn't come into it. She put me in touch with the voices group.

The first one I went to was great. There was a guy talking about a vision that he'd had, not about voices, but things just falling into place. What he was describing was different but I recognised the similarity, the weirdness of it. Other people in the group were saying, 'That happened to me', and it just all fell into place. And maybe it isn't that weird because these folk are alright. That was a good feeling, just going into the group. That night I went home and phoned everyone, my folks and all my pals and told them, 'I hear voices and its fantastic!' That was a huge turning point for me, just coming out about it. Nothing dreadful happened so it was a big weight off my shoulders. No one jumped up and down and screamed when I told them.

I'd been going to the group for a few months when I went along to a workshop that Ron Coleman did. Just hearing him speak made me feel so much hope, I felt 'I can do something about this'. Part of the workshop was about the workbook. I got one for myself and started working through it and making sense of my life. I started to think about my voices rather than them just being there. I started to become aware of them and what it was all about. What were the crows about, and what did I need to do for myself? Schizophrenia and manic depression are hard to fight if you don't even know what they mean, but I knew I was paranoid and I knew I had voices, and I knew I saw crows and that I got panicky. Those four things seemed a hell of lot more manageable than schizophrenia; I don't even know what it is! With these four things, maybe I couldn't get rid of them, but at least I had some ideas about how to work with them.

When I was first working with my voices I gave them the names of colours. Giving them an actual name felt like I was giving them too much power, but I gave them a colour so that it was in my control. A colour is more like a label and that disempowers them, and colour influences mood, and voices are related to mood.

Blue voice is the voice of a guy who abused me when I was 8. One of the things that I did to try and work with that, was to support Aud Jnr to confront the blue voice. It took quite a lot of supporting her to stand up to him and to tell him that what he did was wrong. He never said, 'Yes, what I did was wrong', but he did back off and she became stronger, more confident, and felt less like she was wrong. That was a really big breakthrough and took a huge amount of power away from that blue voice. I realise that he's a bastard and I'm not putting up with him. Again, now that I am more confident in myself, that is less problematic.

Aud Junior was the white voice, but when I was working with her to fight with the blue voice, I gave her a name rather than a colour; it seemed to make sense for her to have more identity, and to acknowledge who she was. She is the voice of me as an 8-year-old child. When I started working on my voices – trying to work out what they were about and challenging them – abuse raises a lot of issues in your head. One of the big ones is guilt. It may not be that rational but it seems common amongst folk. I was able to say; 'Well I did nothing wrong.' I was just a little girl and I did nothing wrong. What seemed more important was not that I'd done nothing wrong, but that the 8-year-old girl knew that she'd done nothing wrong.

Red voice is the voice of a woman that I worked for. How I dealt with her was to use the things she said as a sounding board. If she picked up on something that I'd done and said, 'You did that wrong', I learned to rationalise it to myself and say: 'Well, maybe that wasn't the best thing to have said, but I'll see that person tomorrow and I can check it out with them.' Or I would say: 'What I said was true, and the person is fine.' So I was able to use that critical voice to analyse what I was doing and to find more confidence in myself. I learned to critique the criticism. I occasionally hear her voice if I'm feeling insecure, but I'm much more confident in myself and I can say: 'Well, I'm not going to fret over every single thing that I've done.'

The green voice I've always heard. She ages with me. She can be quite jealous of me. When Maria and I got together she was very, very jealous. She felt very threatened by Maria, but she has moved through that, and has now backed off and accepted that I needed to get on with this life. She's supportive to me, and she is a good support to Aud Jnr. Her and Aud Jnr have conversations that I don't hear. They seem to know things that they have spoken about between themselves. It can be quite surreal when they both come through and say the same things. They can have a relationship that is independent of me.

When I was first working on my voices, one of the things that I used to do was to give them time slots. The red voice and another voice would come in the evening and I'd do this thing of weighing up the criticism. The blue voice more often came at the weekend. It took a long time to build up that process where Aud junior could confront the blue voice. He'd come on a Saturday, and it probably took three or four Saturdays to build up, to stand up to him. I spent a lot of time during the week talking to Aud Jnr, supporting her and building her up during the week, so that by Saturday I tried to support her to make him back off. It was a really draining, difficult time, but I was really fired up. I was very angry and I was cutting down my medication at the time, so I felt like I was waking up. I had so much more energy and felt so much more alive. I also found that, whilst I was on medication, I couldn't hear so much the two positive voices that I'd always had. They were there but the medication just seemed to dampen them down. When I came off the medication, the positive voices became stronger and got louder, so I got a lot of support from them, and lots of good ideas from them. The positive voices didn't really talk to the negative voices, but they did support me and helped me to feel that what I was doing was right. The positive voices supported me to support Aud junior to confront the blue voice.

My paranoid fears seem to come from something small at the beginning, and then they spiral and I get into this huge scary, wacky place which can make perfect sense to me, but if they are true then there isn't much I can do about them; so I've just learned to accept them. I have realised that I am powerless to control things. If aliens are going to come down and take me away in a space ship then I don't know what I can do about it. There is no point in worrying about it.

The crows: I have a few theories about the crows, probably the most sensible is where I was abused; it was near the woods, not far from my home. There were really tall trees with crows in them. I'd forgotten about the abuse, I had shut it out of my memory, and I think the sound and the sight of crows were messengers saying: 'There is something here that you need to deal with.'

There was a big chunk of time where everything started to make sense. The crows, the voices and the abuse were like pieces of a puzzle that I started putting together. Things started adding up. I can remember a point when I had the jigsaw half done and I could see what it meant, and I felt quite powerless in knowing what to do. It was hearing Ron Coleman speak that led me to see what I could do to help. It took lots of steps. I couldn't think well with the medication, so I slowly started to cut it down just to be able to think and to do the work, especially as I was only hearing the negative voices. I came off my medication altogether eventually. It was probably easier for me because I'd never found the medication helpful, so I didn't have a big backlash. If anything, as I started to come off it, the positive voices became stronger and I started to feel more and more well. I had to do something to deal with not sleeping. I hardly slept for three weeks, but slowly a good pattern came back. I've felt angry ever since; that such a big chunk of my life was stolen by the drugs. I got better despite them, not because of them.

CAROLINE

WITH DIRK CORSTENS

Caroline is a 30-year-old married woman who has heard voices since she was 4 years old. When the voices started they were supporting her and positive in expression. As a child she was lonely and a victim of sexual abuse.

She consulted me because her voices were very destructive and negative from when she was 21. A hospital admission for four years and high doses of neuroleptics didn't succeed in pushing the voices to the background. When she decided not to harm herself anymore by order of her voices, she was then able to leave the psychiatric hospital, and started living on her own with her husband-to-be. Her day though was still flooded by her voices and negotiations with them. They commented on every action, her thoughts, and they frustrated every decision. Her diagnosis was borderline personality disorder. She didn't dare to decrease her dose of medication although it sedated her too much. The effect of the medication was that she felt less fear, but it didn't change her voices or their attitude at all.

From the Maastricht Hearing Voices Interview her therapist discovered that she heard four male voices. She permitted the therapist to talk to her voices. In the first conversation the four voices gave their names, something that Caroline didn't know herself. They said they wanted to push Caroline to kill herself. When asked for the reason they said they were angry with Caroline. They said that when she was 21 Caroline joined a religious Christian sect. The members of the sect told Caroline her voices were an 'instrument of the devil', and if she wanted to join the sect, which she did from desperation, she should first do everything to abolish the voices. The voices said that before she entered the sect, Caroline had accepted them as protectors against abuse and neglect, and the voices were allowed to support her. But from then on Caroline had started to fight them and they had lost their influence on her. They were angry about that. From the moment Caroline rejected the voices they had started to fight against her. They commanded her to kill herself, which was the reason for her four-year hospital admission, because Caroline couldn't cope with that and started to seriously self-harm. What the voices said they wanted now was to get respect and get their influence back. Caroline herself wasn't aware of what the voices told the therapist, but it opened her eyes to the motives of the voices.

A month later, when she met the therapist for the second time, two of the voices appeared to have withdrawn. With the two remaining voices the therapist had a new conversation. Again they said they wanted to regain influence, though the two voices had changed their attitude towards Caroline because she approached them on a more equal basis. She started to acknowledge the voices and paid them respect. Between the sessions Caroline had started her own conversations with her voices. She kept a diary of her voices and negotiated every day with her voices at a fixed time. These scheduled conversations gave her the opportunity to neglect them at other times and focus on the things *she* wanted to focus on. She worked hard with the voices, who changed their attitude, and after the fourth session with the therapist Caroline said she had enough material to discuss with her voices on her own without the therapist. In the meantime she was supported by her case manager who didn't speak very often about the voices. A new balance existed between Caroline and her two voices.

Then she became pregnant, and her medication was tapered down drastically without a detrimental effect on her voices or the level of anxiety. She consulted the therapist once again, to show her baby, and for advice on some practical matters. A few months later she wrote a letter to say the voices had disappeared after she'd had a spiritual experience. About two years later she wrote another letter and said that she used a very low dose of antipsychotics, and heard one positive voice that supported her in making difficult choices. She didn't want to get rid of this voice. In the meantime she was divorced, had moved to another part of the country, found a new partner and lived a happy and satisfactory life with her two children. The negative influence of the original voices had definitely disappeared.

DAAN MARSMAN

WITH MARIUS ROMME

Daan was 13 years old at the time of the first interview for the children's study. Together with his real brother, he lived with foster parents at that time. Daan hears about ten voices. It started with three voices when he was 7 years old. From the beginning he hears the voices in his head. These are the voices of others, because they make a different sound than his own voice and he himself would never have said the things they say.

Daan recognises the voices. Marjolein (his biological mother), Evert (her current husband), Tineke, Marie, Ans, Jan, Floris, Johan and Janny. These are all relatives; slightly more male than female voices. It is particularly the voices of Marjolein and Evert, and those of a brother of his father and his wife that are most negative. All voices are sweet when Daan does as they tell him to (annoying his foster mother) and are mad when he doesn't listen to them and when, for example, he is nice to his mum. The voices are there every day. The voices sometimes come when he is at school or when he walks the dog at night. After some searching, Daan remembers that he started hearing voices when he was still living in Wijk bij Duurstede with Marjolein and Evert. They had hit him really hard and subsequently put him in the shed for a couple of hours. Until two years ago, he had a very miserable childhood with physical abuse. It was then that he was put into foster care. For the last two years, Daan and his brother have been living with their current foster parents, who are like real parents to Daan. He sometimes sees his biological father on a Sunday. He very often feels that he is not wanted. He feels safe at home and at his new school. The voices are always nasty and they nag. They mainly talk about his current mother and about Daan himself, for example, 'Why don't you leave that cow?' The voices tell him to do things; they won't let him have any contact with his foster mother; swear at him (dickhead); tell him what he can and cannot do; cause him confusion, so that he cannot concentrate at school, cannot do his homework, looks for fights and does things for which he gets punished. The voices scare him as they make him do things that he doesn't want to do, for example, chase his brother with a knife. They make him feel ashamed and guilty. The voices are never helpful; they are predominantly negative. Therefore, Daan only thinks of them as nasty. Daan is not always that happy with being alive. On a regular basis he still wants to die, despite the fact that he is enjoying life with his foster parents.

Daan visited a RIAGG (regional institute for mental welfare) psychiatrist twice, because of the voices. The psychiatrist told him that he did not know much about this subject and would ask for more information in the Radboud hospital. That was four months ago and he has not heard from him since. His foster mother is going to make an appointment with Dr Landman, a homeopathic physician. We (the research team) know that he handles children who hear voices very well. During the conversation, Daan does not behave according to his age, he is very needy. He either sits on his foster mother's lap or lies on the couch.

Conclusion after the first interview: Daan hears voices of relatives who swear at him. This means that Daan still has the impression that he is bad and he has not come to terms with having been treated in this way. Therefore, he only sees the negative side and not the incompetence of the other person. He relates the swearing to himself instead of seeing it as someone else's behaviour that involves the other person and not him. Therefore, therapy sessions often address his responses, but he will have to adopt a different image about himself as well as the other person. It is not his problem.

During the second interview, a year later, it turns out that his young foster mother (32 years old), has found it difficult to cope with all the stress. She developed arrhythmias and underwent surgery. Daan's voices do not get involved in these problems. The voices have not changed over the past year. These are the same voices as last year. All the voices are angry. Daan hears some of the voices less often than the year before. Daan himself has grown and deals with them in a different way. Last year Daan was scared when the voices appeared, now he gets angry at them. He says: 'I'm able to do more, I feel better within myself.' Sometimes, he can send the voices away. When he ignores them, they start to squabble. It helps, when he thinks of something else. Swearing does not help.

Last year, he also found decision making difficult, but that has changed now. Daan does not find that difficult any more. An example is choosing what to eat: 'I like chips and therefore I am choosing the menu that comes with chips.' He has also developed slightly more insight which becomes apparent when he says: 'The voices come from the past. They crept into me.' Daan sometimes enjoys his childhood now. He feels safer at home, on the street and at school compared to last year. When he listens to the voices and does the wrong things, his foster parents simply set normal limits. For example, he is not allowed to go out to a party if he has not behaved as desired. Dr Landman, (homeopathic physician) has given him medication against the voices. Daan says: 'The voices are destroyed by the medication. It feels like I'm flushing them away.' [Dr Landman does not just work with medication as a technical tool, but also as an aid to get more control over oneself. This is an advantage of the homeopathic approach which is more holistic and if the physician also knows a little about voices, this will lead to better opportunities to connect.] During the past year, Daan has seen Dr Landman about five times for treatment.

At the end of the interview, Daan says: 'I've faith in life again', and this is noticeable. He is feeling better, but he is not ready to come to terms with things yet. He prefers to suppress everything that is related to the past. He has discovered that he is a talented cyclist. He wins races and his foster parents support him in this. He has become muscular and as he says himself: 'not fat any more'.

During the third interview, two years later, Daan claims to hear an additional four voices. This does correspond to some extent with the expansion of his network, with Ria, the mother of another voice hearer etc. Last year, Daan was more in control. The negative change was caused by his foster mother's regular absence due to the illness of Johan (Daan's brother). Last year, both his brother and foster mother were seriously ill. The voices have become more frequent and increasingly negative. Things are not going well at all at school either. There is talk of him being expelled from school. The voices are making Daan angrier again, sadder and more frightened. His responses to the voices make the situation untenable. By order of the voices, he chases his brother with a knife and he behaves unacceptably aggressively at school. Last year, this was less so. His relationship with the voices has changed too, because the voices have become more dominant during the last year. According to Daan, both he and the voices are in charge. His foster mother is under the impression that he is lazy. The voices are also used as an excuse to not have to exert himself at school. His coping style has become more passive too, 'Listening and just not bothering about things'.

The support network is coming apart at the seams a bit: his brother is often ill and therefore gets more attention, which Daan finds difficult to cope with. His foster mother goes a long way to accepting Daan's experiences, but her husband is not able to do so. This sometimes causes friction between them too. His foster mother really does her best, but does not see any results. Last year Daan and his brother ran away to their real father and that was a real downer for her. There are major differences in terms of upbringing between the foster mother and the real father of the boys whom they visit every weekend. The foster mother says that dad (biological dad) is not always that nice. He chased her once and hit her when they had an argument. The father wanted to take the boys away from her. The foster mother is not the legal mother and that is difficult, as the father has already sent the child welfare office after her.

A year later, during the fourth interview, Daan is at boarding school in Belgium and spends weekends with his foster parents and brother. He still hears voices, but recently, far less often than last year. They are still the same voices. They swear at him, but Daan gets less upset about this. He has become far more laconic. He is even sensible when he explains to his foster mum why she should not get upset over all this family gossip. The voices try to make him do things, but he is better at avoiding these. The voices try to impact on daily life, but they are succeeding increasingly less often. Sometimes the voices have an impact at school, but that depends on how Daan feels. He is more in control again, 'They know I'm in charge.'

Last year he visited the Radboud hospital (University hospital in Nijmegen) for a consultation because of the voices. The psychiatrist examined him and advised that Daan should be sent to a boarding school as he finds it difficult to cope with closeness. The voices are regarded as functional and not psychotic. In addition, Daan is prescribed granules by Dr Landman. These granules help control his aggression better. He takes these every other day. His foster mother notices every time he needs them again. He takes magnesium silicata MK Slob 1.5 mg, 10 granules.

At home there are fewer arguments. Daan had a cycling accident and could not train for a while. He was admitted to hospital. He has been at boarding school since last year. Initially he attended a boarding school where things did not go well. The voices became progressively more negative. His foster mother took him out of this school. A month ago he switched to another school and they are both enthusiastic about this one. This school offers more discipline and structure.

His interpretation of the voices has become more differentiated. They are related to physical abuse by his biological mother and her boyfriend. In his exceptional position, he is unlike other children, more of a loner. He finds it difficult to talk about emotions. He really thinks that the voices are related to his problems. In the meantime, he has been accepted in the national training programme for cyclists and that offers a strong identification and compensation. He looks like a real he-man with his bleached hair. It is clear that he is doing well. He says that he has made a number of decisions. He has decided to be kinder to his foster mum, to care for her, as she is suffering enough as it is. He has emotions again, something he did not have a year ago. He even sounds sensible when he advises his foster mum on her behaviour. He has decided to try and make the most of school. He is in love, but also carries around the picture of another girl. If only things could continue like this for him!

DEBRA LAMPSHIRE

My first recollection of voice hearing was when I was very young, around 6 years old. I would hear a very soothing maternal voice telling me that everything was alright, 'they' would 'protect me' and 'not to be afraid'. It was around this time, shortly after starting school, I found out, quite accidentally, that I was adopted. This voice remained during my early years and was always a great comfort to me. The adoption, however, came to affect me more and more. Everything I had felt so certain about seemed destroyed. Within my family the adoption was considered a secret and was only known to this circle. It was also made very clear that it was an issue which was not to be discussed at any time.

As I approached adolescence the range of voices increased and I was visited by four or five of differing gender and age. They now took on a much more critical tone and made disparaging comments regarding my actions. Still the maternal voice remained to soothe and mitigate the negative impact these voices were having on me.

Over the years I was to gain by subterfuge snippets of information regarding my adoption which added to my sense of loss, betrayal and rejection, as well as undermining my self-esteem. I was to discover that I had been sent back to the adoption agency by one couple as it was believed that I was defective in some way and possibly brain-damaged. In later years I was also to become the victim of abuse. I believe that it was not one specific traumatic event that made me susceptible to voice hearing but a succession of significant, distressing events which established a vulnerability to the repeated trauma I experienced, of being worthless, defective and unlovable.

Upon completing my schooling, the voices became more active and far more intrusive; they invaded all parts of my life and I felt I had no privacy and was constantly being observed and scrutinised. I lived in fear of the barrage of abuse that would follow any action of mine. I became increasingly anxious about mixing with others. I retreated into a solitary world as I endeavoured to make sense of what was happening to me. A complex and mystical explanation developed in which I believed that I had been chosen to receive a message from God. This message would relieve mankind of war and conflict and peace would prevail.

What I had to do was stay home and be ready to receive this message.

In the meantime I was being tested by demons and the devil (the voices) to prove I was a worthy recipient of the message. I stayed in my house for eighteen years, not leaving except in the most exceptional circumstances. The voices exposed secrets that only I was privy to.

I began to study the Bible looking for references to myself, and my beliefs became more entrenched and even more fanciful. I was seduced by the notion that my suffering and miserable existence had some purpose and meaning to it.

Constantly I failed. I was unable to demonstrate the qualities required of me. The battle was becoming more and more difficult and I started to doubt that I would ever measure up.

I reached a point where I felt I could no longer continue the quest. I had no option but to kill myself. Surely God would grant me peace and then I would no longer be tormented – I would be free. While the desire to gain peace was overwhelming the will to live was stronger. With the help and assistance of a friend I decided I was going to have one last crack at getting the voices under control and, if that failed, I would know I had done all I could. I had been under mental health services for several years and although I was heavily medicated the voices persisted and my body was lethargic and yet agitated all at the same time.

RECOVERY

I decided that everything I was doing so far was not working for me, so doing the exact opposite made sense to me. I began to reflect and to critically analyse what was happening and I concluded that the demons had made a mistake in choosing me. I was not up to the task and if they had made a mistake in picking me then perhaps they were not as infallible or as powerful as I'd initially believed. In this process my friend was of great importance. My friend always allowed me to drive the process and come up with strategies to confront the voices. This demonstrated to me their belief that I was resourceful, competent and able to drive the recovery process, that I did in fact have the courage, resilience and capacity to heal myself. I had not been able to get this validation from clinicians. My friend's support was hugely affirming and established a sense of control within me that had long been missing in my life.

I decided to test this out. One of the first things I did was change my attitude towards them, so, instead of being fearful of them and bowing to their every whim, I embraced them as friends and welcomed their intrusions, greeting them with kindness and respect. As a consequence, my fear reduced, which in turn alleviated the distress I felt. Now when I heard a voice my anxiety level didn't increase.

I decided that I would set the demons some tasks. I gave them a simple task of washing the dishes unaided. They were unable to achieve this and so the seed of doubt as to their actual power was sown. I realised that the only power the voices had was the power I gave them. They needed me to perform tasks and to speak to certain people; without me they were impotent. It was me that held the power. This was a moment of enlightenment and the beginning of my own journey of taking back control.

It was never my intention to get rid of the voices. They had been such a large part of my life that the idea of living in a silent world scared me. I still had a few that were positive and comforting. I decided that they could stay, but the ones that caused so much distress would have to learn some manners if we were going to coexist.

Now I began the process of reclaiming my life. I approached the voices as I would approach any relationship and began to put parameters around how and when they could contact me. I also began exploring other areas of my life. I thought about the role the voices played in my life and discovered they fulfilled a need in me — a need to feel connected to someone, a need for a friend, a need to belong. As unkind as they were, they were only telling me the truth about myself. The voices kept me so busy I had no time for any other relationships and they also spared me the pain and hurt I had experienced by numerous rejections from people in the past. At least they did not desert me. As the voices receded, feelings of loss and grief filled the void.

I decided I needed to take the risk of inviting real people into my world and cautiously and clumsily this became my new quest. It proved to be pivotal to my recovery. Developing relationships and being exposed to people who showed they could be kind, caring and flawed, just like me, freed me from the need for voices. As I put more time and energy into these relationships, the negative voices receded further and further back.

I devoted my time to just getting my voices under control and it took approximately nine months before I felt completely confident that I had mastered this. I eventually got to the stage where I began to venture out from my home. I continued my education, went to university, made friends and gained employment. Instead of having a life totally consumed by voices, now I began to devour my ordinary life.

It was several years later that I decided to work in the field of mental health as an advisor and educator. I was approached by a clinician who wanted to start up therapy groups for voice hearers. She discussed her ideas and we talked about my understanding of the process and the key points I'd learnt from my own process of dealing with voices.

On reflection, these key points were as follows:

- The voices have something important to say, but they only know how to communicate in a negative, clunky way.
- For me to make sense of the voices I needed to interpret what it is that they are truly trying to tell me.
- I realised that what they have to say is important, so they won't let me ignore them.
- There is a strong relationship between voices and stress. Often they are trying to tell me I'm stressed or worried about something and I need to do something about it.
- Arguing with them doesn't help; they always win.
- They can't always be trusted to tell the truth so I need to evaluate what they are saying and see if there are other possible explanations for what they have said to me.
- The only power they have is the power I give them. I'm in charge here, I'll decide what I do as it is only I who must face the consequences, not the voices.
- They react to the way they are approached. Instead of being fearful of them and bowing to their every whim, I have embraced them as friends, greeting them with kindness and respect. As a consequence my fear has reduced.
- They might fulfill a need in one's life; for me, a need to feel connected to someone, a need for a friend, a need to belong.
- They might fill a void of feelings, of loss and grief.
- They might represent the demons in one's life. For me, I took back the power of my demons.

The mind is a powerful tool and I identified my personal strengths and worked with them. I found it almost impossible to change my emotions but I could change the way I thought about things; I could change my attitude to the voices – which influences the way I think, feel and respond to them.

By drawing on my own experience of getting the voices under control, together with the clinician, we extracted the skills and knowledge that I had acquired and converted that understanding into the basic content for hearing-voices group sessions. Then, after feedback from the participants, we refined these skills further. These are the same skills and approach that I use today in order to function and thrive.

I have found my niche. I have had the opportunity to take what was a catastrophic event and turn it into a positive life-affirming vocation. I am surrounded by people who are as passionate and committed as I am about working with people to enhance their well-being and their lives. I have found where I belong.

DENISE BOSMAN

INTERVIEWS WITH SANDRA ESCHER AND DIRK CORSTENS

Denise took part in the children's study (Escher, 2005) from 1996, and it was during this study that she was referred to Dirk Corstens for therapy. Denise agreed to this. Dirk Corstens also worked on our project and took part in a research project for psychotherapy for people with borderline characteristics. Denise's difficult childhood had caused a strong acting-out of her dissatisfaction. At the first interview in 1996 Denise is 18 years old and lives with her father and sister. Her parents are divorced and she seldom sees her mother.

Denise has heard voices all her life and has experienced trouble with them since the previous year. She is afraid of them and they confuse her. Because of the voices she is unable to pay attention at school. They comment on her life and on things she experiences during the day. They make her argue and want to run away. If she is angry or sad the voices say 'death is better'. When the voices make her afraid she becomes aggressive towards them in order to regain power.

It was after a very stressful period in the previous year that the voices had given Denise trouble. Six months previously she had become pregnant and had an abortion as suggested by one of her teachers. She says, 'That's why the voices came: I didn't want an abortion.' Then, on holiday with her mother, an argument had led to a fight and Denise had left early and gone back home.

Her relationship with her mother had always been problematic. Her mother had had a psychiatric illness (manic depression) with regular outbursts since Denise was six years old. Then, when Denise was 13, her parents divorced. She lived briefly with an uncle and aunt and then moved from Rotterdam to Maastricht to live with her father. The problems in the family were huge with high levels of aggression. Denise tells how she once tried to strangle her sister and was consequently beaten up by her mother. Furthermore, between the ages of 8 and 10, unbeknown to her parents, she had been sexually abused by her piano teacher.

Apart from the voices, she doesn't feel well. She is very anxious when outside on her own and afraid of being followed. She doesn't dare go out at all except with her friend, often staying in bed and watching television instead. When her friend visits she becomes aggressive towards him, calling him all sorts of names, and he accepts it all. She expresses suicidal wishes and, as a means of warding this off, she sometimes cuts herself.

In 1995 and 1996, because of her aggressiveness and the abortion, she had psychiatric outpatient treatment and it was only when she visited the outpatient clinic that she realised she heard voices – before, she had thought they were ghosts. Then the treatment stopped. Denise thinks that this was because she was too old for the youth department and too young for the adult department.

RECOVERY

By the third interview Denise had moved on to live with her friend and his parents. She had begun to study economics at university and hadn't heard voices for six months. She says that the voices disappeared because of her therapy. In therapy she has learned to deal with her emotions. If she is angry she shouts or hits a cushion, then she starts talking about her feelings. She still has arguments but she can express herself and feels more secure. She is still afraid but only when she feels alone, and that is less often now because of her changed social situation. She cries more easily and, although she can talk about it, she still finds this difficult. Because she is now talking about these issues, she sleeps better and is less often tired; she feels more secure and is less doubtful. The voices used to have a strong influence on her concentration and she still has concentration problems even though the voices have gone. Making decisions is still very difficult and she prefers to leave this to other people. If Denise doesn't agree with something, now she will talk about it whereas last year she would have been more likely to start an argument.

During the fourth interview Denise is 21 and living with her father and younger sister again. She has left her boyfriend. She is in her third year at university. She hasn't heard voices for eighteen months and puts this down to her treatment, acknowledging that she has become much calmer as a result of it. She is less afraid and, when she does experience fear, she starts to think about something else. When she is very anxious, which is seldom, she reads or listens to music.

The voices confused Denise but this is no longer the case, as confirmed by the dissociative experience scale. She is much better able to concentrate. The voices made her seek arguments, now she avoids these by talking about her irritations instead. She used to harm herself to ward off the voices, now she doesn't even think about self-harm. She used to find it very difficult to be alone but now she is more independent. She still attends the borderline therapy project. For two years she had intensive therapy twice a week. The frequency of the sessions was then reduced and she now sees her therapist once a week. Soon this will be further reduced to once a fortnight.

About the voices she has learned it is something she can deal with from within herself. She doesn't have to be scared of them. She need not allow them to make choices for her. She can control her own life. Looking back, she thinks her voices had something to do with her parents divorcing; the often aggressive relations at home; the sexual abuse of her piano teacher from which she couldn't defend herself; her moving from Rotterdam to Maastricht when she was 12; the abortion when she was 16 and the damaging relationship with her boyfriend.

DESCRIPTION OF THE TREATMENT BY DIRK CORSTENS

In fact, we didn't pay much attention to the voices. When the stress diminished they didn't show up anymore.

The therapy is called 'schema-focused cognitive therapy' and uses a clear model of borderline disorder. The model differentiates several schema modes that have come into existence through difficult life circumstances and adapts to overwhelming feelings caused by rejection, unpredictability and transgressions of personal integrity. These schema modes can be very rigid and are in conflict with each other. This is the reason why an individual can feel so torn apart, because these modes present themselves in such a variety of ways. The strong changes in mood and self-esteem are explained by these schema modes. This model is explained to the individual extensively and he/she often recognises these modes. The modes are:

- The protector: very closed down, feeling nothing, feeling and appearing detached, not saying much about feelings, appearing 'as normal as possible'. This mode is very present with Denise. She is unable to talk about the overwhelming feelings she has experienced in crisis, in fact she cannot describe what she feels at all.

- The punitive parent: accusing oneself, accusing everybody else, callous and punitive. When people are in this mode they behave and speak with self-loathing. Often they harm themselves. With Denise this mode is active when she is in crisis situations. She harms herself mainly when she is in the angry-child mode.

- The angry child: in this mode the individual is extremely angry, enraged about the perceived injustice of what has been done to her. Stamping with rage, accusing, distrusting everybody. In such a mode Denise threw herself out of a moving car.

- The abused and/or abandoned child: alone, sad, rejected, demanding, inconsolable. Denise persistently denied this mode.
- The adult: capable of thinking through cause and effect, acknowledging the benefit of emotions, but mainly reflecting, incapable of feeling. Denise was not well able to reflect about herself.

The attitude of the therapist in this situation is very important and informed by what Jeffrey Young, who developed the therapy, calls 'limited reparenting'. The therapist adopts the attitude of a substitute parent and is available for patients to call in the evening or at night when they are in crisis. The frequency of the sessions is at least twice a week, temporarily increased when necessary. It is important to meet all the modes in the sessions and to work with them. The past plays an important role: it is carefully analysed, which events and persons played what kind of role in the development of the modes; what people and events caused the modes. Important therapeutic – so-called 'experiential' – techniques are imagination and role plays. Perhaps the name 'cognitive therapy' is a bit misleading but emotions do play a pivotal part in this therapy. People are supported to learn to think about their emotions and use them in a more effective and satisfying way. By imagining stressful situations from the past, strongly supported by the therapist, these situations are re-experienced, but now the image is manipulated to show alternative conclusions and to create imagined situations where the individual experiences power and no longer feels powerless. Conclusions which the individual has reached in the past, determining their reactions, are tested and changed in role-plays with the patient and therapist exchanging roles and exercises with new behaviour.

What was important for Denise, I think, was that I supported her and made sense of her sometimes extreme behaviour by explaining it in the context of rejection and neglect by her parents when she was a child. Denise agreed with this at the end: she had been a very lonely child in an unpredictable and aggressive environment. Her behaviour, feelings and thoughts were justified by this early environment. These difficult feelings had a cause and a goal: to survive. Denise didn't call me after official office hours, I had to stimulate that. She didn't expect much support; she hadn't experienced much support during her life and she was afraid to attach herself to anyone. In our conversations she talked from the protector mode most of the time. It was extremely difficult for her to act from the other schema modes, to bring them into my consulting room. Making sense of her feelings was what most helped Denise to change her self-image. The voices disappeared because she learned to understand her emotions better and to express them. Fundamental change didn't appear though. The work with the imagination, necessary to promote change, she didn't dare engage in. She remained very dependent on her parents, not capable of living on her own. Her father, in particular, prevented her becoming independent; he needed her presence because he was very alone. She chose boyfriends far below her own intellectual level and had very restricted impulse control. These boyfriends encouraged her negative self-image. She remained vulnerable to (supposed) abandonment through which she could then react extremely. She didn't bring this mode to therapy and so we were unable to work with it.

Six months after we ended the therapy she came back in crisis. As a result of conflicts in her relationship with her boyfriend she expressed suicidal tendencies in a very dramatic way. She seemed to be good at choosing the wrong boys. She never complained about voices anymore. I don't think they came back. We started therapy again. She improved quickly once we had sorted out the relationship problems.

DON DUGGER

INTERVIEWS WITH DIRK CORSTENS

Don, born in 1938, was brought to me by his wife Rinske for a consultation because *she* suspected he heard voices. She had visited a hearing voices conference where she concluded that the experiences of psychiatric patients could be taken seriously. She was dissatisfied with the treatment that her husband had received. She knew him to be a very intelligent man who was interested in life. He liked to read and to teach, he was involved in the developments of his profession and she felt that these aspects of her husband had been neglected. Her objections to Don's treatment had not been taken seriously, in fact she felt that there had not really been any treatment at all.

Don had been admitted to hospital in 1984. He had a psychosis and was mute for quite a long time. The diagnosis was schizophrenia. In the first years he couldn't talk, a condition known as 'mutism' in psychiatric jargon. He was treated pharmaceutically and prescribed Clozapine and Lithium. Initially he was perceived as psychotic. Later he showed more resignation but closed himself off from his environment. Nobody asked him about his life. Rinske was clearly perceived as a 'symbiotic spouse' and not taken seriously either. Don had stayed on different wards in the psychiatric hospital for some years but for the last seven he had lived in sheltered housing. He spent most of his time sitting in a chair staring out of the window. He didn't say much but when he did try to speak it was very softly with an American accent, and difficult to understand. He took little care of himself and led a very restricted life. He had become like a shadow, almost invisible. His wife and three children visited him regularly. Only his wife persisted with the image she had of him before he was admitted.

So Don had already lived in psychiatric institutions for fifteen years when he and his wife visited me in 1999. That they were prepared to travel 200km to Maastricht proved how persistent Rinske was in her belief that somewhere the old Don still existed, and also how motivated she was to rediscover him. I talked mainly to Rinske as I could hardly understand what Don was saying. He listened attentively but often seemed very tired. He told me he didn't hear voices or, to be more accurate, he didn't really know whether he did or not. Together with Rinske, and in Don's presence, I reconstructed his life story and tried to find the cause of the dramatic behavioural change that had resulted in his admission fifteen years previously. After two conversations, I asked the GP who prescribed Don's medication to reduce it, guessing that Don's speech impediment and lethargy were partly related to the medication even though he was not on a high dosage. To my surprise, the GP cooperated; I imagined how difficult it would have been if a psychiatrist had prescribed the medication! Gradually, Don became more talkative. He started to make contact with his environment and even described a period when he felt 'harmonious'. He started to read again, spent more time with Rinske and was better able to take care of himself. We didn't meet any more after 2000 but some months later Don became very ill. He appeared dehydrated and had Lithium poisoning. He was in a coma for three weeks, his life in danger. When he finally regained consciousness he became hyperactive. He lived with Rinske again but she found his behaviour manic, although he felt himself to be reborn. He twice fell off his bike and, after breaking his legs, was admitted to a general hospital for surgery where the psychiatrist in charge prescribed him Olanzapine 5mg. Then began what Don called his 'stable period' – 'More stable than ever before'. Don and Rinske were very satisfied with the psychiatrist and kept in regular contact with him. About four years after our first encounter I wrote to Don and Rinske asking them to write down the essential elements of their recovery story; then they visited me again so that we could look back together and share some insights. I will summarise what they told me.

Don said: 'You talked to me as a person. I found an identity. You showed an interest in the play I wrote when I was still working at the school.' (This was a play about an Egyptian goddess). 'That challenged my identity. All that time I had been treated as a patient. I had been in no man's land for years.' Don trained as an anthroposophist and for years he was a teacher at an anthroposophic school. One of the reasons for his derangement in 1984 had been a conflict with one of the intellectual leaders in that field, a conflict that estranged him from the people he belonged to. 'My astral body was on its own. I observed everything but I had lost my 'I', my identity. My emotions had stagnated but I became much clearer when the medication was reduced. Gradually, I rediscovered my identity and found harmony. When I woke from that coma, my bodily crisis, I rediscovered my 'I'. I didn't feel this mist around me anymore. My identity reconnected to the other parts of my being. This manic episode I perceived as a breaking out. The I-forces took possession of me again. I wanted to do things for myself again. It all happened in a tearing rush. The last fracture of my leg, together with the medication probably, had a restraining influence on me that made me find an organic rhythm. The advantage of this manic period was that my wife was drawn back on herself. She distanced herself from me. I needed that. Later on we were able to come together again. Now everything is going well and I have made a very important decision.' Don had decided not to go back to his native country any more because the urge to go back to the United States had always meant a good deal of stress. This had been the direct cause of his admission in 1984. In his opinion he suffered from an inner conflict related to his ancestry (too complicated to describe here) and he discovered that it was necessary to close down his past in a well-balanced way.

Compared to 1999, Don was a completely different man. He spoke clearly, was easy to understand, made contact easily, exhibited facial expression, made jokes and was able to put things into perspective. He obviously enjoyed life. He had conquered the diagnosis of schizophrenia. To me, it was like seeing a man who has escaped from sixteen years of imprisonment. His perspective was different: 'I don't look at those sixteen years as something coincidental. I had to go through specific things, this was my fate. Now I have taken up the thread again.' And Rinske said: 'In psychiatry one only talks about illness. Don lived under continuous pressure from his fourth year on. His anger went underground. People who are ill shouldn't just be written off. Don's background was always important to me. In those sixteen years all our friends gradually disappeared. We became isolated. On the one hand I experienced Don as very distant but on the other I could see how powerful he was. He had to go through it all. I was astonished after all those years of isolation to see that everything he had learned before still was there!'

Don could now tell that he hadn't been suffering from voices in those years but he recognised some inner voices who said some nasty things. We didn't talk much about it, though in our last conversation he told me an impressive story. Once he did hear a voice, the only occasion in his life. At the age of 35 a commanding voice told him to jump out of a window. He did it and broke both his legs. He never heard that voice again. During that period his employer was trying to force him to return to America but his wife and children would not be allowed to accompany him. This presented Don with a huge dilemma: if he wanted to stay in Europe he had to leave his job, but he couldn't afford to do this. The accident made it possible to stay! In some way the voice had forced a decision.

Through her stubbornness in retaining that strong sense of her husband, Rinske had made it possible for Don to regain his identity. Talking about who he really was and tapering down the medication that had imprisoned him for sixteen years had also opened the way for Don's recovery. His wife's persistence and the acknowledgement of him as a person had proved to be Don's escape route from no man's land.

ELEANOR LONGDEN

INTERVIEW WITH JACQUI DILLON

Eleanor is a 25-year-old woman who lives in Bradford. She is a psychology undergraduate at the University of Leeds. She works for the Early Intervention in Psychosis service in Bradford as a service-user development worker, as well as teaching and training on mental-health issues. She enjoys socialising and hanging out with friends.

I've always had a dominant voice and that has been constant throughout my experience. He has named himself and he has given himself an identity. He has a physical form, Machiavellian and rather grotesque. He is the archetypal horror-film figure. The other voices come and go and change but he has been present throughout the whole thing.

I went to university when I was 18 to do a degree in English. I'd never been away from home before, I was quite naïve and I was accruing a massive debt. The group I got into at university were very different people to the kind I had known prior to going. They were very hedonistic, very outgoing, they didn't take their work very seriously and I felt torn between wanting to follow that path and feeling that I ought to be working hard and taking it seriously, being a conscientious and diligent student. The thing that made it more difficult is that I did not have relationships that helped me to develop my sense of self, to help build up self-confidence. I felt that I didn't really know who I was anymore.

It was around that time that this voice turned up. It was very banal, very mundane, it just commented on what I was doing. The way that I understood it at the time was like the voice was, or I was, reprimanding myself for my lack of assertion. Then I made the fatal mistake of mentioning to one of my friends that I was hearing this voice and telling her about the impact that it had on me. She was absolutely horrified, saying that hearing voices is not a good thing and that I should get some help. So I made an appointment to see the GP who referred me to a psychiatrist. I presented myself as a confused, troubled 18-year-old who didn't have much self-esteem or confidence in herself and who was worried about the future. The psychiatrist disregarded all this and honed in on what she perceived as a developing psychosis. The next time I went back she said to me, 'I'd like you to come into hospital voluntarily, just for three days or so.'

It was a savage and terrifying experience. I was the youngest person there by about twenty years. The psychiatrist equated voice hearing with insanity and I got a diagnosis of schizophrenia. With this I got the message that I was a passive victim of pathology. I wasn't encouraged to do anything to actively help myself. Therapy meant drug therapy. It was hugely disempowering. It was all undermining my sense of self, exacerbating all my doubts about myself. The devastating impact just served to make the voices stronger and more aggressive because I became so frightened of them. What started off as experience became symptoms. When I heard the voice I would get very agitated. I went from hearing one mild, rather banal voice, which then became three, became eight, became twelve, and then this dominant voice shows up taking on this terrible physical manifestation.

This all happened in a shockingly short space of time. I went into that hospital a troubled, confused, unhappy 18-year-old and I came out a schizophrenic – and I was a good one. I came to embody what psychosis should look and feel like. They did not send me back home but just let me go to the university halls. It all escalated. There was this terrible domino effect because the more people polarised and victimised me the more bizarre my behaviour became. I was spat at outside the students union and I became this really sad and lonely figure who would drift around campus on her own and sit on her own in lectures. I'd walk into a room and hear this flurry of laughter. People started calling me 'psycho'. My family, they mourned for me like I had actually died because the person that I'd been had gone. It absolutely devastated my family, my mother particularly. In one of my rare moments of lucidity, I saw there were tears in her eyes. I was suddenly struck by this sense that my mum was fighting for me.

RECOVERY

I went back to Bradford and my new psychiatrist was Pat Bracken. That was a massive help. The very first time I met him he said to me, 'Hi Eleanor, nice to meet you. Can you tell me a bit about yourself?' So I just looked at him and said, 'I'm Eleanor and I'm a schizophrenic', and in his quiet, Irish voice, he said something very powerful: 'I don't want to know what other people have told you about yourself, I want to know about you.' It was the first time that I had been given the chance to see myself – not as this genetically determined schizophrenic who was biologically flawed and mentally deficient like a degenerate. He was so much more humane than that, and he didn't talk about auditory hallucinations, he talked about hearing voices and unusual beliefs rather than delusions, anxiety rather than paranoia. He didn't use this terrible mechanistic, clinical language but just couched everything in normal language and normal experience.

So, after seeing my mum is trying, Pat Bracken is trying, his team is trying, my sister is trying, my dad's trying; 'Who's not trying here?' The only person not fighting for me was me. It was a real wake-up call. I sat in my front room, I looked in the mirror and I looked pretty bad. Part of me was saying, 'look, look at yourself' – not in an aggressive way, but this little compassionate part of me was saying, 'Look, is this what it's come to? Aren't you going to do something about it?' I'd got to the absolute lowest and I couldn't go any lower. It was at that moment that I suddenly thought, 'Right, you *are* going to do something about this. You are not going to let this go on any more. This is as far as it goes and you are going to do something about it now.' I was very assertive with myself.

I realised that the psychiatric system had made me a victim, but it was me who was keeping up that victim role. I knew then that what I had to do was to take on this voice because it was him who was running the show. He'd say, 'Jump', and I'd say, 'How high?' I asked myself questions. Why had I sacrificed my sanity to do this degree? 'Think of the ambition you had, think about what you wanted to do. Are you just going to let that go?' But there was one big barrier between me and the future, and that was this voice.

Pat told me about the philosophy of Marius Romme and Sandra Escher and about the Hearing Voices Network and that this is just normal human experience and the importance of conceptualising it in your own way. These experiences are so complex and so meaningful – it doesn't happen in a social, emotional or spiritual vacuum, there is a context to it and a meaning in it.

I spoke to Julie (Downs) on the phone one day and started reading about HVN and thought: 'Whoa! Maybe I can be a part of this.' I then asked Pat if I could come off medication and he agreed to support me in that process. I knew that I needed a clear head to negotiate this weird subconscious world in a constructive way. The first thing I wanted to do was overcome the fear that I felt towards this dominant voice. I was terrified of him. I realised that the fear of him had created this vicious circle of avoidance and isolation and dependence on services and my family and that I needed to break that circle.

I tentatively began to test out what the voice claimed. I began to realise that nobody else could see or hear him – what does that tell me? Having realised this, I decided to try and push it a little bit further. Does he have the influence that he claims? He says that he can do all this stuff, that he can kill my family. Can he though? The voice got wind of this, so he began upping the ante. He had a real survival instinct and he didn't like this potential shift of power. One night he said, 'I want you to cut off your toe and, if you don't, I'll kill your family.' It was the hardest thing I've ever had to do but I said,

'Go on then, just do it.' It was really eerie because during these instructions his voice had been painfully loud and I could hear this phantom choir of his in the background, giggling and talking about me, and his terrible maniacal laughter. And when I said, 'Just do it', it was like a switch had been flicked off and there was silence. It was really frightening. I sat there thinking 'Oh my god, what is he going to do?' But I kept to my word and, what I did was, I sat outside my parent's room all night, from nine at night to seven in the morning, and nothing happened. My parents were absolutely fine. I thought 'Right, I've got you.' You could almost hear his desperate back-pedalling and he was still saying that he was going to do it, but I now doubted him and I began to question him further.

I began to put boundaries in place, saying things to him like, 'Do not talk to me before eight o'clock in the evening because I will not talk to you.' Over time I began to have more control of the times and, again, it made me question 'How powerful is he really if he's willing to wait until after EastEnders to talk to me?' Realising these things made me think 'Well, where is he coming from? He's not coming from outside, he can't be, it can only be from me.' I was very intrigued by this idea and I began to slowly realise that, yes, he is a demon but he was a personal demon. Everyone has their private demons and his demonic aspects were the unaccepted aspects of my self-image, my shadow – so it was appropriate that he was so shadowy. He'd always been dismissed as this psychotic hallucination yet even his physical form did have meaning to it. What I have learned, and the only way I recovered, was by learning that this grotesque aspect of him is superfluous. The contempt and loathing that he expresses is actually to do with me in that it reflects how I feel about myself. He is like a very external form of my own insecurities, my own self-doubt, and that is the part that is relevant and does need attending to, does need taking seriously because it is meaningful. What he says is a very powerful statement about what I am feeling about myself and, in that respect, I do relate him to me by learning to deconstruct this figure and learn what is relevant and what isn't. He has a lot of relevance and a lot of personal meaning and he is capable of making very powerful statements about issues in my life that I need to deal with. It is difficult because voices are often metaphorical and it's about finding the literal meaning in a figurative form of speech and then finding the personal relevance to it. For instance, when he talks very violently about mutilation and death I see it as a barometer and realise that I need to take better care of myself and attend to my own needs more. It sounds like a bizarre thing to say but he is useful in that he does provide insight into conflicts that I need to deal with.

Having realised that maybe I could trust him and be more trusting of him, in turn, he became more compassionate towards me. Rather than being abusive back to him I became more gentle, even loving, towards him and that vicious circle that we'd gotten into of antagonism, hostility and malevolence began to diminish. I realised that he could be a positive force if I would let him be. It took a long time but it got to the point where my demons could be cast out. While he is still around – he has never left and he is still there – he has lost his power to devastate me. I listen to him now because I see that he's listening to me. I don't catastrophise him. I see that – like when my mum gets very stressed she gets bad headaches – when I get very stressed I hear really bad voices. I now show respect to him and he is now more likely to show me respect.

Because everyone responded so negatively to the first voice I heard I learned not to trust my voices. If I'd never entered the psychiatric system things would have been very different for me. This is what has given me this imperative to go back into the system and try to make a difference. I think that the ownership of psychosis belongs to those who experience it. Psychiatry has to accept that. I haven't taken medication for years and I haven't been in services for years. I live a high-functioning, high-achieving life. I am weary of romanticising psychosis and, although what happened was terrible, I'm glad it happened because, emotionally, I was stuck and it gave me the chance to move on. It wasn't a breakdown, it was a breakthrough. My experiences have given me a believable strength. I have had to look down into that black hole and my mind has taken me to some of the worst places that a human being can go to, but I got through that and I am still here and I am still a voice hearer. But I am more than that – I am proud to be a voice hearer. It is an incredibly special and unique experience. I am so glad that I have been given the opportunity to see it that way because recovery is a fundamental human right and I shouldn't be the exception, I should be the rule. That is why I want to be a part of this movement to change the way that we relate to human experience and diversity.

Your soul can't breathe when your mind has been colonised.

ELISABETH SVANHOLMER

WITH TREVOR EYLES

My name is Elisabeth Svanholmer and I was born on 15th August 1981 in Skagen, Denmark. I am single and live alone. I have completed a Danish student exam and I began my training as a physiotherapist in 2008. I am involved with the Working with Voices Project in Aarhus, Denmark. I enjoy painting, writing, dancing and reading.

I have heard voices all my life, which means that I cannot recall a time when I did not hear voices. My sisters and mother tell me that I probably heard voices even before I started speaking. I think that as a baby I would withdraw into my own world or seem to be communicating without having contact with other people. I didn't question my experiences and I cannot remember being afraid of them. I think I communicated with them on a daily basis, although not constantly. My voice-hearing experiences started to change when I was 7 or 8 years old, after we moved to Aarhus and I changed schools.

The five voices that have influenced my life the most are: Søren – an invisible friend who has been with me for as long as I can remember. He represents everything that true friendship means to me: support, respect, honesty, trust, a deep unspoken understanding and the ability to love without wanting to possess. He is a fairy and a boy. ISC – an inner surveillance camera; a function of consciousness that enables me to be very observant and gives me a sense of control. Neither negative nor positive, just constantly registering and verbalising everything that happens inside me and around me at a very high speed. Mother – the voice of my mother representing my difficulties in dealing with my emotions towards her and the fact that I am her daughter. A pessimistic, critical and negative voice. Xhabbo – Sea-God. Can take any shape he wants: human, creature, spirit etc. He is my inner father figure, passionately desiring me, watching over me, teaching and supporting me. Domina – my suppressed sense of self, of value, of being something unique and deserving the best of everything in life. She appeared as several different voices – a process of increasing dissociation. The more I suppressed her, the more voices I attained and the more destructive and violent they became.

From birth until I was 17 I lived alone with my mother, even though I have 3 older siblings (a half-brother and two half-sisters). We have never had any contact with my father and he has never tried to contact me. My mother chose to raise me alone and she has not been in a relationship since she got pregnant with me, so I grew up with no clue as to what men or relationships between men and women were all about. Until I was 8 we lived in Skanderborg and I attended pre-school class and then 1st grade in a Rudolf Steiner school. I experienced my first real friendships and had a boyfriend who I had a deep connection with and strong feelings for. I felt accepted and appreciated. At the end of my 1st grade year my mother told me that she had decided we would move to Aarhus and I was to change school. I clearly remember how I felt: I was angry and in pain; I could not comprehend why my mother would take me away from everything that was good in my life and, for the first time, I questioned the way we lived – just the two of us and the moving around. I realised that my mother, for all her good intentions, did not make choices that were meeting my needs. But I just resigned myself and somehow did what I could to accept the situation. Changing schools was not a positive experience for me. The children in my new class had already found their places in the social hierarchy and I missed my old class, my boyfriend and my close friends from Skanderborg. I became very self-conscious in the attempt to adjust to the new social situation.

During the following years I started hearing voices that were very different from those of my childhood. Since moving from Skanderborg to Aarhus I had begun to have very mixed emotions regarding my mother and I had got to the point of hating her and blaming her for everything that was wrong with me and my life – and hating myself for hating her. I longed for a man who would set things right.

From the age of 12 until I was 22 I was living with increasing inner chaos where I had no feeling of any connection between what I felt, what I knew, what I hoped for, what I sensed, what I wanted, what I needed, what I felt I should do and what I thought I could do. I put all my energy into surviving, getting through the days without damaging myself too much. I found strategies to escape the internal battle and attained an incredibly high level of self-control. I escaped my mind by focusing on how to live a 'normal' life – at school, in relationships. But escaping was always time-limited and, when I returned to my mind or body, I found that everything was even worse than when I left – like coming home to screaming and arguing voices. The worst thing imaginable was that anyone else should feel just a hint of my pain and chaos and for a long time I believed that I would manage to work through my problems by myself.

I was often physically sick: I developed allergies to food, dust and animals, I suffered from headaches, migraines, reoccurring bladder infections and so on. I had violent nightmares, was in a more or less constant state of anxiety and became increasingly insecure – afraid of not being able to control the impulses to mutilate and kill myself and, later on, acting out aggressively towards others. I only felt a minimum of safety when my mother or my ex-boyfriend was close by, sort of taking turns looking after me.

My mother went with me to the psychiatric hospital and managed to convince them to admit me, which was a great relief for me. They diagnosed me with schizophrenia and immediately took me off antidepressant medication and put me on Zyprexa. The medicine helped me to gradually restore my normal sleep pattern, going from three or four hours disrupted sleep to eight to ten hours of deep sleep. After six months I stopped taking the medication and have not taken any since. Since I was still suffering from severe headaches, physical restlessness and feelings of uneasiness and nausea more or less constantly, I asked to be referred to a physiotherapist.

RECOVERING

I began receiving physiotherapy when I was 22. The first period of weekly sessions lasted for six months. A year later I returned to the same therapist and, for another six months, we worked with a Body Awareness Therapy consisting of exercises and massage.

During a two-year period of on/off physiotherapy I experienced building a relationship with a man, based on trust and mutual respect, for the first time in my life. He was capable of giving me all the attention, affirmation and physical care that I needed without me being afraid of losing him or being taken advantage of. I was literally in good hands. He helped me experience my body as a safe place and I realised how tormented I was by anxiety – like a deer always ready to take flight.

For the first time in a long, long time I felt able to be in my body, feel my emotions, think my thoughts, hear my voices and feel that whatever I was experiencing was all right and that things were going to be OK. Experiencing that someone I trusted had faith in me, cared for me and wanted the best for me, helped me rediscover a feeling of self-confidence and self-esteem that I thought I had lost forever. Being embraced made me able to embrace myself.

Discovering that I could live through a whole hour without having a single self-destructive thought or impulse, and once in a while even enjoy being me, was very unfamiliar and quite scary. Maybe I deserved to live after all and live without constant fear and pain. Perhaps there was a way of healing after years and years of separating myself from myself and others. Together we restored my faith in finding someone who dared to relate to me and my world and who could help me make sense of my chaos and support me through my journey.

When I was 24 I met Trevor Eyles and Pia Annat who were working with voice hearers in social psychiatry in Aarhus. Their acceptance and curiosity made me open up and gave me the courage to change my own attitude towards my voices and myself. I chose to start working individually with the Maastricht Interview together with Trevor. I knew that in order to change the way I related to myself I needed a close relationship with a male therapist – one who I felt connected to and could trust – so that I could work through the deep fear of loss and the feelings of abandonment connected to the absence of my father.

The Maastricht Interview helped me to start listening to my voices again – really listening and not just registering that they were there. I also began realising the importance of how I listened: whether I doubted everything they said; if I chose to ignore, disregard or even ridicule what they said. I realised how many ideas I had about who they were and what they wanted without having asked them. Some of the voices responded almost immediately to my new attitude towards them and changed completely from being aggressive, controlling and intimidating to guiding and supporting me, showing me great confidence and respect but also persistently keeping me on this new path. I was able to describe nine regular voices and connect them to my life story. Some of my voices were very uncertain how to respond and one refused to be categorised as a voice.

Three months later I participated in a three-day voice-dialogue course in Odense. It was a very rewarding experience where I found that many of my own thoughts about my experiences and their origin were confirmed, and where I realised just how essential it is to be able to communicate – that everything I experience is in one way or another communication, or an attempt at communication. My voices responded very protectively during those three days but they also seemed threatened and worried. I think it became clear to them that I had begun to take care of myself, act responsively and was able to meet my own needs. This meant that they might lose their reason to exist and that they would have to let go of me and I would have to accept that I could live without them. A tenth voice, Domina, surfaced and I began to understand my fundamental desire to separate everything in order to survive, and I realised just how dysfunctional this mechanism had become.

One month later I joined a self-help group for voice hearers. I had been quite uncertain whether or not I would feel comfortable sharing my experiences in a group. I was ashamed and afraid that it might have a negative effect on others to hear what I had been through and how I treated myself. I was afraid of saying the wrong things, giving advice when it wasn't asked for, of misunderstanding, talking too much, taking up too much space – of somehow not being enough and being too much at the same time. Having done the Maastricht Interview, at least I felt some certainty that I was capable of expressing myself in connection with my voice-hearing experiences. The fact that Trevor was a facilitator in the group gave me a feeling of safety; that I could talk to him about the feelings of uncertainty that occurred in different situations in the group and I could gain a better understanding of how I was interacting with others, verbally as well as on other levels.

As it turned out, the group quickly became a natural part of my life, something I would not want to be without. The possibility of sharing, listening and expressing; seeing how the group and every individual in the group moved, changed and developed; learning to give and receive support – and just being together about something that is so essential to each of the group member's personal perceptions of themselves and the world. Creating a 'fellowship' around voice hearing gives the experience the recognition, the weight of reality and the value that it truly has to every voice hearer.

Again, only one month later, I agreed to appear on television with Trevor Eyles and Johnny Sparvang in a fifteen minute program on voice hearing and the 'making sense of voices' approach. Shortly afterwards I began telling my story at conferences and other educational events within social psychiatry in Denmark. It has been very rewarding and I believe it has helped to pace my recovery process: to hear myself tell my story again and again whilst living my story; to feel my own approach change and to experience my voices changing; to constantly confront and stay conscious of where I have been and where I am going; to remember my difficulties, my sensitivity, and the pain, how I survived, what I have learned and who has helped me along the road.

When I started working with the 'making sense of voices' approach I had ten regular voices of which nine were mainly negative and creating problems for me. This changed quite quickly and, at some point, some of my voices asked if I would let them go. This was actually the hardest part for me – to realise that as the relationship became positive I would end up not needing my voices. It has taken me over a year to let go of all my regular voices and to accept that I can stand on my own two feet. It has been especially difficult to let go of Søren and Xhabbo. It is an ongoing process that will take some time but as I am doing it I realise that I will always hear voices and have extraordinary experiences that could be described as hallucinations – losing my voices is not the same as losing my sensitivity and all that comes with it. Today I am not afraid of what I experience. I know that I can handle my sensitivity, that it is a gift and that I can help others if I use it carefully and with awareness.

MY LIFE NOW

Am I a recovered mental patient? Am I a schizophrenic? Am I a voice hearer? Yes and no. To me, these are all just words, labels. They describe something superficial. I am recovered and recovering. Being me and being human is a process of constantly experiencing, reacting and changing.

The diagnosis 'schizophrenia' has opened doors within the social and psychiatric system in Denmark and it has helped me understand and respect my sensitivity. I see how, when I do not take it seriously and expose myself to stress, or neglect myself, it becomes an area of vulnerability and a hindrance. I have learned to be aware of my needs and how to meet them in the most constructive way in any given situation.

For me to think of myself as a 'voice hearer' is just as much of a diagnostic approach; this label is just more specific and less influenced by years of taboo and stigma. As a voice hearer I have been able to work with my problems in a way that makes sense to me. It is now possible for me to relate to emotions in a very concrete way and to integrate qualities and parts of my personality that I had been distancing myself from. I am gifted, sensitive, schizophrenic, a voice hearer, or a mentally disabled person, depending on who I am talking to and how they perceive the world. I don't mind, as long as I can sense that there is a mutual acceptance and that this is just a concept to make communication easier. It is not who I am. My life now is as it has always been: filled with fear, joy, anger, sorrow, loss, gain, disappointment, frustration, confusion, surprises, trust and satisfaction. The difference is that, now, I believe that the only way to live is by accepting, relating and interacting and I have people around me who help me to keep believing.

FERNAND CHAPPIN

WITH DIRK CORSTENS

Fernand completed our questionnaire in response to the letter requesting stories for this book (see Appendix).

PART 1 – EXPERIENCE, HISTORY, INFLUENCE

Please describe briefly who you are
I am a 37-year-old male, not married, did lower general secondary education and intermediate business education and like athletics and singing.

Can you tell something about the characteristics of your voice-hearing experience
The voices are not mine. I hear three voices outside and two inside my head. The voices outside I usually hear when there are other noises or voices. The voices in my head give the assignment either to save the world or to destroy the world. They are a good and a bad voice. They comment on what I do, say and think. The voices from outside criticise me. I believe these voices connect to each other.

Previously I heard them all day, when I was psychotic. Since seven years I don't hear them daily anymore, but only when there are noises when I am alone. The voices from inside my head can come every moment. Maybe three times a week on average. That can be half an hour, but can also disappear immediately.

Would you describe briefly the characteristics of the five most important voices for you
God and the Devil, in my head, religiously tinted. The voices from outside don't have names. There are two male and one female voice. These are of my age, approximately. The voices comment: they say if I am good or bad. They say I have influence on the world because I am clairvoyant. They say I have an influence on world events. That I am God or the Devil.

Their history
I was 28 years old when I heard the voice(s) for the first time. I was playing guitar in my room, when a female voice said: 'You play guitar beautifully'. I'd lived independently almost two years. I had a busy temporary job where I had to prove myself continuously. I played the guitar fanatically, at a high

level. I also practised sports a lot and also at a rather high level. I had my first girlfriend. With that relationship I began very late. I had nasty experiences with sexuality in my childhood, she probably too. She was very passive during making love. She came from a very different culture (Eastern Europe) and lived a long distance from me. The trigger was when I heard her stepbrother, who laid in bed with his (and her) parents, crying. This probably reminded me of my own childhood. Shortly after that I became psychotic. When I was hospitalised she suddenly broke off the relationship. The first voice was neutral, outside of my head, but soon more came and started to criticise me, and I didn't feel safe in my flat anymore.

The triggers and content
Noises, mood, being alone. I particularly hear the voices when I am in my bedroom. If I talk somewhere about the voices then they want to talk too. If I feel depressed or have negative thoughts then they go along with that.

Their influence
I believed the voices and carried out their assignments. For example, I had to go to Bosnia and save the world. I went out in the middle of the night to go to Bosnia.

Your relationship with them
In the beginning I was completely powerless. Now I've learned to cope with them. They aren't are in charge of me anymore.

Most people have an explanation of their voices. What is yours?
The sexual abuse in my childhood I didn't deal with. The voices represent bottled-up emotions like sadness, mistrust and anger that I can't express. I missed safety.

How important is this explanation for you?
Previously I thought that I had power, that it was God. The voices said I was the Antichrist or, on the contrary, Jesus Christ, a saint or a sanctimonious … etc.

Is this still right?
I doubt if this explanation is still right.

Do you, and others, accept this explanation?
Yes, especially the first.

What did you do when the voices became troublesome?
I tried to have control, but I carried out their assignments. I believed that

they were sincere, that their objectives were good. For the remission of my sins I did it too. I thought bad things, and I did bad things.

PART 2 – MEETING THE 'ACCEPTING VOICES' APPROACH AND ITS APPLICATION TO YOU

How did you know about the Accepting Voices approach?
I was approached by Monique Pennings (a co-worker of the Hearing Voices project in Maastricht).

Who showed interest in your voices for the first time?
Annette Hofman and Dirk Corstens (professionals at the community mental health centre in Maastricht).

What was your reaction to that?
It was a relief that I could talk with someone about the voices. I wasn't declared mad, as I was everywhere else.

What did you do with this information and how did you work with these persons?
I tried to talk to the voices and work with argumentation. I challenged the voices. The professionals helped me with it. I was asked to think about the voices and to imagine what I wanted myself.

Professionals, family members and friends
I learned to think for myself. My family told me I shouldn't withdraw, but stay active. I could talk with my brother about the voices. I talked with my friends about it and they accepted it, at least some of them.

The possibility to talk about the voices and other extrasensory experiences
- My experiences were accepted as normal and not negative
- I learned to know different opinions and coping strategies
- This was the first step to handle the problem better
- I became less isolated, because I could talk about my voices more openly
- I wasn't obliged to keep my experiences secret anymore or to attack it
- I felt supported
- I came in an open atmosphere without prejudice
- I did get positive support for the little steps I made
- I recognised the relation between the voices and my previous life
- I could handle normal daily things better, though I still have the inclination

- to withdraw
- I started to work again
- I reached a level with running that I didn't expect
- Medication supported me too

What helped me was not blindly obeying anymore; that I had my own opinion, and that I learned to recognise when to expect them. I was prepared. That's why they stayed away more often. I could relate between the noises and the voices. I learned to talk about what I had experienced and got more trust in other people, especially professional workers. I came into contact with other voice hearers; I wasn't the only one.

PART 3 – HOW DO YOU LIVE TODAY?

How do you feel generally?
I still have doubts about myself. Sometimes still I want to withdraw, because I am depressed or gloomy. I can start something new enthusiastically but change into passivity fast. Sometimes I feel very cheerful and can enjoy nice moments.

Do you still hear voices?
I can cope with them rather well. I don't have control over the time they come, but I can send them away, I can refer them to another time and then discuss with them.

Did you become more self-assured?
Certainly.

How are your life circumstances at the moment?
Many friends but no partner. I work in a supply room at the sheltered workplace. I still live with my mother and my brother. Sometimes I don't like that because I am not able to invite people spontaneously. I want to live independently again at some point, but I find it difficult. To be alone and getting voices again, and that I will withdraw too much and neglect myself.

Are you financially independent?
Yes. I am still dependent on professional care for supportive talks and still use medication.

Are you active in the hearing voices movement and in what way?
No. Probably in the future, if I was asked again.

FLORE BRUMMANS

INTERVIEW WITH MARIUS ROMME

Flore Brummans is 55 years old, married with three children. Flore is actively involved in women's support groups. She founded the 'Wilskracht' (Willpower) association, for women for whom there is no psychiatric support. Through her association and with the help of subsidies, she bought a caravan for these women, where they can stay the night without others knowing of their whereabouts; a kind of runaway refuge. Furthermore, the association organises self-help groups, for example, a group for voice hearers as well as social events such as parties, Christmas festivities and holidays.

Flore was sexually abused from the age of 6 by a friend of her father. She suspects that her father knew about it. She started hearing a voice from the age of 14 onwards. This coincided with her change in attitude and behaviour. She threw herself into rebellion. The voices instructed her to perform certain tasks, which gave her a kick too. This rebellious behaviour also ended the abuse. She smashed up all sorts of things by order of the voices and she got a kick out of that.

Flore says: I came alive at night. During the day I slept and I would get up at 8pm and then hit the streets til dawn. I lived like this for 30 years, even during my marriage. I then fell in love with a woman who heard voices too and she got me involved in a voice-hearers' group which was run by her. This was the turning point. I was 48 at the time, seven years ago now. At that time I kicked my (prescription) drug habit too. Over a period of seven weeks, she counselled me. Every time one less tablet, I admit it was hell for me; trembling all over; there was nothing I could easily hold in my hands; I could not sleep either any more. I persevered, being in love motivated me to go on. On 12th May 2001 I quit for good.

It was only after I had given up the prescription drugs that I started to live, I could feel again, cry again and laugh again. The self-help group gave me more self-confidence. Your strengths, they build up your self-confidence. Counselling does not primarily focus on your strengths.

I was prescribed drugs from the age of 14, first Valium, followed by all kinds of drugs made by Jansen Cilag and towards the end, weekly Haldol injections. These turned me into a complete zombie. On Fridays and weekends I stayed in bed, apart from that I just walked around a bit, but I was not with it at all. Come Thursdays I would feel faintly human again, but then on Friday I would get another injection. Despite the fact that it had no effect on my symptoms, it was simply continued. Nobody ever asked what was behind my aggressive behaviour. No solution was found, which later turned out to be such a simple one in the accepting and explanatory self-help.

How did your voice hearing take place and what did you do?
There has never been any confusion in my case at all. I recognised the voice, it was the perpetrator. I admit that the voice scared me and it rendered me powerless. After a while I knew what I had to do if it bothered me too much: jukebox at such a high volume that I did not hear the voice. Apart from that I just did as the voice told me to do. During the 34 years that I took prescription drugs, I simply listened and did as I was told by the voice. When I enjoyed something or laughed the voice would punish me. Self-mutilation was my punishment. In the self-help group, I got recognition and support. Then I started to think things over, with the help of others, started to tell everything. Now I am able to talk about it frankly and openly with women.

How did you end up with the self-help group?
Psychiatry did not offer me anything. The conversations were mainly about the weather. That changed when I met a psychiatrist who got angry as she realised that I was wearing different masks. The fact that that psychiatrist became angry was a good thing. I simply let everything happen and was drugged up. A second change happened because of a nurse who kept on nagging me to go to a self-help group. I went and discovered that I could be myself there, which helped me a lot. By the way, I have a very good psychiatrist now. It depends very much on the person.

Since Flore's recovery mainly happened through a self-help group, I am reproducing her experiences on self-help here, as they were discussed in the Expert group study (Corstens et al., 2008) In this study the advantages of support groups for voice hearers were discussed. (Not all the questions were answered.)

1. The opportunity to talk about voices and other experiences in a frank and open manner
I did not dare to tell my counsellor, I was scared to be admitted. In the self-help group I had the courage to do that, others had that courage too there and that is when I thought: 'I'm not the only one.' When I started talking about it, it helped me and also, that I dared to admit it.

2. My experiences were accepted as reality
I felt ashamed about that [the sexual abuse] and did not dare to come out in the open with these experiences. I hurt other people. Now that it has been accepted by me and others, I am far more in control of it.

4. That I did not have to keep my experiences a secret any longer or that I had to defend myself
I still keep it a secret and I only talk about it in the self-help group. That has a positive impact. Outside the group I don't talk about it, I daren't. You cannot transfer it to other situations. People in the self-help group experience freedom.

5. That I can work with my voices and that I don't just have to suppress or obey them
That helps me.

10. That I was given positive encouragement for the small steps I made
That applies to me too.

11. That I progressed in my dealings with the voices
I've got them under control and that is encouraging.

12. That I learned to recognise when to expect the voices
Yes, when you think about it, it does help as you are able to do something else, where in the past you just let it happen.

13. That I became increasingly convinced that the voices had to do with me personally
They related to me, as well as having a relationship with my personal history.

14. That I learned not to obey the voices blindly, but to realise that I had my own opinion
That was a very big step, and it only came late, in the self-help group.

16. That I learned to listen more carefully to these voices and to talk to them
In the past I only obeyed, but I never talked to them. I've become stronger within myself. I gained insight into what I was doing.

17. By talking to the voices I started to discuss topics with them which until then I had mainly kept a secret to myself
Not applicable to me.

18. That I can cope with certain activities better again like, for example, shopping, playing sports
I did not live for 34 years. Because of the self-help group, I have become more active again.

19. That I became a member of a club again, which made me less lonely
The self-help groups really work (Time-Out).

20. That I could cope better with my daily activities again. That helped in managing my voices better
Flore undeniably: yes.

21. That I've started a course again
I've given and followed many courses which helped me a lot.

FRANK DAHMEN

WITH MARIUS ROMME

Frank is a 38-year-old man. He gained his nursing diploma in 1989 and then continued his studies at evening school. He achieved A-levels in 1992 and then studied biology for two years. From 1996 to 2000 he went on to study psychology.

I stopped studying biology because I did not want to take part in animal testing. The end of my biology studies was a very negative experience for me and I felt as if I had fallen into a hole; this made me quite depressed. It was in this context, in 1994, that I started hearing voices. I was 27 years old at that point.

I was hearing the voices through my ears. They contain thoughts which are alien to me, that is to say, not my own thoughts, although some of them are also my own thoughts. When I think, the voices talk at the same time and they say the same things that I am thinking. Sometimes they simply repeat it. Something had died inside of me and the voices said: 'Something died'. The voices made me feel suicidal.

The voices are of three little boys. One of them is the commentator: he makes comments about what I think. Another one is the judge: he judges and insults me about what I do. The last one is the distributor: he gives presents, for example, 'You are going to get marijuana'. The three of them can sing together like a choir but the judge is normally the most dominant. According to the voices, they are 10 to 12 years of age, but I know that they are my mother. I asked them and, about three years ago, one answered: 'I am your mother and I can be whichever voice I like'.

My mother would be 61 today. However, she died at the age of 25, when I was 2 years old. My mother was very important to me. I needed a good mother and I was hoping that I might be able to get one. My father remarried after one year but my second mother was very aggressive towards me. She demanded that I listened to what she said and I was expected to be obedient. She often chose not to communicate with me and I was made to feel guilty for everything. She used me as a way of dealing with her own aggression. This was a psychologically destructive relationship for me. The children from the second marriage were better off.

I was hearing voices during two distinct periods: from the end of my biology studies in 1994 until 1996 and from the end of my psychology studies in the year 2000 until today. Between 1996 and 2000, during my psychology studies, I was free of voices. I stopped these studies because I thought that I was not going to be able to sit the exams. At that point the voices came back. In that second period I often became quite angry when the voices were there. I was talking a lot and I would scream out of the windows of my flat and on the streets. On two occasions I was sectioned and sent to a psychiatric hospital. Both times I was discharged: the first time after one year, the second time after two and a half years.

The voices make me angry when they tell me to 'leave your house without the keys' or to 'throw away your keys'. (In Germany the expression 'throw your keys away' is equivalent to 'come out of the closet' in English.) These are very clear pointers for me to damage myself. In the same way as 'drown yourself, you have got no chance'. But they do also say, 'I love you and I am very sorry that things went wrong'. So this does, of course, create confusing emotions or might actually be statements about my confused emotions.

I did not agree with the treatment in the psychiatric hospital because it was not helpful and there was no psychotherapy. In 2002, the day centre and Pinell, a psychosocial institution, which is more service-user centre, told me about the self-help group of the NeSt – the German Hearing Voices Network. Initially, I just took part and talked with others, then I did some studying and started to work actively for the NeSt. I did not analyse this, I just knew: 'You need friends, so that you do not end up falling into a black hole again.' I learned from Antje Müller (coordinator at the NeSt) that psychotherapy would also be important, so I proceeded to arrange this by myself. I called a lot of people up and agreed to trial sessions and eventually I found a therapist with whom I could engage in therapy.

I do not think that my voices are a symptom of illness; I think they are a reaction to what has happened to me. My first suicide attempt was a reaction to my loneliness and feeling of estrangement from others. With regard to the voices, they also represent a sexual problem. The question is whether I am masochistically inclined or not and whether I am homo- or heterosexual.

As part of the psychotherapy I also wanted to get rid of guilt feelings and anxiety in social contexts. I wanted to become cockier and more self-confident and I did not want to fight but to be able to assert myself more. I wanted to be successful, to find out who I am – to find myself.

During the course of therapy, the voices changed and became friendlier. When the voices talk about the present they are a lot less dominant. However, this does not yet apply to when they talk about my future.

I am now working full time again, as a salesperson in an organic food shop, as part of a rehabilitation programme. I like it. However, it does not mean that all of my problems are resolved.

FRANS DE GRAAF

WITH MARIUS ROMME

My first voice-hearing experience happened unexpectedly, unrestrainedly and uncontrollably.

I heard several voices. A formal voice with formal language, somewhat distant, without any emotion, this voice only supplied facts and corrects too. An emotional voice, talked about my feelings, showed colour, can adopt various roles. These first two voices remained the most important ones. When I hear them I am totally convinced that it is true what they say. Apart from these I also hear a singing voice and an internal voice. This was preceded by a period of slowly increasing exhaustion, sleeplessness and built-up stress, one-sided focus on the problem, as a result of which I could not relax any more.

I lost my rational control due to the emotional situation I was in and I was prepared to win the fight in any which way. That meant that I saw images of murder, rape, torture, destruction, it did not really matter any more, the cultural layer surrounding me disappeared and something animal grew in me. This happened in November 1986. I was 27 years old at the time. In the squat, where I lived at the time, I felt so threatened that I was prepared to go out and fight. There were six living groups in that house and I belonged to one with eight people. There was no space left for me any more when Herman moved in. I returned home from my holidays and suddenly there were two new occupants, his entire circle of friends ended up there. I was studying whilst he was partying: parties all day and all night long. I did not sleep any more. The last straw was his addicted girlfriend, who sometimes would run through the house screaming whenever she was trying to kick her heroin habit again. It was decided that his girlfriend should come and live next to me. That really was the last straw. The moment that the decision about his girlfriend had to be taken, it was me against the entire group. I had been first rights. I was going to tell him that it would be better if he were to leave. When I announced that I would fight, there was nobody. The house was literally empty. For three days in a row they were not there. I had all this aggression in me and could not let it out. The fourth day I woke up with voices in my head. The emotional voice presented first. I became detached from the situation. I entered an entirely new emotional space where the problem (in my home) did not exist any more, whilst the voices were controlling my thoughts and emotions. This even went as far as the voices taking over my body and they even letting me enjoy an orgasm to which I was a spectator myself. Initially, I was powerless and defenceless during these experiences; voices forced it upon me, entered my personal space, pushed me aside and were in control. Around this an organisation delusion developed and I felt pretty threatened.

During later voices periods, not under threatening circumstances, the voices were still talking from the same perspective of the first breakdown. The entire emotional load, the anger, fear and aggression of the first incident is then present yet again in the same way, although I don't really notice it outside my voices period. Following this, my self-image had changed for good, sexually too. Whereas up until then I had seen myself as a purely heterosexual man with heterosexual relationships, I was not when I heard the voices. It turned out that besides my heterosexual side I had a homosexual side too then and on both sides a sadomasochistic side as well as a strong female side. My self-esteem disappeared and a kind of shame developed about my inner world. This shame makes talking about it even more difficult if the other person is not receptive to this. Even when the voices are not a problem any more, the experience of losing your subconscious inhibitions is significant. You do not talk about it, you do not write about it until much later with people with similar experiences and until then it is a burden you carry around and with which you avoid confrontations.

HEALTHCARE SERVICES

During the first period I went to a crisis centre and was admitted to a psychiatric hospital. I had a further fifteen crises which did not result in an admission. In the days that I heard voices and came into contact with the healthcare services, my relationship with the healthcare services was problematic and remains so. I had the good fortune to mainly be in contact with a social-psychiatric nurse of the crisis centre then who did not put me under too much pressure and with whom I had a relationship based on a certain level of trust. Since you cannot talk about your experiences, you are on your own. Besides the reality of the voices, at a certain point I experienced my personality falling apart into pieces. I have always considered that as a real experience that I could work with. It remains important to keep on testing to what extent you can rebuild your life with these experiences, if needed against the disease label that the healthcare services project onto you. This process takes a long time. At that time, I continued with my life, finished my physics studies and after that I worked all that time in a full-time IT position for a large company.

My problem with the healthcare services started when I came into contact with a physician. That physician told me the standard healthcare point of view: my experience is psychosis. I need medication for the rest of my life and my voices should not be discussed, since otherwise the psychosis will return. This meant that the voices were not accepted and this lead to a conflict. The conflict develops about the way in which you want to approach your experiences and what the underlying causes are. This conflict takes up so much energy, that you will have to end the relationship.

However, I continued to live with the diagnosis of paranoid schizophrenic and that had a number of consequences:

- No psychotherapy. There is no discussion about the experience of hearing voices, neither is there any discussion about the problems that lie at their roots.
- The advice not to have children because of the point of view that you have a genetic disease.
- When I report my health status to the occupational health doctor, that I perceive myself to be fully capable to work, it is interpreted as fraud.
- After telling the occupational health doctor that I hear voices, I am immediately treated like a child and information is requested from the psychiatrist or CPN about whether it is true that I am able to work.
- At my annual work assessment alarm bells ring – even after having worked for a year full time, a report is requested from the psychiatrist before my contract is renewed.
- With financial transactions I always have to make a written declaration that something is wrong with me, with the consequence that the cost of life insurance, for example, becomes higher.
- When I want to become self-employed I encounter the same problems with health insurance and unemployment insurance. This problem, twenty years later, still persists.

According to clinical opinion in psychiatry, it is correct to classify my experiences as paranoid schizophrenia, however, the subsequent actions of the physician and the consequences for the person who receives that label are totally unscientific and damaging and I can sometimes get really angry about this. The de-personified behaviour of this form of psychiatry is completely at odds with the physician's oath and very discriminating.

I believe that incidents in my past have also made me vulnerable for a breakdown. I think that my mother's psychosis when I was very young and of which I was very scared played a role. After that it was not allowed to show emotions at home. From the age of eight onwards my parents did not touch me any more. I was too old for that. My mother basically condemned everything about me, my hairstyle, the people I hung out with, everything. In addition to that came the rejection of my house mates and the big tension in the squat where expressing my anger was impossible as there was nobody around any more. A homosexual assault, a couple of years earlier, plays a role too. This memory surfaced, shortly before my breakdown and following that, confusion emerged in my sexual feelings until into my psychosis.

RECOVERY

I differentiate between two recovery phases: during the first phase in the eighties I focused on not having emotion and no voices. In the second phase, the last eight years, I focused on wanting to experience emotions and not being afraid of voices any more, since it turned out, voices are emotions.

The recognition of voices as emotions, together with naming and allowing emotions again were the real turning point for me in the past eight years. By recognising that what the voices tell you are your own emotions, your own fears and anger, you take away the traumatic character of the initial voice hearing, as fears dominate and they go right deep inside you. At the end of the day, you were most frightened and influenced by your own emotions which you do not recognise as such. The discovery 'voices are your own emotions', takes away the trauma, since you can consider your experiences to be your own again, something you wrongly do not do when you hear voices of strangers. These you not automatically will identify with aspects of yourself.

Although I could not deal with hearing voices in the first phase that I heard them, I made up my mind after a while to let the voices explain the content of their message, so that I could get a grip on them. Blocking a period of voice hearing with, for example, Haldol, ultimately was not acceptable for me any more. By involving myself with them, I gradually became convinced that the voices were strongly related to me and discussed subjects with me, that until then I had mainly kept to myself. I also encountered the boundaries of the delusions in which I had often landed with my voices by even bringing up subjects myself that were new to me and of which my voices appeared to know nothing. By doing that, a notion developed of the way in which I could get into a complete delusion with my voices and I was gradually able to be more in charge when I heard the voices. The fact is, that my voices had a varying degree of intensity and their identity was strongly related to what I found plausible in my delusion. When I realised the latter, my relationship with the voices changed and I was involved in the identity they adopted. Therefore, my final conclusion was that my voices did not have a specific shape and that when I did not supply them with a specific context, they remained distant. Around that time I had nothing more to say to my voices and by consistently refusing my voices to take shape, they stayed away. However, I did feel weakened after the last voice-hearing episode. A voice-hearing episode takes up a lot of energy and in that respect I benefited from 'Orab' (neuroleptic medication). The effect of Orab is that it tempers me somewhat and it makes it easier to keep my focus on the outside world and less so on the inner world and the voices.

During the second phase, the last eight years, I came into contact with 'Weerklank' ('Resonance', The Dutch Hearing Voices Network). The book *Accepting Voices* had a profound impact on me and evoked a strong feeling of recognition in me. The idea that as a voice hearer, you go through a number of phases with the voices was immediately recognisable to me. Also the idea of working with your voices and not to simply suppress them with antipsychotics was something I recognised in me too.

During the second phase I started working on experiencing my emotions with emotional bodywork, whereby you feel your emotions in your body; in a Zen meditation group during which you consciously review your emotions and in cognitive behavioural therapy, during which I learnt to name my emotions and to describe them. I still do the latter, but nowadays at home on my laptop.

The Weerklank congress also explained that there are healthcare professionals in the Netherlands who clearly enter into a discussion about voices. I have presented my experience with Weerklank and my experience story to the people who treat me at Altrecht in Utrecht. It just so happened that after my first request for a meaningful discussion, somebody else took over my treatment. The person who treated me first who left was surprised about my experience story and had up until then always refused my requests for a meaningful discussion. The people who subsequently treated me were of a younger generation and responded positively to this. On the basis of my stories, we have agreed to 'a psychotic response in a personal crisis' in terms of my diagnosis. The concept of partial dissociation as described in Van der Hart's book *Trauma, Dissociation and Hypnosis* (*Trauma, Dissociatie en Hypnose*) is mentioned too.

The importance of accepting voice hearing and 'Weerklank' is that it provides a voice hearer with a sufficient base to ask for the help you personally want. Apart from *Accepting Voices* I have found very little in terms of relevant literature which would enable a voice hearer to compare with one's own experiences. Even, regarding the longer-term progression, once you can deal with your voices or once they have disappeared, I found hardly any literature.

I still work full-time in the IT sector, but I am also taking a small amount of Risperdal. Without Risperdal I am earlier finished with working and can only go on until three in the afternoon. With Risperdal I just work on for the whole day. I am less excitable.

GAVIN YOUNG

Dear Dr Escher,

I hope you don't mind me using your personal email address to greet you ... I just didn't feel that using Intervoice was appropriate in this case. So, good morning from southern Oregon, USA.

Basically, I wanted to thank you and Dr Romme from the deepest place in my heart for the work you do for/with voice hearers. Reading *Accepting Voices* was pivotal in my recovery. I also bought *Making Sense of Voices* some time ago, and look forward to reading it. You and Dr Romme have a very accessible writing style which works for both professionals and lay people. I can't wait to dig deeper into the mystery of voice hearing ...

If I had written you five years ago, you would have encountered a very different person. I was depressed beyond hope, the voices screamed at me 24/7 (I have evil voices) and I had no idea what was wrong with me. I was a tragic figure in a tragic landscape and everybody around me just kept saying, 'Snap out of it!!' as if I could ... despair, ruin, tragedy, no future at all ... I prayed some days that I would die, that God in His/Her mercy would deliver me from this hideous 'thing' through death (although interestingly, I was never suicidal; there was a spark of hope in me even in the worst of times and I never gave up the will to go on living ...).

The first psychiatrist I saw told me I had 'methamphetamine psychosis' and that the voices would go away. Well, they never did. The second psychiatrist I saw put me on three antipsychotics and dismissed me with 'schizo-affective disorder' – a diagnosis I never bought.

It was only after reading about your work and how voices often correlate with trauma that I began to dig deeper. I was in the midst of serious trauma when I began to hear; I also realised I had had a number of traumatic events prior to this one event that I hadn't 'dealt with' properly; they were just buried.

So you see, you and Dr Romme gave me the 'keys to the kingdom' so to speak, and I began to feel empowered again when I realised that how I dealt with the voices was up to me.

Today, I have a fantastic psychiatrist who doesn't dismiss my experiences, but treats them as real, as I do. I currently take only Abilify and have had good results with it (or is it that I'm just getting better and better the further away from the trauma that I move?).

I still hear today and the voices are as nasty as they ever were, but they're very muted now, easy to ignore, and even easier to joke around with (which infuriates them – it seems they're only happy when I take them seriously and they have me scared to pieces, which is no longer the case, so in a sense, they've lost their jobs! I think of them now as buffoons rather than a serious threat.)

I've also arrived at a place where I consider the voices or 'words' (as I call them now) to be a blessing rather than a curse and this has made all the difference in the world. I have often called them my Greatest Teachers, as the content of what they say has deep meaning for me, inasmuch as it's called to the fore areas that I've kept buried since childhood ... the voices keep me honest about myself. And it was simply a matter of how I chose to react to them.

I also have a diagnosis of Complex PTSD which I can live with and makes perfect sense to me. And the blessings go on: I started my own business; bought a beautiful home; belong to a voice-hearers' group on Yahoo for support and have my West Highland White Terrier, Sprite, to keep me company. I'm also developing a social life, which I thought I'd never have again. Moreover, through CBT, I am gradually working my way back into the world, which feels good, but still scary at times (I'm sure you understand).

The voices stole my self-confidence but I'm gradually getting it back again, because I believe today that I never really lost it to begin with, I just forgot I had it or, put another way, I disowned it and had to reclaim it through putting back together all the dissociated parts of me – it's like a huge jigsaw puzzle called 'MY LIFE'.

I've developed a set of coping tools which I believe to be my salvation. I have you and Dr Romme to thank for that ... you started me on the road back to sanity. If I can share some of that knowledge and hope with other hearers then the whole experience is worth it! In a sense, you've given me a 'gospel' to spread ...

Thank you for taking time out of your busy schedule to read this lengthy and somewhat redundant email (I always get flustered around celebrities <grin>) and please give my best to Dr Romme. You two are my heroes ... thanks again.

Yours sincerely (a real fan),
Gavin Young

GINA ROHMIT

INTERVIEW WITH MARIUS ROMME

Gina started to hear voices after a year of great stress during which she had experienced problems with her job, her boyfriend and her accommodation

I left home after my parents divorced. My mother got a new man friend and I thought, 'I can leave now because there is someone who cares for her'. I think it was also to do with my desire to live on my own and become more independent. I heard from a woman where I worked that a flat had become available in a slightly antisocial neighborhood. At first I liked it very much but, gradually, I heard and saw threatening situations. There was some drug dealing and I became more and more afraid, but at that time I still had my boyfriend whom I asked to stay more often for the night. He officially lived with his mother and her man friend. Also, around that time, the hairdresser's where I worked closed down and I became redundant.

I found a new job but the boss only really hired me because he was lonely. After a short time he found a new girlfriend and tried to make me redundant by becoming very unpleasant. He even manipulated some of my clients to sign a statement claiming that I didn't do my job well. I was very upset about this but when I tried to discuss it with my boyfriend he just said, 'It's your business, you'll have to sort it out yourself.' As soon as I was fired my boyfriend got a job in a nearby town and started to lose interest in me. I couldn't understand why and I couldn't accept it. Then his mother's man friend had a serious car accident and died. I hadn't had the announcement so I didn't know which church to go to for the funeral. We had more and more quarrels. Finally, I became so angry that I packed his clothes in a plastic bag and took them to him, knowing he wouldn't come back. He confessed that he found me stressful and was not up to it. We ended our relationship with a row. For me it became a nightmare. Some time later I heard that he was dating another girl. I thought, 'This is incredible. You live with a person for three years and you still hardly know each other. I had not reckoned on this. He had just waited until he saw an opportunity to leave me.'

After that, I was on my own in the flat and became more and more afraid of everything that was happening around me – people on the walkways dealing drugs, there was even an arson attack on my floor. When I went to sleep I always put some clothes near my bed so I could get away quickly if something happened. [These flats were later demolished because of escalating crime.] I went to the housing society to ask for another flat but they didn't have anything free. Now I couldn't go anywhere.

My mother had a new man friend and my father was living with a woman. I thought, 'You'll just have to put up with it until you find something somewhere else.' I was ashamed of myself because I was on social benefit; I was ashamed because I lived in an antisocial neighborhood; I was ashamed of myself for having parents who had been divorced. I became depressed and started to doubt myself. I thought: 'Nobody wants you, you can't be good enough.' I didn't even dare to apply for a job any more. My mother visited me daily but her man friend thought she was too involved with her daughter. She was always weighing the pros and cons yet she still came over every day. Then, after living for a year with all this stress, I managed to get a very elegant flat, one with security. I was really happy and thought 'Hurray! Nothing can go wrong now. I can really start enjoying my life at last.' My mother helped me furnish and decorate the flat but I was so stressed that it wasn't quick enough for me and I shouted that it all had to be done faster. So we managed to get the flat painted and the walls papered within three days. While moving I was so tired that I thought, 'I can't make it'. My mother was around and that gave me a safe feeling. At a certain moment, however, I started talking within myself. Everything I thought, I expressed out loud– like hanging my clothes in the cupboard – so my mother asked, 'Why are you talking to yourself? You should hear yourself talking.'

Having settled in I just sat gazing for hours and hours. My mother asked, 'What's happening to you. Go and do something. Go into town.' I just sat there. And then those voices started. That's why I sat: I was thinking about what I heard. I didn't understand what was going on. I thought, 'What's happening to me now?' At first I thought, 'This is only temporary, it will go away' but I began to be afraid. I heard a voice that said: 'I will ruin you; I will get at you. I will ruin you mentally. I will violate you. You don't deserve to live in such a nice flat.'

First of all I only heard voices inside the flat but then I heard them in my car too. I thought, 'Now they're starting to follow me.' Then, in between, I would think: 'Tomorrow it will be better. I must keep calm. It will go away'.

That intense anxiety and seeing images in the flat was only in the beginning. I saw someone with tattoos. I saw a very aggressive figure, very real. Even now if I remind myself I can see it again, it's incredible how realistically you can see such an image. Once I was putting up a mirror on the wall in the corridor and I thought that the woman next door could see me from the balcony and I thought I was watched. I told my mother and she said 'what are you making of that?' Thereafter I was thinking that they wanted to violate me. I had the feeling that there was someone around me who wanted to violate me. So I called the friend of my mother. I said; 'John I have to watch out tonight because there is someone here who wants to violate me.' That friend started to laugh at me. I thought this is the limit. They nearly want to kill me around here and nobody takes me seriously. I didn't grasp that nobody believed me while I was in such a distress. It was so realistic, and it became increasingly more extreme.

During that period, my mother made an appointment with the doctor and I asked him: 'What do I have?' He said: 'You're having a psychosis. Where do you want to go, to the psychiatric hospital or the psychiatric department of the general hospital?' I said: 'I'm not mad. I don't need to go anywhere.' I took my bag, because I had taken a knife to defend myself – I felt threatened all the time. My mother said, 'Please stay calm. Just try it for a few days.' When my mother said something I accepted it. And, anyway, I knew I couldn't stay with my mother because her friend John wouldn't agree and I couldn't stay at my father's either, so I thought, 'Alright, for a few days, it might be good not to be in that flat. I'll sleep for a few days and then everything will be alright.'

In the psychiatric ward I was immediately given medicine which made me feel sloshed. I could hardly get up but they came to get me anyway because I had to sit with the group. I thought: 'This isn't for me.' I said: 'Leave me alone, I can hardly get up.' In that group they didn't talk about voices, so I didn't know whether there were other voice hearers there. The voices reduced with the medicine but they never disappeared. After five days I told my mother I wanted to leave. At the outpatient clinic I again met the psychiatrist and asked 'What did you give me? I can hardly sit still.' He said: 'With most people that's a side-effect of the medicines.' I said: 'But I can't live like this.' I was given something else that made me so sleepy that I could hardly dress myself. I mostly just slept. The medication has never really helped me but I have been messing about with it for two years.

RECOVERY

My mother (who owned a hairdresser's shop) knew a woman who worked at the library and this person asked her: 'Is Gina always so absent-minded?' My mother explained, confidentially, that I had had a few problems and was having a psychosis. This woman had read a book on the subject and offered to lend it to my mother, so we both read it too. The book's preface was written by Prof Romme and, indirectly, I discovered his address – it turned out he lived near Maastricht. I read that hearing voices is related to somebody from the past who troubles you– that was what I thought, so I decided that I must go and see Prof Romme.

Prof Romme took my voices seriously, he acknowledged how they annoyed me and made me afraid; he looked extensively at all that had happened to me before I started to hear them and came to understand that I felt very powerless. I would have preferred to get rid of the voices immediately but he said that that this was not possible. I first had to look at ways to cope differently with my voices in order to get more control over them. I had to listen to them, to what they said, and ask myself if it was true; if they were really as powerful as they suggested. Together with Romme I started to look at what I could do for myself. I discovered that I could question the voices. Sitting outside in the sun in an inner yard, screened from the outside world, the voices said: 'Gosh! What are you doing, sitting there in your bikini doing nothing?' and I thought, 'You can't see, nobody can see me and you can't look through the walls', and then I thought 'Alright, I'm just going to stay here, sitting, whether you can see me or not'. I learned to ask the voices, 'Can anybody see me?', and their answer didn't fit at all. Sometimes, when I went out, they'd say, 'There she is, going out again' and I felt that as critical. I realised, myself, that such things were none of their business. I had no job so I was allowed to go out. I told Romme about that and he asked whether I possibly also thought such things myself, for example, that it wasn't right not to have a job and still go partying. And that was right.

I can give some more examples, such as when the voices said 'How awful she looks' on a day I wasn't feeling good and was thinking 'My gosh, I do look awful!' Then I had the idea that everybody knew and was looking at me. It was an overreaction on my part. I noticed more often that it was my own idea that nobody liked me. This made me understand that these were my own thoughts. It is quite strange but somehow these are your own thoughts about quite an understandable emotion. The voices actually talked about things that reflected the situation I was in because it was a fact, I didn't have the money to live in such a beautiful flat. Most people who lived there had a job. I'd got this spacious flat while I was on social benefit. I couldn't see a way out so I thought that it must be the flat. Now I think that at that time so much had happened that I was very unhappy. In discussions with Romme we found out that much had happened before the voices came and I perceived myself as being guilty of it all. Besides the problems with the flat I also think that I hear voices because of an inferiority complex and the voices confirm this when they tell me I am not good enough.

At a certain moment I decided to go and live with my mother again but I still didn't have the courage to find work. With Romme, we also talked about my future and about what I really liked doing. That's when I decided:

'I want a life again. I'll stop making a fool of myself. I'll follow an entrepreneurial course. I want my own business. That has always been my dream.' And the strange thing was that I started following this course while still hearing voices. I felt more secure living with my mother and doing the course meant I was better able take my mind off my problems; I became more convinced that I was not ill. I didn't want to project myself as someone who has an illness. I worked with my mother at her hairdresser's shop for a trial period and found that I was quite capable. If the voices came when I was busy with a client, which was what I had feared, Romme advised me to excuse myself, go to the toilet and tell the voices, 'Not now, come tonight when I'm home'. That was effective.

I have since finished the course and taken on a hairdresser's shop of my own. I have started my own business. It has been pretty tough because I am rather insecure, but I have succeeded. Slowly, I discovered that my voices were my worries fed by my insecurity. In a voice-dialogue session, talking directly to each voice, I realised who, in reality, represented the most awful voice. The time of difficulty with that man I realised was in the past. When I discovered all this and succeeded with my business, the voices vanished.

HANNELORE KLAFKI

A SUMMARY BY MARIUS ROMME

Hannelore Klafki from Berlin, founded the German Hearing Voices Network (NeSt). For many years she worked as the Network's coordinator. She was also active as a member of the board of the Federal Association of (ex-) Users and Survivors of Psychiatry (Bundesverband Psychiatrieerfahrener). Unfortunately she died on 3rd September 2005 at the age of 53, following an aneurysm of the brain.

Peter Lehmann of Lehmann Publishing, where Hannelore had been due to start work, put together a book in her memory containing a collection of her publications and speeches: *Meine Stimmen – Quälgeister und Schutzengel* (*My Voices – Tormenting Spirits and Guardian Angels,* Hannelore Klafki, 2006) and this has turned out to be a valuable collection for voice hearers and other recipients of psychiatry. In their obituary, the German Hearing Voices Network proclaimed her to be 'a friend, source of energy, mentor, realistic visionary and a supportive force'. The following extract is a summary of her presentation at the German Hearing Voices Network (Netzwerk Stimmenhören) in Berlin on 25th October, 2003. 'Yesterday, Today and Tomorrow: Voice hearing – a catastrophe? Yes or no?' (see pp. 59–64 of the above book).

As we were thinking in the hearing voices group about the contents of the paper that I should read at the conference, they suggested to me that I should talk about myself. I will therefore try to use my own story to give an alternative possibility of the development of a person, who is hearing voices.

I am now 51 years of age. At the age of 16 – now 35 years ago – I started hearing voices for the first time. Out of fear of being declared insane, I never told anyone about these voices. After an initial period of great difficulty, I was able to relate with my voices in such a way, that they did not have a negative impact on my life anymore. They were accompanying my life, were a part of me and were giving me advice and helpful hints. If at times they were a little overbearing I could tell them off like naughty children.

In another chapter of the above mentioned book Hannelore describes her stressful adolescent years, with difficult family relationships and the experience of sexual abuse at the age of 16. However, in that chapter she also describes how she was initially able to find a way out of her stressful situation with the help of the voices. (See pages 13 – 29 for details.) Everything was fine until about twenty years after she first heard her voices.

I was experiencing a deep crisis in my life as a result of different life events. My marriage had failed and, as a result of a surety [acting as a guarantor] for the debts of my husband, I was in debt for half a million German marks. At the time I was in a dead-end situation. As a result my voices turned into threatening, tormenting spirits. I sought help from psychiatric services and told them about my fear of my voices. I got all sorts of psychopharmaceuticals which were designed to kill off the voices. However, nothing worked.

I kept on being admitted to psychiatric services where they told me that I was severely mentally ill. During the course of my time in psychiatry, I was given six different psychiatric diagnoses. As a result, I was increasingly isolating myself, gave up on myself, and was unable to get my life back in order. My dead-end situation was made worse through psychopharmaceuticals and diagnoses, and for a long time I was pushed into a hopelesss victim role.

RECOVERY

Eventually there was a turning point in this merry-go-round of isolation, psychiatric hospital admission and always new kinds of medication. Another patient dragged me along to Schöneberg, a district of Berlin. Here I encountered a very active social worker who did not just see the severely mentally ill woman in me but who simply talked to me in a 'normal' way. At first I could barely believe that someone was actually seeing a 'normal' human being in me. For the first time in a long time I felt myself being taken seriously. As a result I slowly started talking to her about my voices.

She was one of the first people in Germany, who in the early 90s, started to look at the phenomenon of voice hearing in greater detail. Psychiatric professionals such as Ursula Plog, Thomas Bock and Monika Hoffmann organised the initial working groups and small events on the topic. They presented research results by Marius Romme and Sandra Escher from the Netherlands, which proved that many voice hearers were in fact able to live well with this phenomenon, and had never become patients of psychiatry. An increasing number of voice hearers were thus encouraged to talk about their experiences. I also started slowly to remember the years with my voices before I came into contact with psychiatric services which had been completely pushed to the back of my mind. Gradually I started to fight back and I founded a self-help group in Berlin.

During the summer I went to an international meeting in Maastricht where I met other voice hearers. There were, for example, representatives of the self-help movements of the Netherlands and from Great Britain; Jeannette Woolthuis and Ron Coleman. Full of new ideas, full of new zeal and almost overly excited, I returned to Berlin. We had to be able to create a network in Berlin as well. But who was going to help? Where was I going to find comrades-in-arms? I plunged head-on into work. I was of course completely exhausted at some point and thus did, one last time, end up back in a psychiatric hospital. However, I only spent a few days there this time. I was simply too indignant at the way that I was being 'treated'.

Since that time I have not been back in a psychiatric hospital, have not taken any psychopharmaceuticals and have not got a new diagnosis. After my discharge I went straight back to work and prepared the first conference at the town hall in Neukölln (district of Berlin). Many allowed themselves to be inspired by my enthusiasm and quite quickly, we became a small but inspired group.

Through all of this, but also through the great support we received from the above-mentioned social worker, her colleagues and other people from Schöneberg who had experienced psychiatric services, it turned into a successful event. We quickly took on board the definitions of the British 'Hearing Voices Network'. This meant that voice hearers were experts by experience and those working in psychiatry were experts by training. The aim of all three groups of the German Hearing Voices Network is to prevent crises in order to avoid or reduce the number of admissions to psychiatric hospitals.

If all of this had already existed when I was first going through this difficult crisis in my life, I am sure I would have been spared being psychiatrised. However, it is also true that if we still had not got all of these things, I would be one of many chronic cases, one of many people, who cannot live their lives without the help of psychopharmaceuticals, support and psychiatric help. Thank God I have been able to get out of this victim role. In this context, Ron Coleman has been and continues to be a great example.

I have evolved from being a victim to being an expert by experience – an expert on my own affairs. For this I am grateful to the German Hearing Voices Network. Without my commitment to the German Hearing Voices Network I would not be where I am today. I always say, in trying to help others I am also helping myself.

Finally, in the hope that many may soon be able to say the same as myself on this, I would like to recite the last verse of my poem:

Whatever was in former days, not so good.
What will tomorrow bring? – I do not know.
Today, I have got new courage
And – standing upright – I can look into your faces.

Honouring Hannelore:
Hannelore was a powerful, principled and a very creative personality. She built up the German Hearing Voices Network and was greatly appreciated by her peer voice hearers. She very much stimulated them with their recovery. We were very lucky to have known her. Having an idea is one thing but making it work in reality and let it grow is a more courageous act. Hannelore did so in Germany. As Peter Lehmann states in his preface: 'Many people have lost a wonderful person in Hannelore.'

HELEN

WITH JACQUI DILLON

I suffered severe abuse throughout my childhood and have always known my voices to be related to this. I am very clear about the nature and origin of my voices. I see them as post-traumatic after-effects of the abuse, natural and normal in the circumstances. I have never and would never attach any pathological labels such as 'schizophrenia' to my experiences. The voices mirror the sorts of things which I used to experience throughout my childhood. The main voice I hear is my father's voice. He criticises me and tells me, for example, that I am 'stupid', 'useless' and 'worthless', that I 'deserve to be abused' and 'should never have been born'. He also comments on what I do, telling me that it 'is not good enough'. This happens, for instance, when I am cleaning the house: I have not cleaned or hoovered up 'every last piece of dirt' and 'must do it again and again until it is perfect'. The voices are there every day and so I have had to develop ways of coping with them.

Throughout my childhood my father made me feel more like an object than a human being. He never provided any sort of love, kindness or support. My brother and I seemed to be useful only in terms of acting as outlets for his abusive behaviour, as punch bags or objects to be used, abused and then thrown away. My father constantly criticised me. Everything I did was 'wrong' and 'not good enough'. He used to beat me, push me around, bang my head against the wall, and he also sexually abused me when I was a young child. All of this led to my becoming severely depressed and having extremely low self-esteem. I really believed that I did not deserve to exist in any shape or form on this planet. In discussing this with a therapist, I used to describe feeling like a piece of excrement under someone's shoe. I used to go to see her and sit with a black bin bag over my head (with a hole in it for my head). This was useful at the time, in terms of helping me to express exactly how I felt about myself – like a piece of rubbish to be thrown away.

I do not remember happy times from my childhood, because it was lived out in constant fear; fear of abuse and of the extreme punishments which were regularly meted out, sometimes for small misdemeanours but often for no reason at all. My father kept us in a tightly controlled prison, in which we lived, breathed and drank fear and even feared for our lives. Even when I was away from him, I was anticipating the next round of cruelty and abuse so I could never relax or enjoy myself. There was no escape from the abuse because no one would believe me when I tried to get help. Family members refused to believe and the police took no notice. My father was a well-respected hospital consultant, an academic and a Fellow of the Royal College of Surgeons. The experience of not being believed is a common one for Survivors.

Throughout my childhood, I dissociated in order to cope and constantly wished for death, although I have never in fact tried to kill myself, mainly because of my belief in God. As a psychology undergraduate at Manchester University, I sought help for my difficulties and was referred to a clinical psychologist. I opted not to tell her about the voices but did describe the abuse which we had suffered. After a few sessions, she described herself as a 'Freudian therapist' and informed me that my experiences of abuse were 'not real' but 'the result of fantasy'. There was nobody around to help me at the time and I felt profoundly suicidal. At this, and other traumatic times in my life, I have found the power of prayer to be invaluable. Prayer led me to my first support group for Survivors of abuse. The support, love, understanding and friendship which I experienced there, as well as through my subsequent contact with many other Survivors in different support groups and settings over the years really have been invaluable.

I have experienced considerable abuse and trauma throughout my life. However, working in the 'mental health system' has easily been the worst and most traumatic experience of my life. The experience of inhabiting two different worlds (i.e., that of the professional and the patient) has felt like a huge and overwhelming burden to carry; firstly, because I have been enabled to see clearly the human-rights abuse which takes place regularly in the name of 'mental health care' and, secondly, because I have been prevented from using my own expertise to benefit the system as a whole. The prevailing 'them and us' culture of stigma and division does not allow for this. When I have tried to do this, I have been ignored at best and bullied. There have been attempts to silence me, discredit me and force me out.

My father passed away suddenly and unexpectedly in September 2004. He had a heart attack and collapsed as he was leaving for work, outside the family home, where he had lived alone for the past nine years. He was sixty-four years old. That day, on receiving the telephone call to say that my father was dying, I left work in tears, but managed to get to my car and drive to the hospital. When I arrived, I was still extremely frightened of my father, as well as being very angry with him. He was in a coma and on a life support machine. The first thing I said to him when I entered the room where he was lying was, 'Why did you abuse us?' Later, as I stood by his bedside, I noticed that, despite the fact that he was in a coma and unable to move and speak, a part of me was convinced that his hand could rise up and strike me again at any time as it had done so many times before. I was gripped with fear, convinced that he might abuse me again at any moment. These feelings of overwhelming fear continued throughout the time that my father was in hospital. The day before my father's funeral, I went to the Chapel of Rest again to say more prayers for him. This was the first time that the fear diminished and I was able to remain comfortably alone with his body in the room.

After my father's death, the nature of the voices changed and, for the first time ever, I heard him say some positive things about me. What a surprise that was! However, the voices soon reverted to being negative and critical again. Perhaps it was too much to hope that my father's passing from this world would make the voices do likewise. It might sound strange, but since my father passed away, I feel that I have a much better relationship with him. When he was alive, I became ill trying to reconcile with him. This was because he stubbornly refused to discuss the past. (Most Survivors do not receive a positive response from their abusers.) I was so hurt by my father's behaviour that I was forced, for my own health and well-being, to stop seeing him. However, since he passed away, I feel that he is in a different place spiritually and I regularly pray for the progress of his soul in the next world.

RECOVERY

The most effective coping strategy which I have discovered over the years is prayer. Prayer has saved my life on a number of occasions as well as the faith which I discovered in answer to a prayer about 22 years ago. The Bahá'í Faith has helped me in many ways, including the following:
- The beautiful and powerful prayers and writings have given me strength, guidance, comfort and hope.
- The Faith provides a positive vision of human nature, society and the future of the human race and
- My self-esteem has increased because I have gradually come to believe that I am a creation of God, a servant of God, as opposed to the degrading and demeaning identity which I was forced to assume throughout my childhood.

Prayer seems to provide strength from another dimension, which then allows me to continue with the activities of daily life. Prayer is the main factor which has allowed me not only to survive but also to study, train and work as a clinical psychologist. This is something which I consider to be miraculous in the circumstances, given the extent of abuse and trauma which I have suffered and the subsequent mental health problems with which I have had to struggle. When I am finding it hard to cope, I repeat a phrase in my mind

'Ya Bahá'u'l'Abhá' calling on the assistance of God and meaning 'O Thou Glory of Glories' in Arabic. I find this to be very effective. Other voice hearers I have worked with who are religiously inclined sometimes find it helpful to repeat a Buddhist mantra, a passage from the Qur'an or from the Bible, such as 'The Lord is my shepherd, I shall not want' or 'God is with me'. More secularly minded voice hearers sometimes find it helpful to repeat other phrases in their minds, such as 'I am in charge and make my own choices', 'I am powerful' and 'I am loved'. There are many strategies for coping with voices and each person must find or be helped to find what is most useful for them.

One of the most effective ways I have found of dealing with the voices and all of the other after-effects of severe childhood abuse is to transform the negative into something positive: 'Service to others' has meant that I am able to use my own Expertise by Experience for the benefit of others. I feel extremely blessed and privileged to have been able to do this. At the time when my father was lying on the doorstep of the family home dying, I was working with a Survivor who hears voices, among other after-effects of abuse. When I received the telephone call from the hospital later that day, I was about to start running a Hearing Voices Group with a colleague. The Bahá'í Faith teaches that 'work is worship' and so work is perhaps also a form of prayer for me.

Other notably positive experiences include my first meeting with Marius Romme and Ron Coleman at a conference in the UK quite some years ago. This I attended with colleagues from work. The conference was different to anything I had ever experienced before. People with experience of mental-health problems were not only respected but they were listened to, taken seriously, and their opinions and views sought out. They gave talks (e.g., Ron Coleman) that were inspiring and inspired and professionals learnt from them and worked in partnership with them. I felt as though I had entered a new and wonderful world that felt like heaven compared to the hell of the 'mental health system'. The atmosphere at this conference was decidedly spiritual compared to the overall lack of spirituality present in the 'mental health system'.

There have been many people who have inspired me and given me hope over the years, including Rufus May and Rachel Perkins, two other clinical psychologists with experience of mental health problems, Patricia Deegan, Daniel Fisher and The National Empowerment Center, Lucy Johnstone and psychiatrists from the Critical Psychiatry Network. I have also been inspired by other Survivors, some famous (Oprah Winfrey, Maya Angelou) and many others who I have worked with and learnt alongside over the years. I have been particularly helped by talking therapies, integrative and eclectic models having been the most helpful ones. I had to pay for these myself as there is insufficient investment in psychological therapies in the NHS. The nature of the relationship with the therapist, their personal qualities, as well as their training, experience and approach are all extremely important. A Survivor friend has recommended that I try EMDR (Eye Movement Desensitisation and Reprocessing), which I am currently in the process of researching and pursuing. I have enrolled for EMDR training myself. I have also been helped by various complementary therapies, such as Reiki, and I am interested in the importance of nutritional therapy to mental (and physical) health. All of these (and other) more humane approaches are likely to prove more beneficial than current ways of working. I believe that new ways of working need to be developed in partnership with the Experts by Experience. I have not come across any 'quick fix' solutions and it may be that healing is gradual and progressive. It is also possible that some after-effects will never completely disappear. This underlines the importance of appropriate ongoing support, as well as wider preventative work to address the causes of psychological distress, such as child abuse, trauma and social inequality.

I have faith that one day people in distress will receive the care they need. My prayer now would be that a more enlightened approach will prevail. The fact that voice hearing is often linked to experiences of abuse and trauma needs to be acknowledged and addressed. Care must become more holistic, ethical and spiritual in nature, more about love, kindness, understanding, respect and choice, and less about corrupt, unethical vested interests, unscientific, stigmatising labels (such as 'schizophrenia' and 'personality disorder'), oppression and human rights abuse. Rather than an illness/deficit model, I would like to see a focus on people's strengths, talents and goals. I would like to see professionals working in partnership with the Experts by Experience and learning from them. I hope that the work of inspiring people like Romme and Escher, Loren Mosher, Judith Lewis Herman, Mary Boyle, Lucy Johnstone, Ron Coleman, John Read and organisations like the Hearing Voices Network and Intervoice will be taken seriously. I would like to see an end to stigma and the beginning of a human rights and citizenship agenda for people in distress. For me, this day cannot come quickly enough!

For the past 16 years I have worked as a clinical psychologist in the 'mental health system'. This system would have us believe that people like me who hear voices are suffering from 'schizophrenia', 'the biological disease of the brain unrelated to interpersonal events of childhood or adulthood', that we should be forced to take psychiatric medication for life and are unable to function as members of society. The prevailing psychiatric worldview offers no insight into the experience of psychological distress and voice hearing. Most people develop mental health problems on account of difficult life experiences, including child abuse and not because of genetic and biological disease processes. This ignorant propaganda has been allowed to flourish because of a lack of moral principles (e.g., profit before people), corrupt financial, political and professional vested interests and a lack of dialogue with the Experts by Experience. Current ways of working are unethical, are based on stigma, prejudice and ignorance and are extremely harmful to the many Survivors of abuse and trauma who become patients in the system. I am very happy that this anthology is being published and I hope that it will contribute towards a process of positive change.

Just last week, I attended a ward round, during which a patient with a diagnosis of 'schizophrenia' bravely described having been abused by a paedophile ring as a child. When the patient left the room, the psychiatrist declared that he was suffering from 'false memory syndrome'. Patients who describe such experiences are generally disbelieved by psychiatrists, their experiences relegated to the realm of 'fantasy', 'delusion' and 'false memory'. Once a person has received a diagnosis of 'schizophrenia', then they are classed as a non-person who deserves little respect, has few human rights and no insight. The fact that a large proportion of people who experience the 'signs and symptoms' of the supposed 'disease' are experiencing the normal after-effects of abuse and trauma, has long escaped the 'mental health system' and those who work in it. As far are the system is concerned, severe child abuse is an irrelevant factor in people's lives, despite research evidence to the contrary. Patients are not asked about abuse at assessment and if they do disclose such experiences, then these are 'not real'. I could write extensively about the abuse of patients which I have witnessed over the years. Society and the professionals and organisations which make it up have long denied the reality of child abuse, there is very little understanding of the after-effects, as well as of how to help people in effective and humane ways.

It is shameful that the very system in society which could and should be trailblazing social inclusion and citizenship, often does the exact opposite in practice.

MRS HUTTEN

WITH DIRK CORSTENS

I am 47 years old and married. I attended primary and domestic science schools and one of my hobbies is making cards.

I must confess that I don't remember everything, but I still know that two voices were in my head almost every day. They were male voices and they were threatening. They gave commands and they ruled my life. I don't know how long ago, maybe five or seven years. I heard the voices outside in the street and also inside the house. At that time I felt extremely burned out and I took much medication. I was depressed. I didn't like life anymore. I also suffered from the voices when my husband was with me. I couldn't bear him touching me, the voices didn't allow that. I wasn't good for anything. When crossing a street I would be run over by cars the voices told me. If someone walked behind me he would be after me according to the voices. Eventually I was so afraid I didn't dare to go outside anymore.

I was punished for everything because I had permitted him [my husband] to touch me and I hadn't resisted it. I felt powerless. I was wrapped up in the voices completely. For a period I was treated by Dirk Corstens but I can't remember much, only what we talked about. It did help though. I believed that I had to talk back to the voices; engage in a conversation. I got much help and support from my husband. He supported me when I didn't dare to go outside or when I didn't want to cross the street.

What I remember is that I talked with Dirk Corstens and my GP (I also got much support from him). My family didn't understand. Things improved because of these talks, step by step, and also because I was at the daycare centre, an organisation of support for psychiatric patients. I was treated there for about two years until the moment came when I thought 'What am I doing here?' I had nothing to tell anymore. My purpose had always been to find ordinary work, to get back to normal life. And I succeeded. Now I am doing fine. I am not bothered by voices anymore. In the beginning I missed it. I felt empty and lonely. But now I have got back to what I want to be and want to have. I feel I am back again. I am still married, have friends and a job I like (I work in a catering business). I have become very independent; I don't take medication anymore and do all this without support.

Dirk Corstens adds: The above was written as a letter in response to an invitation from me to contribute to the book. According to my files I saw

Mrs Hutten four times in 1998. She had to travel 200 km and I met her together with her husband. I didn't make many notes but in my notes I found she heard two voices, one of her grandfather and one of her stepfather. She told me she couldn't have a proper conversation with them. The voices were negative and they forbade her to talk about them. 'I believe that I will be punished – at least, the voices tell me that – that I, or other people, will be involved in an accident, or will die. I'm afraid that I will say too much about the past.' She had heard the voices for three years. She started to talk about her past. The encouragement of her husband and her determination to stop being a psychiatric patient made her choose her own life again. She started to cope with the abuse by the two people who were represented by her voices.

JACQUI DILLON

Jacqui Dillon lives in London with her partner and children. She is the Chair of the National Hearing Voices Network in England. She is an experienced Hearing Voices Group facilitator and has a broad range of experience in working with voice hearers, as well as providing training, consultation and supervision on 'Hearing Voices' both nationally and internationally. She is a published writer and is currently writing her memoirs.

I hear voices, many kinds of voices, voices born from my experience; men, women and children; philosophers, demons and angels; kings and queens; waifs and strays; protective men with sinister voices; a magical, loving mother with a soothing, calming voice; a sadistic tormentor with a wicked sense of humour. There are many frightened children, some who sing and play, others who argue and fight. And a screaming baby who drives everyone mad. Poor baby.

I have heard voices since I was 3 years old. By the age of 7, I slept with a small transistor radio pressed up against my ear to try and block out the roar of voices that erupted every night when I lay down to go to sleep. I still use that strategy sometimes.

My early years were filled with many terrifying and disturbing experiences that literally shattered me into pieces. My family were involved with a group of organised, sadistic paedophiles who abused children and took part in extreme sadomasochistic practices. The consequence of such extreme and sustained abuse is devastating. Its effects are all-consuming, encompassing every aspect of experience. To be betrayed and exploited by those who are meant to protect you leaves a profound sense of terror, isolation and shame.

To survive, I developed a number of self-sufficient strategies. As well as hearing voices, I began to self-harm at an early age. I also developed a complex relationship with food which created an illusion of control over the arbitrary and cruel world I existed in. I became resourceful at adapting to extreme circumstances. I moved between worlds, one where I was at the mercy of sick and twisted adults who blamed me for their actions and one where I was an ordinary little girl, trying to do her best at school. I was creative and had a rich, imaginative, internal world that belonged to me alone. I won writing and drawing competitions and was considered a bright and gifted child. This, coupled with my innate sense of justice, meant that I knew that what my abusers were doing to me was wrong and that I both wanted and deserved better. I imagined a world where I would be safe, free and loved. One day I would escape.

The abuse ended when I was 15 but the consequences of it lived on inside of me for many years. Despite this, I developed a successful career in the media. I was still hearing voices and self-harming throughout this time but I hid it well. I was adept at inhabiting different worlds and used to keeping secrets locked inside me. Those who had abused me threatened to kill me if I ever told anyone about what had happened, so I remained silent.

It was the birth of my first daughter when I was 25 which eventually freed me to break the silence. My daughter was much longed for and the day of her birth is one of the happiest of my life. I gave birth to her naturally and, for the first time ever, I felt proud of my body and prouder still of the perfect baby it had produced. It was like a wondrous gift had been bestowed upon me. She was absolutely beautiful. But seeing this tiny, vulnerable baby also unlocked many horrifying memories from the past. My voices multiplied and intensified. They began saying things that disturbed and frightened me. I began seeing horrifying images of abuse, torture and death. I could feel it in my body. Marks and bruises appeared on my skin like stigmata. My self-harming spiralled out of control and I became convinced that someone would try to kill me and my daughter. I became intensely paranoid and was terrified to leave the house. I felt like I was going mad.

I lived in a dual world. I was a devoted mother, breastfeeding my daughter on demand, and we had a close and intimate bond. She was clearly thriving, yet I feared contaminating her with all of the poison that swirled around inside me. I desperately wanted to be a loving mother and to raise my child in a safe and happy home but I started to feel as if there was no escape from the horrors of the past. I began to think that the only way out was to end my life. In desperation I called my GP who urgently referred me to a psychiatrist. I was admitted to the local psychiatric hospital that afternoon. It felt like the end of the world.

Despite the threats that my abusers had made, I did start to try and talk about what they had done to me. I was desperate to get home to my little girl and I knew that what had happened to me as a child was the root cause of my distress. To my astonishment, the psychiatrists that I tried to tell either denied my experience or told me that I would never ever recover from what had happened. They told me that I had an illness: I was mentally ill. I was expected to be the passive recipient of treatment for this disorder and medication was the only option open to me. I was being told what to do and given contradictory opinions – that the only way to get better was to take medication but that, actually, I would never really get better anyway. No one ever asked me what I thought might help even though I felt that I had coped admirably up until that time. What I was experiencing was never considered to be a natural and human response to things that had happened in my life. The fact that I listened to my voices was evidence of my illness, and wanting to keep them in order to understand more about myself was seen as me being resistant to treatment.

As far as I am concerned, I am not sick. What my abusers did to me was sick. I have had a perfectly natural, human response to devastating experiences. Living with the knowledge of what was done to me, and the way in which psychiatry has added insult to injury by blaming me, is enough to drive anyone mad. My first psychiatric admission in 1993 was my last. I knew then that to be in such a desperate state in such an unsafe environment was potentially lethal. Ironically, the place that was meant to provide sanctuary for me became the place that nearly drove me over the edge once and for all.

I was very fortunate that other people in my life didn't blame me or deny what had happened to me. They were willing to listen to me and my voices and to support me in making sense of what the voices were trying to communicate to me. I worked closely with a counsellor and, later, with a therapist who believed in me and had faith in my ability to recover. With their support and that of my partner and closest friends I started on the long and winding road back to myself. It has been an internal process of truth and reconciliation, of listening, bearing witness and of facing the horrors of the past.

A starting point for me was creating a new paradigm for myself that honoured my resilience and capacity to heal. I wanted a framework which would enable me to safely listen to my voices and make sense of my experiences. I read a vast amount of material and became better informed about the many ways of understanding human experience. I researched the phenomenon of dissociation and began to appreciate the extent to which I had utilised this capacity in my own survival. I also read a lot of attachment theory. I began to comprehend the impact of my early experiences as well as understanding, conceptually, what a good enough parent was. Discovering the work of Judith Lewis Herman in *Trauma and Recovery* had a profound effect on me. Suddenly, my own experiences were put into a wider context. I was not alone in feeling outraged by the damage done by society, in pathologising survivors of abuse. The personal became political. I began envisaging a brighter future. I was a woman on a mission. One day I would show them all.

Having my own personal crisis plan was essential when things were really difficult as I was determined that I would never return to a psychiatric hospital, however desperate I became. So I developed ways of keeping safe and focused on taking life one day at a time. I had a list of twenty things to do when desperate which I kept by my phone in times of crisis. I reminded myself of previous times when I had felt suicidal and what I would have missed if I'd succumbed to the despair. I had mantras that I repeated to counter terror and that helped me to rebuild my belief in myself. If a voice kept saying to me: 'You are a bad mother', I would say, 'I love my daughter and she loves me'. Or, if a voice kept saying: 'You are doomed. You will die a horrible death', I would say, 'I am safe now and I am free.' I would repeat these words of power over and over, both in my head and out loud, and, slowly, I began to believe them. I stopped having contact with people who undermined me and slowly developed relationships with those who supported me, both with friends and, later on, through co-counselling. Over time, I created my own support network. The love and wisdom of both my counsellor and my therapist was essential in guiding and sustaining me on my journey. I could not have undertaken the work without them, yet I have done much of the hard labour on my own.

It was important for me to find structure in my life with ordinary activities which enabled me to take care of myself. Getting enough sleep, keeping my house clean, listening to music, keeping busy or slowing down when things got too much, provided a safe basis to work from. I also found taking care of myself physically really helped. Complementary therapies like homeopathy that work holistically, taking account of the whole person – mind, body and spirit – really appealed to me. My homeopath accepted my voices as part of me and not as some problem that needed to be eradicated. More recently, I have been influenced by new research into psychophysiology and the impact that trauma has on the body.

I also developed my own creative strategies. I began drawing and painting images that haunted me and painting became my alternative to self-harm. I would use paint and my bare hands to release and illustrate intense feelings and, gradually, I stopped hurting myself. I also discovered that singing is a great release and that it's hard to listen to voices when you are singing. Expressing intense emotion like terror, rage and despair was also really important in helping to release my distress and lessen the intensity of disturbing voices and visions. I did this in many ways both in therapy and also by going out and dancing with my friends all night, going to the countryside and screaming on the top of a mountain, sitting by the sea and crying an ocean of tears.

I began writing a daily journal which gave me a sense of order and structure in what often felt like a chaotic environment. Writing became my way of putting the different voices and feelings that were troubling me outside of me. I was able to gain some perspective, which enabled me to make more sense of what was going on. I began to see patterns and triggers and I would ask my voices questions which they would then write or draw a response to. It was at this point that I first began to grasp that my voices were more than simply voices. I began to realise that I was inhabited by different people. These 'voices' had different names and identities. They had defined and distinct personalities. This realisation was a startling relief. My sense of my own identity shifted. I moved from being 'me' to 'we'.

My relationship with my different selves changed over time. I wanted to encourage communication between the different selves and eventually worked towards a mutual collaboration with them. As far as I was concerned we were in this together. However difficult they sometimes were I knew that the voices of my different selves reflected important truths about my experiences. So, if a voice was threatening me, I immediately wondered if *they* had been threatened. Through writing and internal dialogues I was able to ask my voices questions which they began to answer. My curiosity and non-threatening stance was transformatory. Instead of the terror and retaliation that had previously existed, an atmosphere of safety and acceptance was created. I began to understand that my voices were dissociated selves that were internalised representations of the world that I grew up in. These various selves had been born from my experience. Each self was a part of the whole of me. What they really needed was my unconditional love and support, much in the same way a loving parent supports a child. I began to see that I needed to listen to them and understand them and the context in which they emerged and to greet them with compassion and understanding. I began to honour them as they had helped me to survive. Slowly we began supporting and understanding each other and an increasing sense of connectedness and wholeness grew. Life became a shared project. Gradually, I felt less ashamed about who I was and began to marvel at how creative I had been in surviving such monstrous abuse. I became excited by what my mind had managed to invent. At times it felt like I had created a work of art.

It has been an arduous journey, a mission we have dedicated ourselves to for many years and recorded in more than 145 journals to date. I plan to publish an account of my life, as I feel I have an important story to tell about the human potential to destroy, and create; a testament to the persistence of the human spirit to survive in the most extreme circumstances. My survival story is both extraordinary and an ordinary, everyday human endeavour.

Pathologising the creative endeavours of ordinary people to survive the raw deal that life has dealt them is not only insulting but diminishes the achievements we accomplish with so very little. It also colludes in protecting abusers from being held accountable for their crimes. I know for a fact that the man at the centre of the ring that abused me is still operating – for now.

Abuse thrives in secrecy. We must expose the truth and not perpetuate injustice further, otherwise today's child-abuse victims become tomorrow's psychiatric patients. People need to know of the horrific cruelty we human beings are capable of, and of our magnificent and heroic resilience in the face of it. We need to expand our view of what it means to be human. Instead of asking the question 'What is wrong with you?', we need to ask 'What has happened to you?' This sense of outrage is what has driven me in my work.

They say that living well is the best revenge. Well, I do my best. My life isn't perfect but I do live it to the full and, each day, find myself becoming closer to who I want to be. Having multiple selves can still drive me crazy sometimes but that isn't my fault. I am driven mad by what has happened to me but that's only human. And it has become easier. More troubling is my struggle to find meaning in a world that often makes no sense to me. My work helps, both in the connections I make with people and also through my sense of influencing positive change.

For someone who was told by the system that she would never recover, actually, life's pretty good! Personally, I am more content than ever before. I have a fabulous partner and I am privileged to have some wonderful people in my life. I would not be here if it were not for the love of good people. I marvel at my own and at others' capacity to love, despite the odds. I am a loving parent to my daughters, although I received no nurturing myself as a child, and, to my delight, they love me back. They fill me with hope. The greatest truth is love.

JAN HOLLOWAY

WITH JACQUI DILLON

Jan Holloway is a 49-year-old woman. She is married and lives in London. She works as an occupational therapist in an assertive outreach team, a community mental health team which works with clients who have serious and enduring mental health issues. Jan enjoys cycling, dancing, art, listening to music, being a DJ, spending money and drinking Diet Coke.

I hear voices through my ears. The perception is that they are coming from another person or creature or something, although in my mind I think that they probably are from me or part of me. I used to think that something was taking me over and trying to control me. I hear two voices: one of them is the voice of my former therapist; and later another voice came, a voice that I don't recognise which is also female, middle-aged and also an intellectual. They are both have cultured accents and are well-spoken with no swearing or slang, which adds to their authority. They are very moralistic, which makes me feel really judged.

I originally went into therapy because I had been diagnosed with epilepsy and I was finding that hard to deal with. I had been having therapy for six years and it had been reasonably useful for about four of these six years but then the therapist started doing things that made me feel unsafe; she started not charging the bills regularly and allowing the session to go over by 15 minutes one week and not the next. It seemed fairly random as far as I was concerned; it felt like boundaries were being crossed and it didn't feel that safe. At the same time I had just got a job as a manager of a day centre and I don't think management suited me. There were a lot of challenging situations happening in the workplace. Also, through that job I made friends with people who were quite intense emotionally. They talked about feelings a lot more than I did and were quite assertive. I felt quite overwhelmed by those people. So the therapy, the work and the friendships all contributed to me starting to feel as if people could get inside my head. They could take my thoughts away and put theirs in and it felt too dangerous to get too close to people because of that. On the other hand, I'd enjoyed these close friendships and didn't want to go back to the kind of friendships that I'd had before, so it became a dilemma.

I talked about it a lot in therapy but I also started to feel intruded on by the therapist. We started getting into arguments – about the billing and that she was letting sessions run over and whether I should have therapy more than once a week or not. Then, one day, I went into therapy and she said that we needed to have a break, which I wasn't totally surprised about because the therapy relationship had deteriorated, and I asked, 'When does the break start?' I assumed that there would be a month's notice as we had been seeing each other for six years, but she said, 'Tonight is your last session.' I was really shocked.

I was in a daze for a few days and I started to hear her voice about two or three days after that. It started off quite neutral but then it got more and more critical and it said that I should kill people that I was close to because they would try and take over my mind. The dilemma was that I didn't want to do that and the voice was saying that the only other alternative is to kill yourself. That was a stark choice. It just got more and more frequent, louder and more intense, and that was when I needed to go into hospital because I tried to take my own life.

At that point, I didn't tell my GP, the people in casualty or the people at the hospital that I was hearing voices because I was worried about the diagnosis. Also, the voice was saying that if I did tell people she would make sure that my then boyfriend and friends would get hurt or killed, so I couldn't tell anyway.

In between the first and second admissions I started to take some medication and I began some new therapy with someone who was able to deal with the kind of experiences that I was having. It was that that made me realise that I had to tell people what was going on and that I had to trust people more. And, when I did tell them, they said, 'Well we knew that anyway.' They didn't ask what the content was and weren't interested in the meaning, just 'is it commanding you to do things?' They said, 'It's your illness and we've got to get rid of it.' They did tell me that the medication would take the voices away, which it hasn't. When I've been in hospital in the past, not many of the nurses have been very interested. The belief still seems to be that talking about voices will make it worse. I was trained like that as well and that view is still quite prevalent.

RECOVERY

When I first saw Marius and Sandra speak back in 1993, when they had just written *Accepting Voices*, I was really blown away because they were flying in the face of what most people were saying then, which is that voices didn't make any sense. Instinctively, I knew they were right; I had wanted to work that way for eleven years but it had been trained out of me. We were told that it was dangerous to talk to people about their voices – I knew that was flawed, and it was great to hear someone like a psychiatrist and a journalist say what I knew instinctively was right. I felt liberated.

Therapy enabled me to look at what was going on in my life; that led to the start of me hearing voices but also the more distant past, for example, family relationships. My mother was quite a big character and quite controlling and I think that there was a connection there that I made in therapy; my tendency towards wanting to be a good person (my therapist used to call it 'behaving like a saint') and the fear of my less saintly side. We were brought up to do what posh people told you to – well-spoken people seemed to have more authority than people with accents – so there is something from the past which makes me put my voices in a position of authority. They are very critical a lot of the time, but not directly. They talk about me, so it's, 'she's doing this, she's done that really badly…' which makes it harder to challenge. Now that I have got used to this running commentary I don't mind it and sometimes it helps me to focus because I can be a bit fragmented and scattered. Sometimes, when I am trying to concentrate on something and they are describing it, it actually helps. I've learned to allow it to help over the years.

The therapy wasn't supposed to be about understanding everything, but I think I understand now enough to start working on some of the other things. For example, I think my school days had an impact on me, although I have only been thinking about this recently. Infant school was really difficult as they were quite cruel. If you didn't eat your dinner they would hold your nose and force you to swallow it and they would hit us for spelling something wrong and also for what they called 'telling tales'. I got hit for telling my teacher that somebody had messed up my desk so, then, I didn't tell the teachers anything and consequently got bullied by quite a few people because they knew they could do what they liked to me and I wouldn't tell anyone. Secondary school was very chaotic. There were lots of incidents of violence; lots of kids carried knives and one boy carried an airgun. I was also bullied in that school, again, because I wouldn't tell people, so I became isolated. I think that led to me not making very deep friendships.

I finished the therapy more than six years ago but I still use a lot of the understanding and the things that I learned about myself there to help me.

I have found support from a wide range of people, lots of different friends, especially those friends who hear voices; some of the friends that I met in hospital and, of course, my husband, who has a big tolerance for unusual ideas, doesn't get too shocked and is very supportive. It seems to me people who have a tolerance for the unusual and who are able to challenge some of the ideas that are not that helpful to me – that's the theme that runs through the people that I want to talk to when I am going through a bad time with voices and paranoia and stuff like that.

When my voices change for the worse I am now much more aware that I need to change how I am running my life, maybe slow down a bit or change certain relationships with people. But, over the years, I have learned to use my voices as a bit of a barometer, either internally or externally. I get more voices and become more stressed if there are unspoken dynamics between people, or if people are being picked on.

I am more able to ask for help generally since my breakdown and I am able to say 'no' more easily if I think that something is stressing me out. I'm getting better at changing relationships with people, or severing them altogether, if they are not doing me or the other person much good. I value different states of mind and different kinds of people much more than I did. I am more conscious of them now and I build them when I can but I am also trying to be open as well. It's a constant struggle.

I am more in touch with what I am feeling now. There were times not that long ago when I would have feelings and I wouldn't even know what they were called, whether it was anger or sadness. I am more able to name what I am feeling now; I allow myself to feel it for a bit longer so I can name it. Expressing feelings is still difficult. I am better at using paint and paper or drawing what I am feeling than actually saying it. Sometimes I look at it and think 'that makes some sense out of what I have experienced' and it helps me to explain it to other people in a way that I can't do with words. It gets the feelings out so that I am not just trapped with them. Sometimes just painting patterns or clouds or something is very relaxing.

I love listening to music and that helps with voices in a very specific way. I do wear a Walkman sometimes if the voices are bad and it can soften them. Music also helps with the scattered thoughts and feelings, especially if it is something with a beat to it. It helps me to feel more structured. I also like music because I socialise through it by going out dancing. I like playing as a DJ and I enjoy watching other people enjoy music. Spending time with people that I feel safe and comfortable with, sometimes talking about voices but just spending time together, is good for me. Cycling is good because you can't really attend to voices when you are on a busy road. Swimming is good, too, because the water surrounds me and that helps me to feel a bit more contained.

I now feel much more proud and much less ashamed of being a voice hearer which I think is because the context has changed and a lot more people are talking about it. There weren't groups around when I first started hearing voices so there wasn't that culture of acceptance back then, so it was more a context in which to feel ashamed. I just have more pride in the experience having lived with it for fifteen years. I would like to not hear voices, or if I heard voices that were more supportive it would be different. It's not something that I particularly enjoy or an experience that I would wish on anyone, but I am not ashamed of it and I am proud of being able to live with it and of what I have learned from it.

JEANETTE BRINK

WITH MARIUS ROMME

Jeanette, 37 years old, initially heard one and then three voices in her head for many years. And although the psychiatrist told her it was her own voice she heard, it still drove her pretty mad. It made her very lonely too.

I was lying in bed on a weekday evening. I was 18 and still lived with my parents at that time. I was just about to fall asleep when I heard somebody call my name. I got up to ask my parents what it was, but it had not been them. 'What?' I did not understand it at all. As soon as I was back in bed, I heard it again, 'Jeanette, Jeanette.'

'Who is it?' I asked anxiously. 'I'm Jantje,' the voice said. I could not distinguish anyone in the room. It was very scary, but exciting too. I had always been interested in paranormal things and now I was experiencing it myself. The voice and I chatted quite a lot. The voice told me that it had known me for a long time. The next day I was convinced that I had dreamt it. Such a thing just was not possible. However, I was not quite sure and when I got home from school I went straight to my room. 'Are you still there?' I asked in a slightly facetious way. 'Yes indeed,' the voice said. Unbelievable. However, my curiosity quickly disappeared. Jantje was very nasty. And he was with me all the time, wherever I went. I saw him too.

Until then I had been a perfectly normal girl. I was at college, had lots of friends and went out regularly. I was perhaps very shy and somewhat insecure, but there was nothing wrong with me. Suddenly my life had been turned upside down. The voice that I heard started giving me orders. He became more and more commanding. For example, I had to keep on going up and down the stairs and if I did not follow his orders, he would hurt me very much. He was there all the time and knew everything; I could not hide anything from it. I thought I was going mad. How could this just happen like that, what kind of nightmare was this? I kept quiet about it for two weeks, hoping it would go away. In a panic I turned to my parents. They really took care of me, but they were shocked too.

Together with my mum I went to see the GP who reacted in a pleasant way. He told me that I could always ring him, even in the middle of the night. However, since he only knew little about voice hearing he referred me to a psychiatrist who was convinced that the voice came from within me. I 'thanked' him, it was my own imagination. He prescribed medication. It worked well in terms of getting me to sleep, as I had hardly slept all that time. After taking these pills, I slept for three days. However, following that the voices went on as before. Apart from ordering me about, Jantje mainly talked about sex. All these things he wanted to do with me … sometimes I even felt things he did with me. And sometimes I saw him. I saw him in a tree once; a very angry male face. Yes, I know. It sounds weird, but for me it was real. The pills did not work at all and I started to do more and more as I was told to by Jantje. That is when I felt safe.

SEXUALLY FRUSTRATED

When you hear voices, it is usually assumed that you are schizophrenic. However, I was neither psychotic, nor confused, as I was able to think very straight. I understood that it was very bizarre that I kept on hearing Jantje. And when, for example, he told me I could fly, of course I knew it was a lie. However, there was nothing I could do against it. I was often livid at that voice. I would shout hysterically then that he should go away, that I hated him. 'I will be with you forever. You're never going to get rid of me,' he would tell me viciously.

I had stopped going to school. I could not concentrate any more and could not remember anything any more. That was caused by all the medication that I was taking. I was walking around like a zombie. In order to get out and about, they let me do some voluntary work at my former school. Despite this I gradually became isolated. People thought of me as weird; girlfriends did not understand me. Luckily I received a lot of support from my parents. It is only a year ago now that things have been going well for me and since they have told me how difficult a time they had back then. It was terrible for them to see me like that.

I used to see the psychiatrist once a week. I told him about the sexual intimidation of the voice. Every single time, the psychiatrist tried to convince me that the voice was my own imagination. I had never had sex with a guy yet and he thought that Jantje kept on talking about sex, as I suppressed my emotions; I was sexually frustrated. If only I were to go to bed with someone, the voice would go away. I did not really believe him, but hey; he was the doctor and I assumed he was right. I wanted to get rid of that voice so desperately that I tried it anyway. I went out and seduced the first guy that came along. However, instead of things getting better, they got worse. After a while, two more voices even presented. One called himself God, the other the devil. I had to obey God otherwise I would fall into the hands of the devil. They gave me contradictory orders, it drove me insane. This period lasted a year. From a perfectly normal girl I changed into a wreck, with the psychiatric patient label stuck on me. I was very lonely. And I had no idea what to expect of my future.

RECOVERY

I believed that I was the only one who suffered from this, until I heard about the 'Weerklank' ('Resonance', the Dutch Hearing Voices Network) Association on television. They want to break down the taboo surrounding 'hearing voices' and they provide education and advice. I was so relieved that there were people out there experiencing similar things. I attended a meeting. That gave me and strength and something to hold onto. My tactics worked.

During that same period, something very important happened. One day the voices told me that this time I had really gone too far. I had not obeyed them well enough and therefore needed to be punished. During the next night, I would die and I would fall into the hands of Satan forever. I was panic-stricken, but I still managed to fall asleep. The next morning I simply woke up as normal. I was not dead at all.

This night was a turning point. I realised that whatever the voices were telling me, it was nonsense. They were just talking nonsense. I did not need to obey them at all. I was relieved of an enormous burden; my fear. I also felt very ready to fight. I thought: let's see who is the strongest here after all: you or me? I started to pretend not hearing the voices. In order to shut them out, I started to concentrate on my own thoughts. As long I could hear these, they would drown out the three demons in me. With everything I did I started to think: 'This is a spoon, this is a fork. I am putting them on the table as I'm going to eat later.' That gave me control.

Until that moment, I had always felt so powerless. And my technique worked: the voices were less loud, less dominant. I was becoming increasingly convinced: as long as I keep on ignoring them I will chase them away. It worked indeed, albeit that it took me another five years before I had banned them from my life altogether.

In those last years, I pretended to everyone as if nothing was wrong any more. I deceived my psychiatrist into thinking that his treatment (going to bed with someone) had worked after all. I had no faith in him. I stopped taking my medication. In order to keep up appearances, I told my parents that things were going better too. I moved out so that I could escape their glances. Of course I did not discuss this with new people I met.

I had a boyfriend at that time, but I was convinced he would leave me if he knew. It was only when our relationship was over and he accused me of always being so occupied with myself, I told him. It was too late to save our relationship, but he was very understanding. At that moment, I had almost got rid of the voices. It was only at night that they would bother me. And then one night, I was 26 years old, they stayed away. I had won. It was wonderful being free again.

EASY PREY

I still do not know wherever these voices came from. There is no logical explanation for it. Even the experts do not agree on it. It could be that the voices come from within you, as my psychiatrist claimed. In regular healthcare, they are usually convinced of this, but it is not watertight. For example, they measured brain activity of voice hearers at times and in places which cannot be explained at all. However, in psychiatry, they have always denied voices coming from outside. Therefore, the content of the voices was not really discussed in detail during treatment. The objective was: pulling the patient back to reality and the voices of course had nothing to do with reality.

Nowadays there are also psychiatrists who are open to the idea that voices could indeed come from outside. Professor Marius Romme played a revolutionary role in this area. He demonstrated that only one in three people who hear voices are psychiatric patients. His treatment is based on the assumption that the voices are real, since that often has a positive impact on the healing process. However, he cannot explain them either. Nobody can. Personally, I have an opinion on this indeed. I still believe that my voices did not arise from my own imagination. They sounded so different. This could not have been me. I believe that there are many different spirits hanging around in our world and that I was bothered by unhappy, miserable spirits who enjoy tormenting people. They catch people who are very sensitive: easy prey.

However, it is just a philosophy. I cannot prove it. But then again, that is not necessary. Everybody can think what they like. The only thing that I find regrettable is that people immediately think you are completely nuts when you hear voices. Or they say: 'Once mad, always mad.' I know many people who got rid of their voices and who lead a normal life again. . .

Nowadays I regularly talk about my experiences. I am not embarrassed about it any more. It simply happened to me. I now work as a voluntary worker for the 'Resonance' association. I want to help fellow sufferers, since that helped me a lot too. Most people suffer a lot from negative voices. The voices tell you that you are not capable of achieving anything, that you are worthless, they swear at you. I hope that these people will manage to overcome their fear since regardless of whether the voices come from the inside or the outside I believe that to be the only key. I know that voices can always come back. However, I am not scared of them any more. Let's assume they come back to me: I now know how to fight them. They will not get control over me any more.

JEANNETTE WOOLTHUIS

WITH SANDRA ESCHER

Jeannette Woolthuis has been active in the Dutch Patients Society for a number of years, as well as being a board member of 'Resonance', the Dutch Hearing Voices Network. Jeannette was also for a long time the secretary, and then became president. She now has her own practice as a therapist for people who hear voices and specialises in working with children.

I have always heard voices. I must have been 2 years old when I noticed that a plant answered me. It was so normal for me that I never discussed this with others. I thought that everyone heard voices. At one point the voices quietened down, and then they disappeared. I think I was in primary school at that time, busy with other things.

When I was 11 years old I was pulled off my bicycle and dragged into an alcove and raped. Whilst I was being raped, other people were walking past but nobody did anything. That confirmed what I always feared: that nobody would ever help me. I was afraid I would die. That nearly happened – he tried to strangle me and darkness descended upon me, but he stopped just in time.

At the time of the rape I started to hear two voices – adult male voices. I didn't have a name for them and actually I still don't have names for them. I was in so much shock that I didn't quite realise what was happening to me. I was actually watching myself from a distance. The memories of what actually happened are the memories of a bystander.

Even though I was still only young, I went to the police station to put in an assault charge. However, I couldn't describe what had happened to me, I didn't know the words. Nobody responded at the police station – they didn't take any notice. I went home, but I didn't tell my parents what had happened because I knew I was not supposed to be in that neighborhood. I had been late so had taken the faster road through the red-light area, which is why I thought it was own fault. My parents must have noticed that something had happened but they never asked me anything. I had to deal with it all on my own. Apart from that I liked my parents and we had a good relationship.

The voices did not change and become scary from one day to the next. If I look back, the voices slowly but surely started to play a more important role in my life. They told me that they were gods and that they ruled the world; that I was a chosen one – but for what they did not tell me. The voices took me seriously when I was anxious and all alone. They were the only ones who understood me and gave me support and therefore they became more influential and I became dependent on them. But then they started to give me orders. Firstly, very simple ones on the level of obedience, such as: 'you have to be good; children have to listen to their parents'. If I obeyed them they rewarded me. They told me that I was under their control. That was really scary. Slowly, their orders extended and the punishments, if I did not do what they told me to do, became more severe. If I did not do it all right then I had, for example, to run up and down the stairs three times. Sometimes they would threaten me with 'if you don't do this or that, then we will kill such-and-such' or 'we will ensure that this or that person will become ill'. I believed it to be true and found out later that it was as the voices said. It made me very nervous as it made me feel responsible for the health and lives of other people.

I really ended up in trouble when at school during gymnastics class I fell out of the rings; suddenly I couldn't do a whole heap of things anymore. Up till this moment I had been doing very well at school. I received very high grades and wanted to become a doctor and I had the capacities to become one. After the accident I couldn't concentrate any longer; I couldn't remember things very well anymore. My motor skills deteriorated rapidly and I couldn't participate in any sports activities any more. My usually high grades became very low grades and I started to doubt myself and my whole sense of living. I became extremely depressed. After the accident I couldn't apply myself to anything. I didn't understand what I was doing. Even during a conversation, after having only mentioned the first sentence, I had already lost the sense and meaning of the conversation. I became so down, so sombre and quiet, that it became apparent and I ended up with a psychiatrist from the psychiatric ward in the local hospital. She asked: 'Do you hear voices?' After that she asked me, 'What do the voices say?' I totally panicked at this stage and just said, 'I've got to die, right now.'

The voices had extreme power over me. They did not allow me to speak about death at all because, if I did, a lot of people would be in danger. The voices threatened others, something I was not allowed to do because I was responsible for the demise of others. That's where they held me in their grip. I had to become totally emotionless and was not allowed to display any grief or sadness because that was dangerous. I was not allowed to display any anger because that was bad. My whole sensory system died. I had no feelings whatsoever. The voices became louder and stronger and started screaming at me.

After that consultation with the psychiatrist I was admitted to the psychiatric ward of a general hospital and, after ten days or so, was informed that I would be admitted to a psychiatric hospital. I thought: 'This is the end. I'm 16 years old and I'm going to the loony-tune bin'. In the loony-tune bin, however, I quickly discovered that I was not as crazy as I thought. Strange things happened there. I quickly found out that, in hospital, humour does not exist. What held me together and what got me through those years might have been cynical humour but at least it *was* a sense of humour.

I tried to explain to the psychiatrist what my problems were at that time. He told me that voices do not exist and that I was psychotic. He gave me medication for the psychoses. I tried to reason that if the medications worked against psychosis then they should also work against the voices. But that didn't happen, so obviously something else was going on. The doctor said that wasn't true as it was part of my delusion. I then became very angry. I said to him: 'I don't want to talk to you anymore because you don't listen to me anyway, so none of this is of any use.' After this I started behaving myself and tried to stay really obedient, and I didn't mention the voices anymore. Shortly after that I was discharged. In my medical notes was written: 'Manipulative – we will wait till the next one in her family shows up with problems. But she is doing well, and no doubt the voices were just an attention-seeking behaviour.'

After my discharge I went back to live with my parents, however after being in hospital for nine months I couldn't handle living with them anymore. After some time I moved in with a friend of mine. I knew this friend from the psychiatric hospital; he was a nurse there. The relationship didn't work out. I overdosed on my medications so I ended up being admitted to another psychiatric hospital. I made many suicide attempts. At the last one I thought, 'this just has to work', but it didn't. This was so pathetic, so I decided that if I can't die, I'll just have to keep living. I decided for myself that, although I might hear and see things others can't hear and see, my communication skills are still pretty good. I joined the patient's council of the hospital, despite my voices. I flourished there so much that I became the Chair.

One day the director of the hospital approached me and asked to speak to me. He said: 'I think it's a shame you are in this hospital. You have the capacity to do so much more! You don't belong here. You are not crazy at all! You have a problem with acknowledging your feelings ... you've lost your feelings. I want you to call a friend of mine who is a psychiatrist in Amsterdam and tell him I asked you to contact him. Tell him, "I've lost my feelings and I want them back"... here's his telephone number.'

RECOVERY

I left the hospital and went to live in an apartment on my own. After pondering for a long time I finally called the psychiatrist in Amsterdam and made an appointment. When I began my therapy with him it was horrible! It was the most difficult period of my life. He slowly but steadily investigated what the voices were saying to me and when they had started to appear in my life. Very early on he said: 'The voices are saying things that come true. You are acknowledged in what they say.' By formulating it in this way he concurred with me that a large part of me was not psychotic. I often knew what was going to happen in the future. That made it even more difficult. The voices could predict the future but they were also there because of the strange way I dealt with my emotions. The big question was this: why had I decided what were positive and what were negative emotions? And why had I set myself up for failure? The perfectionism of it all, without my realising it, had brought me to utter despair. The requirements I demanded of myself that I had to act altruistically because otherwise I was a 'good-for-nothing'. The black-and-white thinking I had towards myself, I didn't have towards other people. I was measuring myself against two different standards; I set myself such high limits and judged myself so harshly, constantly sticking horrible, nasty labels on myself, on my thinking and my actions, but not on others, only on myself. Actually, I was very high-handed, arrogant – as arrogant as hell. That's what the voices continually have been saying to me. This made sense. As strange as it sounds, they were actually right in a very strange way.

The voices responded neutrally to the psychiatrist, as if he wasn't actually there. Sometimes I wasn't allowed to go to see him, although they didn't say this outright. Afterwards, I could reason that it was subconsciously forbidden. Through that, they ensured that I became half-way psychotic again. For example, I had the delusion that Amsterdam had been bombed and that my psychiatrist had been killed. Then I wouldn't attend my appointment.

He would call me and say: 'Hi, where are you?' I'd tell him, 'But you're dead, aren't you?' Then I'd attend my appointment, bright red with embarrassment and say, 'Oops, sorry, my mistake.' He could laugh about things like that; he had the same sense of humour that I had. And he was someone who understood what you were saying when you've only mentioned half of it. So, actually, I could talk and think with him at my own pace. I didn't continually have to adapt and adjust to someone else's thinking and understanding patterns. I'm very fast-paced in my thinking and speaking. He continually said to me, 'Don't you have any idea how clever and intelligent you are?' 'No,' I replied, 'because other people don't understand me.' He said, 'Don't you understand others, or do others not understand you?' I would think about that and notice that there was actually a difference. He then said, 'If you think and reason so fast then you are skipping instead of walking, and missing steps. Have a look at what you are doing.' I didn't see any of that. I thought I was stupid, extremely stupid, because I couldn't even communicate with people. I knew I was different but I tried to adapt myself to others so that I wouldn't stand out or be sidelined. I pushed myself too hard.

Looking back, I realise I made a number of choices. The first choice was to stay alive. That was an important decision because I stopped thinking about not wanting to live anymore. If you don't want to live any longer, then you don't make plans for the future. So I decided to start living again, and that had a number of consequences. I had to start looking after myself and doing something about my appearance. The next step was to look at myself and find myself OK or not, because the psychiatrist felt that I was fine – even more than fine – and had said: 'I don't understand why you think so negatively and why you have such low self-esteem and opinion of yourself, because if there's anyone who has the capacity to do more, then that is you.' Because of that, I reasoned that it must be so, but why am I a nobody? Because of that conversation I slowly started to rethink what I was actually doing to myself. And why do I set myself such high expectations? What was actually so bad about me? Why don't I have any rights? One day the psychiatrist asked me, 'Who are you, actually?' I totally flipped at that question. I reached total panic state. Later I started thinking about why I totally panicked at that question. Then I thought, 'I am totally nothing … that's what's happened to me. Who I am now is my own voices … it's not me any more.' I didn't know who I was any more. I didn't know what my feelings were anymore and, what belonged to the voices and what belonged to others.

Through the tolerance of the psychiatrist I learned to feel that emotions such as anger and sadness were my own emotions and that they were allowed to be there. He said: 'I would be angry about what has happened to you, so why am I not seeing your anger? How is it possible that you are angry and I don't see your anger?' I answered: 'If I display my anger then I'm going to be so angry that I am going to snap. I am petrified of my anger and I don't dare go there. I'm scared that I might hurt someone else or that I'm going to smash this whole place to pieces. I don't want to do that. There's such an unbelievably great volcano inside me, I can't do it. I learnt that at home already, that I was never allowed to be angry.' He said: 'I believe that you are really scared of your anger. There are so many things that have happened to you that you are angry about. You are indeed a volcano, ready to explode.' To teach me how to deal effectively with my anger and to display it properly, he sent me to a four-day workshop. He said: 'You are going there to work on your rape experience. You are going to sort it out.' And I did. I fought with all kinds of therapists. I went through the whole experience all over again. I discovered that if I felt an emotion I wasn't going to die. I could stay inside my body and I could keep on living.

After that I was able to make new choices. I was not the offender – the girl that lay there was the victim. That was me. I could finally feel the pain that I felt at that time. The extreme fear and anxiety of dying was my anxiety. That was the first time that I was in my body, feeling my whole body without missing a part of it. I had been living too much in my head. I sometimes felt only my head and the rest of me felt nothing. I could feel again because I had experienced my anger and nobody got hurt.

After that I finally dared admit to myself that I could well be the one who was very angry, instead of my voices. But I could only make that step forwards after I had identified other emotions as my own feelings instead of making them part of the voices. It had been a very handy excuse and survival mechanism to link my anger to the voices instead of to me.

Before attending that workshop, I relied totally on my psychiatrist. He believed in me but I didn't believe in myself. He was my hope for a future. I was terrified that I would attack him in anger, because I cared a lot about him at that time. After that workshop, I totally relied on myself. I became my own boss. I realised that there was nobody who could hurt me and therefore the next person to attack me was going to be dead. That was a good decision to make. It was a very definite decision. I have the right to be boss over my body and therefore also over my mind. That was a good one for the voices – they didn't like the new me. After that workshop one of the voices said to me, 'Ta ta! I'm off!' But there was still one voice left.

When I went back to my psychiatrist I was still pretty agitated and distressed as the 'can of worms' had well and truly been opened. I had a lot of flashbacks but the obstacles were gone. I could become angry again and took responsibility for that and for any actions as a result of that anger. Because of what I've learned throughout this therapy I've also had to say to myself: 'You are responsible for the amount that you get hurt. For example, it's not the way in which someone annoys you but the amount that you allow it to affect and bother you and apply it to yourself.' Because of that, I've re-established my boundaries. What I find important I will accept and, even if it is true, if I don't feel like accepting it, then I don't accept it, even the right for me to be there for myself. I don't need to disappear any longer. I am not dependent on someone else. I also don't need to place myself above others. I am just there because I want to be there and because I am there – people need to take me into consideration.

After that, I started to think about what I wanted to do with the rest of my life. I started studying. Now, I'm not just qualified by experience, I am also a qualified therapist. This meant that I had to stand up for myself. That message was clear. Emotionally I had to change a lot of things. I had to rediscover myself and, above all, to accept myself.

JO

PART 1

My name is Jo. I am 30 years old, female and single. My main education has been attending a further education college and completing a social work course. My main activity at the moment is caring for my five animals. My hobbies are sport and reading.

I hear eight voices, mainly in my head, but have experienced voices from outside, through my ears. I have one voice which is the strongest and this one occurred due to early traumatic life events; this voice is part of me, but my other seven voices are also part of me through other stressful events in my life. I have been hearing voices for twenty-five years. I hear my voices most of the time, sometimes all day and all night. They get more frequent when I get stressed-out.

The first of my five voices is male and has no name. He is nasty, very dominant, likes to be in charge and is very aggressive. The age of the 'nasty' one has gone from a young man to middle age. The second of my voices is female and her name is Joyce. She is also aggressive but tends to be dominated by my first voice. Joyce can be bossy, vindictive and very hurtful when talking to me. The third of my voices is a child's voice, aged about 7 to 8. I refer to this voice as 'squente', because that is how he talks. Squente can make very disturbing comments. The fourth of my voices is really two because it splits into two people at times; the voice/voices are female. I refer to these as F1 and F2. They bitch with each other about me and can be very derogatory. The fifth of my voices is a female voice and is 28 years old. I refer to her as the 'lady' because she talks very correctly in the Queen's English, so to speak. She is bitchy and nasty.

I first started hearing voices at the age of 5, and for twenty-five years they have always been consistent. I first started to hear a voice after an early traumatic episode of abuse. I remember my first voice so clearly because it took on the identity of the person who had abused me. But then I thought everyone had an imaginary friend so at first I didn't think it was anything out of the ordinary ... anyhow I can remember it being in the school playground. I was 5 years old and I asked a friend if she heard a voice in her head. She looked at me and called me a 'nutter'. Then I knew I was different.

My life changed at one point very dramatically. I had never told anyone I heard voices and, as soon as I did, I was treated as abnormal. My voices have influenced me in all my everyday experiences; for a long time they controlled what I could and could not do. I know that due to my life-events my voices have varied according to what has happened in my life. My personal development has been inhibited because of the impact of the control they have had in my life and on what I have been allowed to do.

When I remember things that have happened to me it makes me feel angry and frustrated. This triggers my voices, providing them with ammunition to annoy and pester me. When I am frightened my voices act on this, they wind me up and subsequently make me more frightened. My voices have told me repeatedly that I am a worthless person … I have been persistently told this when growing up by the person who was abusive. My voices always use the expression 'I am right, you know I am right'. Sometimes I end up thinking they *are* right and other times I think 'No they're not right' and I will be quite adamant about it.

In the past, when I heard my voices all time, I was almost completely controlled by them. Sometimes they would say: 'If you don't do this something really nasty will happen to you.' My voices used to make me act impulsively, bordering on the uncontrollable. They prevented me doing the most basic everyday things, such as having a bath; they controlled what clothes I wore and whether I brushed my teeth or not. I now have more control over the impulsiveness and I can reassure myself that I am a worthwhile person. My voices can still control whether or not I can do everyday activities, which at times is very frustrating.

Looking back, my voices rendered me virtually powerless to control what I did as a response to them. I learned to control them better because I wanted my life back and I know now that I can influence them by the coping techniques I now use. My explanation for my voices is that they are due to traumatic life events. I have accepted this and use it to explain the way the pattern of my voices works. People involved with me both professionally and personally also accept this explanation. The coping strategies I use when most bothered by my voices are: listening to music, being with my animals, sports, talking to people, taking care of myself, counting things down.

In the past I have been violent to other people due to what my voices have insisted I do; I have attempted to take my own life and have self-harmed. I was totally consumed by my voices; I felt I had to get on with them and do as they said because I was afraid of them. They rendered me virtually powerless, so I did as I was told. I believe that I have a different relationship with them now; I can control my feelings about what they say to me, I no longer act on impulse and I accept responsibility.

PART 2

I was introduced to the accepting voices approach by my psychiatrist while I was an inpatient in hospital. The first person who really talked about my voices with me was the psychiatric doctor; my reaction was 'God somebody is actually bothering to talk to me about my voices.' I worked with the doctor with the information he had introduced me to and together we did the Maastricht Interview. Meeting with the doctor was, and still is, a positive experience. He gave me the opportunity to talk about my voice-hearing experiences and, perhaps just as importantly, I was treated as an equal. I also met another service user who accepted voices, and speaking together was a very uplifting experience … at last I was not alone; this person showed me that you can use your voice-hearing experiences positively. She is another person who has always helped me, and she has done so in many ways. She has shown me what true friendship is all about and has never treated me as a second-class citizen.

I have now got my life worked out in perspective and can do many more things. I can concentrate on other things in my life, like relationships and am able to live independently, virtually medication free. I can read again, go swimming and perform some sort of normal role in society, and I can communicate my thoughts and feelings a lot better.

PART 3

My life now is more stable, and all the people who are of concern to me think so too. I still hear my voices but I have a lot more control over them, instead of them over me. I have various ways of coping: sometimes I talk about them; I write about them or I do things to distract them, such as listening to music, reading and sports. Sometimes I have bad days and my voices can be troublesome. This I have accepted. I found that once I had accepted my voices I could also manage them better. I have a fairly good quality of life. I live in this house with my best friend and soulmate, three cats and two dogs – at times the only things that keep me going. Finances … well I'd like more money I suppose … but I just think, 'People are worse off than me.' I plan to return to writing. I am a strong-minded, independent woman who now accepts help and support when needed.

JOHN EXELL

PART 1

My name is John Exell. I was born in mid-February 1949, am male and single. I have an honours degree and a postgraduate diploma, both in architecture. I studied for these after my hospitalisation (twice) with schizophrenia. I worked in architecture for a while but have now taken early retirement. My main activities and hobbies are the service user/survivor movement, writing, poetry, sculpture, crafts, art, reading, meditation and an increasing interest in exercise. I am a member of Mensa.

Most of my voices come from outside. I hear them with my mind. They seem to come from other people – friends, family, acquaintances, strangers, near or far. It is as if I am in ESP communication with them. They seem to know all about me. This was what I thought was happening. But I have recently realised that I create my voices; that they come from my mind, my unconscious, as dreams do. I started hearing voices at the age of 19, at university, when my schizophrenia started. They have been with me ever since, in varying frequency. Since realising that I create them, they have more or less stopped, except when I am stressed, and have become much easier to deal with.

As I said, my voices seem to come from others. They bear the characteristics of the person I believe they are coming from so they are extremely various; they can seem to come from anyone with all their characteristics. The voices can be very critical, telling me what to do, etc; these seem to come from authority figures in my life. I believe these are an outcome of my low self-esteem. Some voices can be very loving and seductive; these seem to come from young, attractive females in my life. I think these voices are just wishful thinking on my part.

I was 19 years of age, nearly 20, when it started. I was at university. This was in January 1969. It was during a student strike that I took part in. There were a lot of other things going on for me too; it was a very stressful time. That Christmas I had taken my second acid trip, which went disastrously wrong. The day before I first heard voices I had spent a very strange day. I woke up wanting to think about it all, which I started to do, then something prompted me to go into the university main square (I lived on campus). I went there, completely untogether, and another student simply laughed at me. This must have been the last straw. I had something like a panic attack, and the voices started. They seemed to come from the student who laughed at me. It was all very confusing and extremely stressful. This, no doubt, brought on my schizophrenia. I went to see some friends but couldn't talk to them. They tried to help me. I then went to my room, on my own, and quietly went crazy, hearing more voices which seemed to come from another student. I stayed in my room for a while, acting even crazier; then wandered around the university, hardly talking to anyone. I believe I stayed there for a couple of weeks, I don't remember going to lectures – I don't remember, I don't know if the strike finished while I was there, I was completely out of it. I wasn't aware that I was ill, I thought it was all natural, hearing voices, etc. I just accepted them as part of reality. After a while I left, and things began to get a bit better.

I completely dropped out; wandered around; lived in various flats with various friends, many new found ones; read a lot of strange books, listened to music; took more drugs, LSD and cannabis, to escape from what had happened at university; had many strange experiences, including voices and visual 'hallucinations'. I didn't talk much at all. I did take up a bit of art, which was good. I got into a real fantasy world, didn't really relate to others, but was a lot happier than being at university. No one realised anything was wrong. I think I must have been very annoying.

I ran out of money and returned home to my parents thinking everything would be fine, but it wasn't. I had an argument with my mother about my lifestyle; she didn't realise that I was 'ill' at the time. I had another 'panic attack', went crazy again, had a very strange 'reincarnation experience', was 'visited by a spirit' who spoke to me, and I ended up believing that I was Jesus Christ. I ended up seeing a psychiatrist and was asked to go into hospital, which I did. This was about August 1970. I was put on antipsychotics and given ECT, and came out after about two months, returning home, where everyone, especially my mother, was extremely nice to me. As far as I can remember, the voices had stopped for the time being, but I was heavily doped-up with medication, with all its negative side effects. I was depressed when I came out of hospital – I had been a lot happier, though a bit crazy, before I went in. Looking back on all this, I can truthfully say that something was wrong with me, that I was 'ill' and a bit stupid, or rather, extremely uninformed.

Before the student laughed at me, I had heard no voices. As a child, I had on several occasions seen white light coming from my mother. At the time I thought that this wasn't unusual; it didn't in any way disturb me. In fact I really enjoyed it and told no one. At the age of 6, I had an extremely traumatic and devastating experience which deeply affected me. Before that, I had had an extremely happy childhood.

As I said, the voices vary. If I am feeling guilty about something, I may hear accusing voices. If I have low self-esteem, I may hear critical voices. If I am feeling good, I may hear nice voices. They go with my mood. If I feel good, they can make me feel even better, if I feel bad, they can make me feel even worse. Their frequency is in direct relationship to the amount I am stressed: they are at their peak the more stressed I feel, so they increase the stress. So, to break the cycle, I simply stop what I'm doing, drop everything, go to bed and take a nap. Depending on the amount of stress, the nap may last for days. Luckily, I am in a position to do this. An orthodox job would be the death of me.

The first voice I heard seemed to come from the student who laughed at me, seemed to be the student telling me what to do. Looking back at this, if I separate all the elements and just see that it was myself or my subconscious 'ordering me about' and exploring what it said, it does seem that it was my 'subconscious' giving me some very good advice – and it now all makes perfect sense. The voices I heard in my room shortly afterwards, seeming to come from another student (who was important at the university) could, in fact, be interpreted as my unconscious telling me what he was really like. This all makes perfect sense now as well.

Looking back at all the voices I have heard – the ones I can remember – some definitely had something to say to me. But this does not appear to be true for all of them. At the time I heard them, some were deeply disturbing, some I believed in, some seemed nonsense. Now, having realised that they come from me, from my unconscious, I am beginning to make more sense of them. Sometimes it is more fruitful for me to just ignore them, which I do sometimes. When I am stressed, I sometimes get caught up with them without realising it.

In the past, I have told some voices to go and they went. Once, when trying to make a difficult decision, I conjured up some voices to ask their advice. I was very calm and relaxed at the time. But most of the time I have had no control over them – but then I didn't try to control them. Now, when I remember to simply ignore them if they are a bother, they simply stop.

I used to think that I was hearing people's ESP messages to me. I have now realised that I create the voices; that they come from my unconscious, my subconscious, or some, even from my intuition. Further analysis showed me that the voices were what I thought the person involved would say if I talked to them, they were my idea of what that person was thinking. So my voices could be used as an insight into someone's character. Most people, especially mental health professionals, agree that I create my voices. Realising that I create my voices was a major breakthrough – it was extremely liberating, it was a 'eureka' moment. I still agree with this, that I create my voices. I feel that they are similar to dreams, dreams we have while awake. Some dreams are really profound, while some are garbage, and many are in between.

At the onset of my schizophrenia and before hospitalisation, before I was aware that I could be 'ill', I accepted the voices and believed in them. Luckily, they did not tell me to do anything really bad. If they had, maybe I would have stopped believing in them … I don't know … but they did say some very stupid things. After hospitalisation, after I realised something could be wrong, sometimes I talked to the voices, sometimes I ignored them, sometimes I told them to go, and sometimes I thought that they might be trying to tell me something.

When I am stressed or 'ill', I tend to believe in the voices, they tend to overwhelm me and take me over, I tend to obey them. However, as I said previously, they have not, as yet, asked me to do anything really bad, and if they did, I may have stopped believing in them. Since realising that I create the voices (this was just over a year ago), I have not been seriously ill with schizophrenia. Maybe I never will be again. So I don't know how I would react. I sincerely hope that I will remember that I create them myself. And I sincerely hope that I don't get over-stressed like I have before.

PART 2

A Hearing Voices group started at my local Mind, which I attended. It was run by two mental health professionals. It was extremely liberating being able to talk about my voices openly and freely. I had never done this before. Before this, the very mention by me that I was hearing voices, even to 'warm and understanding' counsellors, bought on the reaction: 'I think you had better see your psychiatrist.' And if I told my psychiatrist that I was hearing voices, he would simply up my medication with its awful side effects. So I had learned to keep extremely quiet about my voices.

One reaction to the Voices group was for me to think very deeply about what my voices were. Talking to other voices hearers, swapping stories and experiences was highly stimulating and positive. The idea that voices were our own creation was talked about. I couldn't accept this at the time. I still thought that I was getting ESP messages from other people, which is what it seemed to be. The group folded after a while, but it left a very positive mark on me. There is an attempt at present (which I am involved in) to resurrect it. The group also left its positive mark on the rest of the local mental health professionals. I was able to mention the fact that I heard voices to others without fear of being whisked off to see the psychiatrist. And when I did see the psychiatrist, I was able to talk more freely about my voices, and my medication was not upped. However, I was still not able to talk as freely as I had done at the group. Other things at the group were discussed to do with schizophrenia and our experiences which I also found extremely liberating.

Some time after the group had folded, I wrote a letter to the wisest person I know about my voices (particularly as I thought that some came from him). He replied that there is nothing wrong with hearing voices but that they are very unreliable and that the best way to deal with them is to ignore them. I took his advice and the voices disappeared. But I missed the nice ones, and the nice ones came back.

About a year ago, I was alone in my flat, listening and talking to a nice voice, which I thought was coming from a woman friend of mine, when I had the profound realisation that I was creating her voice, just as I was creating my reply. This was extremely liberating and a major breakthrough. Thinking about this, I decided that the voices came from my subconscious or unconscious, that they were similar to daydreams, but, as they all seemed to be nonsense, I simply ignored them and this worked very well – besides I had the rest of my life to live.

I must add that, shortly before realising that I created my voices, I became a client of the Institute of Optimum Nutrition. I saw a nutritionist there, Lorraine Perretta. I place her second to God and my mother in helping me with my schizophrenia. Needless to say, psychiatrists and doctors are way down the list.

PART 3

Then I was asked to write this story. Writing in detail about what happened when I was 19; I looked at this and the voices extremely closely, and realised that some of my voices had something very important to say to me. I now see some of the voices as a positive asset and something beneficial – but all this is very new to me, and my attitude may change over the coming weeks.

Inside us is heaven and hell and all the regions in between. The voices come from inside us, from any region. It can be extremely difficult to tell which region the voice comes from. So maybe, to be on the safe side, it is better to completely ignore all voices, I don't really know. At least, don't take them too seriously.

But I must repeat that it was through relating to a nice voice that I realised that I created my voices and was enabled to write all this. I think that the individual voice hearer must weigh up all the evidence for themselves and act accordingly with their voices: ignore them, relate to them, even enjoy them, or whatever.

At present, the voices are no longer external, they are in my head. They are extremely nice. They say things like, 'Don't you think you ought to tidy your flat' (and my flat is very untidy) and 'Time you had something to eat, John' (I've forgotten to eat all day as I've been totally absorbed writing this story). So, really, that's all I can say at present – besides, I'm hungry, and I want to tidy up my flat.

JOHN ROBINSON

INTERVIEW WITH JACQUI DILLON

John Robinson is a 57-year-old man. He runs the Deptford Hearing Voices service in south London. Apart from being very committed to his work and his own personal development he also enjoys Five Rhythms dance and attends a drama class to be 'like a child with other children'.

I've always experienced voices in my head, although it was only after I had started the Deptford Hearing Voices service that I realised I was hearing voices. It was only after reading and reading and talking to client after client that I came to realise that I'd been hearing my voices for a very, very long time, since I was a child. I've always experienced them in my head.

There are a group of them almost speaking like the same voice. Sometimes there's more of a single voice and sometimes there is what I call the God voice. It is a really, really wise voice that hardly ever comes. The most consistent thing that the voices have done is big me up a bit.

So there is 'God', and this babble of voices who often say positive things but who sometimes send me down paths that are questionable, perhaps because they are mischievous or maybe naïve, like a child. At those times I've had to really keep my feet on the ground. As my life got better those voices have faded away because I think I have less need for them. One particularly nasty voice that came for a very short time, a very loud threatening scary voice came in the past five years. I had a very strong feeling that I had to destroy this voice very quickly. So what I visualised was that the voice, the entity was dissolving into bubbles so that it was literally fragmenting before my very eyes. I was deconstructing it, diffusing it, breaking it up and sending it into the ether. It came back a couple of times and I forced myself, really forced myself to keep on visualising it and it hasn't returned. It was a really frightening experience but I just sensed this threat and had to destroy it because I didn't want it to become part of my internal world.

There also used to be this destiny feeling where all this stuff that I'd gone through was preparation for a greater future, a greater destiny, I was going to be the ambassador general of the UN! The voices were very encouraging, they thought very highly of me. I know now that those thoughts would be considered grandiose but I know that it was my sustaining delusion. It taught me how good delusions can be and how powerful. That was the one delusion that kept me feeling OK despite some of the rubbish that I went through in my life.

I can't separate how I am feeling and how I work from my past, so I need to say something about this. Describing my past often leaves many unanswered questions of why?

I was born of mixed parents in 1950. My mother born half Malay, half Chinese; an illegitimate child, brought up an orphan in a convent. Her education was basic and left her somewhat unskilled and unprepared for the world with little sense of who she was; my father, who was the first man she'd met, was English, born in Malaya (now Malaysia) and a merchant seaman captain of a small ship, perhaps the size of a coaster or ocean going sea trawler. As a seaman he spent most time absent at sea. Their marriage, in 1948, did not last more than 2 years, breaking under the strains of first an unwanted birth and then from the strains of coping with the unremitting demands of a child, and went together with living in cramped conditions. Severe family and cultural prejudices over mixed-race marriages present in those colonial times created additional strains, as did my father's inevitably long absences at sea.

My background was made up of a lot of extreme isolation. I used to be locked up in a room for quite long periods of time, sometimes without food, perhaps overnight for one day, two days. There was lots of gratuitous and vicarious cruelty because my parents were poorly resourced. There was a sense of constant threat. I never seemed to get it right, I never seemed to understand. What I didn't realise is that I was never going to get it right because my parents didn't want me. It was only a few years ago my mum told me that they tried to abort me.

At no time in the first twenty-nine years of my life was there a permanent abode called home. In my first years of life I was in turn brought up in a series of cheap mouse-ridden hotels in colonial Singapore (my mother's description), then brought into the care of Iban Dyaks in Sarawak (Borneo) for 18 months after an incident in which my father, in one his many drunken rages, threw me out of a first-floor window. After that I then found myself living and sleeping with many adult crewmen in my father's tramp steamer for three years before being placed at 7 years old in boarding school in Singapore. At boarding school I was assaulted by many older boys, then by the school caretaker's son and finally a teacher; actions that caused me to attempt my first unsuccessful suicide (out of three) before finally running away to live with various gangs in Singapore. During my two years with the gangs I was an accomplice in many criminal activities, experienced violence and witnessed violence and sometimes death visited upon others.

At around 9 years of age I started working as a child labourer in a chicken farm in South Western Australia until just after 12 years old. After that I was returned to Singapore more or less unschooled where I started to make a vicarious living from working in the markets. At 12½ I then found myself in an orphanage in Hull before being sent to foster parents, paid to look after me at age 14. After living two and half years with them I then, with their encouragement, enlisted in the Army as a junior soldier at 15½, where I stayed until taking my own discharge at age 29 to go to Sussex University.

After Sussex University I stayed in a rented house in Brighton, becoming in turn a clinical nurse teacher, a qualified nurse tutor, an insurance salesman, before moving into general management in the NHS for four years. I left management to become a psychiatric nurse and later a community psychiatric nurse. I would say the beginnings of self-reflection started in dribs and drabs when I was at University but only started to gather pace several years after I started my psychiatric nurse training (age 40) under the old system of nurse education.

Many years later when I was asked by a psychiatric nurse tutor why I had applied for the registered mental nurse course, my answer was that I wanted to learn about myself as well as learn about people. And in this respect working in mental health has indeed helped me learn a great deal about myself and people, a process that continues to this day. The learning is always reciprocal between me and the clients I work with and something I am always happy to acknowledge.

I started up my Deptford Hearing Voices service in April 1996, on All Fools' day. When I started this service I knew nothing. I was the average staff nurse. The prevailing wisdom at that time was that you didn't encourage people to talk about their voices because you were encouraging them in their delusions and you got them to do distracting activity instead. My immediate way of doing the research was to get in touch with the Hearing Voices Network and they gave me a list of existing projects around the country, so I started to make a lot of telephone calls. The service has been running for eleven years now.

It was rather late in my life that I came to realise that my personal experience, the kind of stuff I had in my head, was voices because I'd never had a dialogue with anyone about it. It was only after reading and reading and talking to client after client that I came to realise that I'd been hearing my voices for a very, very long time, since I was a child. For a lot of people when they first get their experiences, it's for the first time so it makes it more shocking, but of course I never had that.

A lot of my life has been about a search for meaning and trying to make sense of myself and my existence. I've never talked to anyone about my voices. I've had counselling and psychoanalysis but that's more been about the things that have happened in my life. This is still work in progress. I am now seeing a therapist and I will continue this work because it will make me a better person and also it will make me a better therapist for my clients. I'm still on a journey.

I never understood that I was dissociating up until very recently. I actually caught myself at it because, for the whole of my life, it has been so seamless. I'd been doing various kinds of bodywork and one night, I had been to this party and it was about midnight and I was waiting for a bus home. I was reflecting on the evening and I realised that it had been different. I felt more immediate. I didn't feel cut off. And all the way home I was thinking, 'My God this is what has been happening to you all of this time.' The spacing out, feeling far away from things, far away from people, feeling disembodied.

I don't think it's any surprise that I'm doing the work that I am doing. A client said to me recently that I am very creative and that I make really good use of metaphors and analogies. She said that you are also good at making sense out of nonsense and I thought, 'Yeah! I do think it's about making sense and trying to have a dialogue that helps people to find coherence.' As my life got better those voices have faded away because I think I have less need for them. Now that I have something valuable in my life they have faded away. A sense of a self has only begun to emerge in the past five or so years. Before that I was just fragments. Life has never been better than now. Today is the best day.

JOHNNY SPARVANG

INTERVIEW WITH TREVOR EYLES

I am 39 years old and live in Aarhus, Denmark. I am a single male and I live alone in my own apartment. I have a state school education and I am now in part-time employment. My main interest is chess – I am an active team player – and sport in general.

I have always heard voices inside my head. Initially I thought they were the voices of other people but then considered them as a part of myself, although I didn't understand why. Since the onset, I have heard the same two voices – one male and one female. They are both about 40 years old and have always been that age. They have also both been extremely negative from the outset; commanding, threatening and bullying.

I first heard the voices at the age of 15, during the school summer holidays. Both voices were negative. During that time, and leading up to it, I had been extensively bullied at school due to dyslexia and a slight speech impediment. My childhood and family life with my parents and younger sister was happy and secure, but the bullying seemed to be carried on by the voices, although I didn't connect the two things at the time.

The typical themes for the voices are that I am stupid, ugly and worthless. I have always felt very hurt and saddened by the things the voices have said, but actually began to believe them more and more as time went by. I was also frightened of the voices because they encouraged me to commit suicide, and at the same time I was scared of the reactions of other people, so I didn't tell anyone about them. Not even my family.

I felt I had no control over the voices whatsoever. I just tried to tell them to go away and used all of my strength to resist them. They ignored me and intensified their efforts. In the beginning, I thought that I was mentally ill because the voices were in my head. I later learned that there was another explanation connected with my life experiences.

To begin with, and because I felt isolated with the voices, I began to drink alcohol quite heavily. This was quite a normal development amongst my peers at the time, anyway. For me it quickly became a habit and I found that if I became drunk enough, then I had a little respite from the voices. Over the next few years I became an alcoholic and was finally drinking 50 to 60 alcoholic beverages each day. Eventually, my parents insisted that I get help and I went into a treatment program in my early twenties. Still nobody knew about the voices. Having been cured of the alcohol problem and back in society, I was suddenly faced with the fact that I still had the voices and no way to cope with them.

I was eventually admitted to the local psychiatric hospital, but still told no one of the voices. I was diagnosed and treated for depression in the first instance. During the third or fourth admission I finally told a student nurse that I heard voices. The relief was immense – I felt that I had been released from a huge burden.

However, my diagnosis was quickly altered to that of schizophrenia and I was heavily medicated. The dosage was increased over a period of time because each time I was asked if I still heard voices, I said, 'Yes.' During the next ten years I became more and more socially isolated. I managed to continue living alone but with massive support from the social psychiatric home help. Inhibited by the voices and dulled by the medication, I slept sixteen to eighteen hours a day and ordered junk food so that I wouldn't have to go out or cook for myself. My only outside interest was chess, which I continued to pursue but found difficult due to interference by the voices.

RECOVERY

Finally, in 2003, one of my support workers, Trevor Eyles, told me of a conference he had attended. Marius Romme, Sandra Escher and Ron Coleman had spoken of a new approach to hearing voices. We were both excited about the ideas and were keen to start a group. Imagine my amazement when I was told that some people actually heard friendly voices. It became my dream to have a positive voice, at least just occasionally.

Over the following months I continued to ask Trevor when we could start the group, but he was always extremely busy with his work. Eventually I think he was tired of listening to me plaguing him, so he managed to find a couple of hours a week in the evening where we could meet. The group comprised three voice hearers to begin with, and one of Trevor's colleagues, Pia Annat. This quickly developed to a larger group and soon other small groups were formed in the area. As the word spread, more and more people became interested.

The importance of joining a group and speaking with other voice hearers cannot be emphasised enough. After the first meeting I felt almost elated at having spoken openly about the voices to people whom I'd not met before.

I was now extremely motivated to work with Trevor and explore the voices, although still very disturbed by them. We decided to complete the Maastricht Interview and go to the Netherlands together and partake in a voice-dialogue course in Maastricht. Marius, Sandra and Dirk Corstens worked with groups from Denmark and Sweden. I recall it as the toughest few days of my life. This was also a turning point for me as I began to relate my past life experiences to the voices and could see how they had affected me. On the way home to Denmark, Trevor encouraged me to make a deal with the voices for the first time, that I would talk to them when we got home if they left me in peace to sleep throughout the night. To my amazement it worked! This too was a turning point for me as I realised I had some form of control over the voices. It became a strategy that I used on a daily basis.

Talking to the voices and questioning what they said also gave me further empowerment. In the group one evening I was disturbed by the voices and Trevor asked if they wanted to say something. They said that he (Trevor) was a liar and a cheat and I shouldn't believe him. Later that night the voices began to argue violently in my head. I called Trevor and, luckily, he answered the phone. He asked what the voices were arguing about and I told him that the male voice still said he was a liar and a cheat, but the female voice now thought differently. Trevor encouraged me to gradually build an alliance with the female voice and together we changed the male voice.

Over the next year the voices both diminished, became less intrusive, and finally on 13 December 2005 they stopped altogether. During this period I had begun to join Trevor, lecturing about voice hearing. I started very nervously with a five to ten minute account of my life as a voice hearer. Afterwards the female voice complimented me and said I had done really well. I finally had the friendly voice that I had dreamed of in the beginning! I have heard her nine times since December 2005 and always after lecturing. Today I can talk for one and a half hours!

Following the trip to Maastricht early in 2004, I slowly began to reduce the medication. At that time I was taking 26 tablets a day, a cocktail of various medicines whose only real effect had been to dope me up and make me gain weight. They never had an effect on the voices.

Today I am pleased to say that I no longer take any medication (apart from an occasional sleeping tablet). I have a part-time job, minimal home support, which will soon cease altogether, and am presently zooming up the national chess ratings. I have a hectic social life, have great contact with my family and relatives again, and am always busy helping other voice hearers. In Aarhus, I am part of a small group of voice hearers that have started a local network in an office with a telephone help line. Later this year I plan to start a course in social psychiatry as a worker with user experience.

JOLANDA VAN HOEIJ

WITH SANDRA ESCHER

According to me my voices are part of me, but I mostly experience them as coming from someone else as I hear them. I realise they are part of me, but this has not always been so. My ideas have changed over the past few years – following my first training on voice hearing with the Maastricht Interview, together with the approach 'talking to voices'. I became curious about them. I started talking about them with my psychiatrist and she explained them to me. When I began to hear voices I did not give much thought to the 'why' and 'how'.

I hear three voices and they all have names: Hannah, Eva and Nina. I hear them through my ears. All three are female. Nina is about 7 years of age. She is still a child. I think Eva is 18 or 20 years old, and Hannah stays about the same age as me. I have never experienced voices giving me a compliment.

Nina cries a lot but is also immediately present when other people, or I myself, want to have bodily contact. At that moment Nina sets the rules. She does not get angry but she takes control over me and behaves like a 7-year-old child. I might even say things that come from Nina. If something happens that I do not want, I hear Nina crying. It might also be that Nina starts singing, as she did during the abuse. Nina originates from a long time ago and she is connected to the sexual abuse. Nina is always there, but I do not want to talk about it now.

Eva is a voice that always has comments. Sometimes she talks about what other people do, but mostly about me. Eva cannot talk decently. She uses vulgar language. Eva also thinks that I have to harm myself. She thinks I shouldn't exist. Eva came when I was 18 and my family withdrew the formal complaint to the police about the person who had sexually abused me. Actually, with her scolding and cursing – something I started to do as well – Eva has done me a favour by making me more defended from others. Eva wanted me to act sturdier. That wasn't such a bad idea, for managing to live at that moment it was the best attitude.

Hannah is the voice that got older with time. She was always there. I was a bit of a loner and Hannah was my mate. I can remember, when I worked in childcare, a little boy in that group told me that he had an imaginary friend. That is about how Hannah is. She was just there, and maybe that also had its advantages. I was a lonely child. I went to school, I had my friends at school, but I never took them home. I did not feel in need of them. I wasn't pestered as a child. Nearly every day I spent with my uncle and Aunt Hanny who lived opposite our house. At that time my mother worked. That is normal now, then it wasn't. My father worked as well. So, after school, I was at my aunt and uncle's house. I went with them on their holidays and I stayed with them every Saturday. Eventually, I spent more time with my Aunt Hanny than at home. However my uncle could not keep his hands off me – that is why Nina came.

The voices have had influences in many ways on a lot of things: they took over things I had trouble with, like Nina taking over my intimacy, Eva my defensibility, and Hannah putting my thoughts into order. Hannah is very practical, in a matter-of-fact way, and has a good overview. Eva's scolding was not only meant for me but also aimed at others. She gave me instructions. Others became afraid of me. I am not proud of it now but, then, I was proud. Later I became afraid of that voice as it had so much influence on me. At that time I became more and more stressed, my eating habits changed and my self-harm extended. At a certain moment I became very depressed.

I was 25 years old. I realised that I could no longer live on my own. It began as a slow process but, after I was admitted to Assen (psychiatric hospital) it all speeded up. Eva, especially, changed a lot. She first killed other people with her language and later shifted to me. I really felt sorry to be in Assen. I felt I'd been handed over to psychiatry. I didn't have any other possibilities any more. There was nothing else I could do and I felt I could not survive it. In a way it was my own choice to go to Assen – but one's choices are so limited; if you look for help, hearing voices gets interwoven with the assumption that 'only schizophrenics hear voices' and you become a 'mad person'. My treatment consisted of medication and trying to find the correct dose. In the end, I went to live with my parents again. Later on I began living on my own and I found a job – that was quite nice.

RECOVERY

I discovered the relationship between my voices and my traumatic experiences (sexual abuse) when I lived in Apeldoorn. The voices were hindering me a lot. Things were not going well for me. In the end I got therapy from a female psychiatrist (Iwona) and, after three months, I was admitted to hospital again. There, the voices caused a lot of trouble and, one way or another, the psychiatrist saw this. When she asked: 'Do you hear voices?' I thought, 'It's now or never.' Then she said, 'It doesn't matter.' I can remember that when she said this, it was so completely new to me that, in my confused state, I didn't know how to deal with it. She (Iwona) talked about it so lightly and as if something could be done about it. I had never thought this myself. What Iwona said gave a turning point to my thoughts about my experiences.

For a very long time I'd felt very powerless, as I didn't think I could do something about it myself. But when I followed your [to Sandra] training I realised that I could have my own say in things as well. I will give an example. During my pregnancy, Eva started to say I was going to be a bad mother, but when she said: 'It must be a very bad child that you are going to have', I became so angry that I told her off. After my anger at Eva, the voices have never said anything negative about my son. This event showed me that, when I am really convinced I am able to have my way. But to do it I have to be sure of it myself.

I think I have created the voices myself as I needed them badly in order not to become stressed out. Don't ask me how I did it. I think it was my survival strategy. This explanation is very important for me. My psychiatrist, who helped me enormously, has accepted my explanation – none of the other therapists did. Out of the twelve therapists I have seen, only one has accepted my explanation.

I never talk about my experiences with my parents. They don't want to know about them. They know I hear voices and have found it reassuring that I got medication, but how I came to hear voices they do not want to discuss. Even my mother does not want to do this, even though she is very supportive. If I need something practical she is there. She is there for my child, too, but she says: 'I can't help you with those other things.' My father does not have a clue about what happened to me. He blocks it from his mind. According to him, my illness is now cured.

How did your psychiatrist help you?
I have been quite often in psychiatric care and no one talked about my voices. My psychiatrist, Iwona, is the only one. That was eight years ago. She is worth her weight in gold. The difference between Iwona and the others is that she makes me feel equal. She stands beside me, and together we look at what can be done differently. If I said, 'I don't want medication', that was clear to her. We didn't have to debate about it; together we looked for other possibilities, other solutions.

I will give an example. I worked for Pandora, a Dutch organisation that offers mental health education to users and professionals. There, I saw a small advertisement about your [to Sandra] training, I showed it to Iwona and she agreed with it and told me to find out the details – she just came along. The training was on my own initiative. What Iwona does is listen to my reasoning – something others had not done before. She really was interested in what I wanted to do. That was quite a relief as I was a bit afraid of my future. Iwona taught me that my voices came because there was a reason. Then I saw a future. If you know it has to do with behaviour and not with an illness, it makes it much more open to discussion. For example, medication might help for a few hours, it might help me to sleep, but it does not help in the long run. My experiences must be taken seriously and in my case this meant talking about my voices and to my voices in order to learn to understand them – understanding that they have everything to do with what happened to me.

It was Iwona who related my voices with the sexual abuse. My other therapists had never done that. They said, for example, that I had a slight psychotic disability and I was vulnerable to psychosis. Because of my contacts with Iwona I realised I was not ill. That was an eye-opener. I reasoned that, if I am not ill, I must be able to do something about it. If it isn't in my genes, if I wasn't born with it, then there must be other ways.

Iwona also taught me to cope with my voices in a different way. She taught me to invite my voices for a meeting. Then I needed her help to learn how to chair the meeting. Look, if I chaired the meeting on my own I couldn't handle it because either Eva or Nina were too strong or too rude and then I didn't know what to do. Iwona was the one who made it clear to me why this was happening, or she could make it more relative so I could get a clearer idea about what was said by the voices.

Another example. I knew I really wanted to have a baby, so I had to reduce my medication as much as possible. When the voices were hindering and I knew the origin, I thought there must be other ways to deal with them than medication. If you try to get relief from pain by medication, it doesn't mean the cause has disappeared.

Can you mention other people who have helped you?
Yes, Heeltje was a big help, but she is not a therapist. I met Heeltje when I was 20 years old and living in Hoogezand. She had a kind of foster family. She was a kind a foster mother. She was always there. She was my home. I always went there during the weekends, even when I was admitted to the psychiatric hospital. To her, it did not matter what I had done, I was always welcome. She even accepted that I harmed myself. I think if it had not been for Heeltje I would have ended up living on the streets.

Have you learned to cope differently with your emotions?
Yes, I now dare to think more positively about myself. I dare to allow my anger about what has happened in the past, but I can also handle it differently. I might drown myself in it but I might also put it aside. I can now control

when I want to keep certain activity out of my consciousness. I know I can choose; in the past it happened automatically and that wasn't too practical.

Have you regained personal power?
Yes, I have learned that I am my own boss and that I have grown up. I now have to take responsibility for myself again.

Have your ideas about your future changed?
Education didn't change anything. I noticed that an education cost me more energy than the other people in that education. Because of the voices I took more time to do things. By the time of the final examinations I had used all my energy. I was finished. What has given me my future is my son. I am so proud that I have such a lovely time with him and that I can take good care of myself. I make choices now. My son is the most important one, therefore I have to take care that I stay in a rhythm because then I can handle it. The other thing that has been part of my recovery was that I feel that my abuse is recognised, that my honour is restored. That has helped me to become the person I am today.

KARINA CARLYN

I am Karina Carolyn. I am 37 years old, female, single and a graduate of Latin American Studies. I do voluntary work for the mental health charity Mind and the Hearing Voices Network. My hobbies include creative writing, arts and crafts.

I don't hear voices now but I did up till a year ago. I heard voices for more than ten years without taking medication. Now I take medication that suits me, at a low dose, and I hardly hear voices at all now.

Experience
When I used to hear voices, they appeared to be coming from outside of me, through my ears. I knew that they were part of my subconscious, when I could rationalise it, but whilst I was actually hearing them, they seemed very real. I couldn't always tell whether they were real or not. They were always in the third person, talking and discussing me, in groups and in choruses.

Characteristics
I heard many different voices. The strongest and most negative came from the people I used to go to school with. These were a mixed group. I was bullied at school and a lot of the content came from this time, like I was carrying past voices around with me in the present. These voices were full of hate and disgust, teasing, mocking and belittling. The second group of voices were of the students from the university I went to in Portsmouth. These were pretty negative too. The next group of voices I heard were from my surroundings, my neighbours. These were mixed, negative and sometimes positive, but mostly commenting on what I did. The worst of my neighbours were two teenagers who lived behind us. I find teenagers quite difficult, probably because I was bullied so much at school, especially by a group of boys.

A couple of the positive voices I heard were from a male Indian psychologist and a male Indian doctor who lived in our street. There was another Indian doctor who I only heard negative voices from; his voice was full of hatred and disgust. The last was my next-door neighbour's (Jackie, a woman), which was a mixture of scorn and pity for me.

History

I was 26 when I first started hearing voices. I was in Mexico in the bathroom of the house I was sharing with three other students and they were talking behind my back, or so I thought. At first I thought that I was hearing things, then I thought people were really out to get me, and then I thought my ears needed syringing. I stopped trusting people because they seemed to be constantly undermining me and slagging me off. After I came back from Latin America, I became more withdrawn, more reclusive, frightened and paranoid.

Triggers

The most important triggers were going into crowded places such as restaurants, pubs, busy streets or on buses. The voices were constantly there but were worse when I went out. They would sometimes become overwhelming. I would hear them in my house, but they weren't as bad or bothersome or uncontrollable as when I was out. I found going out difficult, so I spent a lot of time at home.

Content

The voices would say things like, 'She's a nutter', or a 'loony', or 'she's disgusting' and 'she failed her A-levels'. They said worse things but I don't like to say them.

Influence

The voices made me afraid and fearful, they had the ability to strip me of my dignity and self-respect. I would react to my voices by trying to ignore them, like when I was being bullied, I would try to ignore the bullies. I was never sure if they were real when they were happening, so I didn't want to make a scene or appear mad. In the early days of hearing voices, when I didn't know I *was* hearing voices, I was on a train in Turkey, hearing voices all night, making me feel disgusting, hellish and totally distraught. The next morning I shouted at a train full of people because I had had enough. I really believed that the people on that train had been horrendous to me all night, even though the majority of them were Turkish, they sounded English to me – what anxiety can do to a person.

Control

I didn't really have much control over the voices. I couldn't make them go away when I was out. When I was at home I only had to put the radio on, or music, or the television, to get rid of them. When I was out they would have a go at me.

Explanation

My explanation for my voices is simple – the voices were me. Although they didn't have my voice, they were my thoughts and my life experiences, and part of my subconscious. Because of my negative past experiences and the trauma I have suffered in the past, my voices were negative. Because of what I have been through, they are like a tape recording of what people have said to me in the past. Other people have accepted this explanation as it is a common psychological model.

Coping

The coping strategies I used to cope with the voices were distractions. As I have mentioned earlier, I would play music at home or on my Walkman, turn the radio on, watch TV or read. I used aromatic oils – as I learned that the more stressed I was, the worse the voices would be – so I used relaxation techniques such as self-massage. I also took lots of baths in essential oils. And I would only go out with someone accompanying me because it helped not being alone when I heard the worst voices. Towards the end of hearing the voices, I did learn to go out a little by myself and not take a taxi everywhere.

RECOVERY

I came into contact with the accepting voices approach in the early 90s when I joined the Hearing Voices Network and it was in its infancy. I started to read all the literature by Romme and Escher, Paul Baker and Nigel Rose, etc. I used to go to the group in Manchester every month – it was my only lifeline to sanity then. I talked to the group (Helen Heap was running it and Terence McLaughlin was attending then). I used to share my voice-hearing experience with the group and it felt great to be able to talk about it to people who understood what I was going through, and even to have a laugh about the strange things voices sometimes said.

I also went to a psychotherapy centre, in 1994, called the Red House. Here, I met other people in therapy and could talk at length with the therapists about the voices, and they would help me find a meaning for them. This made the voices less threatening and frightening. Sometimes I would try the techniques that the psychologists taught me: repeating things to myself more positively in order to counteract the negatives. This worked some of the time, but not always. As time progressed and I had more therapy, I was going out more, even travelling on buses by myself a little, so that I was gaining more control. My world had expanded, even though it was still difficult and could be a battle sometimes. Later, after having psychotherapy, I wasn't afraid any longer. I rarely heard voices saying they were going to murder me, like in the early days. They could still make me feel tearful and lower my self-esteem but I did have days when I could cope.

I started doing voluntary work for the Hearing Voices Network. That helped me – being at the centre of all the knowledge about hearing voices and meeting lots of people who were involved. I was editing the newsletter, which I enjoyed. I gave a few talks, which I found difficult because I am not a natural speaker – I write better than I talk. But I found that the interest that people and professionals had in my experience helped my self-esteem, so I didn't view myself as totally mad and irredeemable.

Since then, I have joined Start (an arts base for people with mental health problems in Salford) where I do creative writing and crafts. I am also a member of the Transitional Employment Project (TEP) that sends people on job placements. I have done voluntary work with TEP, Mind, the Citizens Advice Bureau and the Hearing Voices Network. I have been active over the last ten years despite hearing voices. I also have a boyfriend whom I met at the Red House and who gives me a lot of support and love.

What helped me was the support I got from the Hearing Voices Network. Support groups helped at first but, afterwards, I didn't find them as useful. I felt I had grown out of them, although I still liked to keep in touch, feeling a part of something and being accepted for who I was. I felt the support I got from the people at the Red House was invaluable. Doing voluntary work helped increase my self-esteem and gave me a focus and something to do. Being creative helped me, as it gave me a really important focus, belief in myself and an outlet for my self-expression.

There is a difference with accepting voices: it does help you cope better with life, but life is still a struggle and an everyday battle. Life is never easy and I have had to accept that, too. My life is now in a state of change but I feel more positive. Today, I hardly hear voices, so I feel freer and more able to do the things I want to. I don't have any professionals in my life anymore. I used to have a support worker, a psychologist and a psychiatrist. Now I see the psychiatrist every six months, just to see how I am doing.

LISETTE DE KLERK

WITH SANDRA ESCHER

In 1995 Lisette gave a lecture at a conference organised by Maastricht University in connection with the research project, Hearing Voices. This chapter is based on that lecture, first published in the second edition of *Stemmen Horen Accepteren* (Romme & Escher, 1999) by Tirion in Baarn. The experience described dates from a period before 1995. Sandra Escher interviewed Lisette in 1998.

I want to tell you how I learned to cope with my voice in the hope that it helps me to silence the voice and because I believe it is important to give other people courage. I have a real nasty past and an equally nasty voice. Now I have a good female partner and a 4-year-old daughter. I live in a nice house. I am standing at the beginning of a life that I choose myself now.

I was 17 years old when I started to hear the voice. At a certain moment, completely unexpectedly, I heard a remark, laughter or a single word. I actually looked back to see where it came from. Gradually, I learned that there wasn't anything there, wherever it came from. In the beginning it was only a word or a laugh and the voice said positive things. But these positive remarks only lasted for a short period, then the voice became more negative. Everything I did was criticised, everything I did was a failure, I wasn't worth anything, I was ugly, I was good for nothing. The voice forbade me to do my homework, for example. Then, afterwards, I began to be criticised in three ways: at school, by my parents and then by my voice again. I don't believe anybody saw what happened to me, but I suffered much, especially when I had lost pieces of time. For example, I could walk on the beach; I didn't know how I had arrived there, but suddenly I was sitting on the beach. I even heard the seagulls and could smell the sea. If the voice believed, it was enough. Then, I didn't know how, I came back and all at once I was in the room where I was supposed to be, for example, in the classroom. In that period I didn't understand what happened to me at all. I felt it was strange and I felt very different too.

I still lived with my mother and stepfather at that time. There was much tension, especially at home. I was wrestling with my past: the divorce of my father and mother when I was 9 and my incest history. At that time I wasn't very much conscious of the incest. I suppressed that with all my power. From 12 to 15 years of age I was sexually abused regularly and in a very extreme way by my stepfather. It always happened in the evening while my mother was away. At that time she was giving demonstrations for skincare products and was away three or four times a week. I don't want to talk about the kind of incest I experienced. When I was 15 we moved from Zeeland to Brabant and because my mother had lost her job she wasn't away as frequently as before. My stepfather didn't get the opportunity anymore and the abuse gradually stopped, but the entire incest problem didn't stop until I was 28.

I didn't speak to anybody about it until two years ago. Then I wanted help. It started when my stepfather hit a little niece at my daughter's birthday party and I suddenly remembered the incest. It seemed as if the sound of that slap awakened me (*until that moment kept out of consciousness by dissociation and voices*). I started to experience strange things like blackouts and flashbacks of the incest. I became extremely scared. I felt depressed. I didn't like anything anymore. I was scared in advance that things would go wrong. I didn't do well. I didn't dare to go to the shops or walk in the streets anymore. And I was very worried about my daughter who had just had her second birthday. At the same time I felt that I didn't want to live like that anymore.

I had never talked about my hearing voices because my voice didn't allow me to. He had scared me so much that I really hadn't dared. He had said that I would get extreme punishment if I told. When I began to talk about him for the first time two years ago he started my self-harm. He does it, the self-harm. I am not aware of it; it is kept out of my consciousness. (Brainwashing is not only effective in the long term in wartime). I have often lived outside my consciousness. When I awoke, in a manner of speaking, I felt as if I hadn't been away. I only became conscious again when I hurt myself or when my little daughter walked towards me and bumped against my legs. Then I would feel pain and automatically know that it had happened again. With the self-harm, the voice would tell me afterwards what the punishment was for.

RECOVERY

When I asked for help two years ago I ended up in day therapy. I won't say it was no use. I did get a kind of daily structure but I didn't proceed with the voice. To me, that was fighting a losing battle. After I had been in day therapy for about two months I met my present therapist. With her I did talk about the incest and the voice. Very quickly, I felt able to trust her. I really had something with her although it was a long time before I could open up completely to her, in fact I still can't entirely, maybe because my stepfather forbade me to talk about what happened.

The voice is male and called Stefan. *My therapist made it clear that there was a similarity between my voice and my stepfather.* As soon as she told me that I got a flashback and saw my stepfather. I also understood that they are not really similar but that the voice resembles him and asks me to do the same things. For example, the ban on eating: my stepfather loved good meals but would say to me: 'Don't eat too much because it will make you fat.' The voice forbids me to eat too. When I became aware of the similarity between Stefan and my stepfather I could start to complete the puzzle. It was chaos in my head. The voice, the flashbacks and my incestuous past were all mixed up. One moment I was 15 years old and the next I was 9. *From my therapist I learned that specific images were connected to specific ages.* I couldn't place all these things at first. I believe the main reason I gained power over the voice was that I worked on myself. *I dared to become aware of things from my past.* This wasn't at all easy because when I started to talk about the voice for the first time it became worse for me. I became incredibly frightened. I received several medications but nothing helped. I got a numb feeling and bodily reactions like a dry mouth, headache and terrible tiredness. You start to see the world as a mist around you. The voice certainly didn't leave although there was some medication that reduced the fear. *The nice thing about my therapist was that she sometimes said things that the voice had said. Her recognition did a lot for me.* For example, if I am not allowed to do something by the voice, she will not say to 'do it'. I am already forced by the voice in that way but she will try something different, get me to a stage where I will see things from another perspective. *My fear wasn't a sign for either of us to stop.*

The processing of the incest, with which she helped me terrifically and still does, has already provided some reinforcement to my own 'I'. *I learned from her about the way I react, why I react and how I could react.* This has given me much more power and made me better able to cope with the voice. There are still some periods when I am afraid and think, 'Oh, I won't succeed', but that is pure anxiety, the severe panic has gone. I know now that I can fight it. At present I think that the most important thing is my own little 'I'. I can be proud of myself nowadays, for example, and praise myself, and say to myself, 'You did this well.' Previously I could never have done that.

What the voice says didn't change over time; what has changed is how I act towards the voice. That change has grown. Although I'd heard about the book *Accepting Voices* it was a long time before I ordered it and when I actually got it I left it unread for a couple of weeks. The title alone, 'accepting' voices, I thought, 'I will never accept that voice.' But now I do accept it. I still find it horribly annoying but think now 'So be it. It belongs to me.' My only hope now is that it will eventually become quiet. That hope I have. I have already experienced it once, after the lecture about voices I gave three years ago.

Then it was quiet for three days. I still experience time gaps regularly but, at least for now, nothing more happens. I mean no self-harm. My therapist tells me that losing myself is related to my past. When something connects me to a memory there is this mechanism through which I have learnt in the past to detach myself, to be away.

As of 1998, Lisette and her partner have a daughter, Sanne (8 years old) and a son Gebriel (2 years old). Lisette still hears the voice. He never disappeared completely. She says: 'I hear him during the day and in the evening, but he doesn't get me down anymore.'

MARION ASLAN

A SPIRITUAL AWAKENING

At the age of 39 life seemed sweet – I was happily married with a young son, co-owner of a thriving business and had opportunities to travel to Europe and Asia on a regular basis. At 40 it all came crashing down. I had experienced some postnatal depression immediately after my son was born and, on seeking help, had been offered antidepressants (which I rejected) and told by an impassive male GP to 'pull myself together'. Over time, I thought I had succeeded in doing just that but, within a year or so, my marriage had ended and I had become severely depressed as I was frozen out of the business and experienced financial difficulties, in addition to fighting for custody of my son. I retreated into my own world pretty much, managing to care for my son until he was in bed asleep and then seeking some solace in music, wine and my own thoughts and memories.

I was not particularly surprised when I first experienced hearing a voice as I had become interested by now in all things spiritual, though as yet did not have a strong faith or religious belief, just inquisitiveness. On that particular day, a Saturday afternoon in November 1994, I had said to my friend, Paula, 'I'm just going upstairs to listen to some music.' I hadn't seen her for over ten years, since my wedding party in fact. Now I was about to be divorced. Upstairs, I put on some relaxing music (dolphin sounds), lay down and let the sound wash over me. Ten minutes later I was kissing Paula goodbye and leaving my son in her care. They were still making the cakes in the kitchen that we'd all started ten minutes earlier. She later told me I had a determined, almost robotic, appearance and pushed her away with force when she tried to stop me leaving. I grabbed the car keys and started my journey, just as the voice had commanded me to. I can't remember the first instruction; I just knew it was taking me somewhere. This voice was inside my head, though I knew it not to be me or my own thoughts. It never occurred to me not to listen, communicate and respond. I believed this to be a gift, sent to assist me in my time of need and despair, and was grateful that it had come. It didn't have a gender as such, it just was.

It was a game, like Hide and Seek. If I listened carefully, the voice told me which way, where to go: 'Left ... now right ... go to the shopping centre.' I parked and wandered into the shopping centre, into familiar shops. No, he's not here. I had to find Paula's brother, Pat. He'd been a good friend to me over the last week or so. I'd been Pat's teacher when he was young, now he would guide me. And I was being guided to meet him. I never questioned who the voice was, simply accepted that I was tuning into a higher power. It felt comforting, and I remember feeling a sense of exhilaration that I was seeing the world through new eyes. After months of deep depression it felt as if I was gaining new meaning and purpose to life.

'Okay,' I reply, returning to the car, 'so he's not there, should I try a friend's house?' But I drive past because I know by looking at the house that he's not there. I'm tempted to go in and see them anyway, but the voice tells me to keep going. I begin to feel a sense of excitement and anticipation. I know something wonderful has been arranged … just keep following my instincts and the instructions. But the further I get away from Coventry, the weaker the voice is. I get as far as the airport … hot? 'No, cold, very cold,' says the voice, 'go back.' So I turn round and go back. Suddenly, I'm confused. I can't hear the voice any more. Why has it deserted me?

As usual, there are roadworks. I remember seeing the faces of the workmen. I know they are saying, 'Who is this crazy woman?' I'm driving in and out of the cones, on fresh tarmac. They are angry. I drive on a bit then stop abruptly on the kerb. I get out of the car, and in front of me is this scene of terrible devastation – dozens of cars piled into each other, their occupants bloodied, all dead. Death flashes before my eyes. But then the voice returns: 'God doesn't want you yet, you can turn around'. He's allowing me to go back for my little boy. My son needs me. I wander in and out of the carnage. I'm a survivor. I probably have the dazed, glazed look of a trauma victim, but I'm alive – not like these other poor sods. Carnage all around – how come I'm the lucky one? The voice says, 'Turn around, go back.'

I come to and I'm alone on the main road, but there's a pub nearby … that must be where Patrick is waiting … so I'll be OK, I will have won the game. Run, run over the grass … the car park … just leave the car … into the pub. 'Is Patrick here?' … pitying looks. Oh shit … reality is seesawing. I'm aware enough to feel embarrassed … play it cool … no money … can't get a drink … phone … 'Is there a phone?' People point out a phone booth … I go in but I can't remember how to actually use the phone, let alone reverse the charges. I'm really pissed off that Patrick hasn't been tuning into the voices like I have. If he'd done that he'd know where to meet me! Pitying looks when I come out of the booth. I hear the word 'police' mentioned, and then they are there. They are quite sweet to me really. I proudly show them where I have 'parked' the car on the bypass, assure them I haven't been drinking and that I'm not on drugs. I follow them out to my car and point out my rose-quartz crystal in the glove box. It's important that I don't lose it – more important than the car, really. I tell them about the game, why I'm here. It sounds mad even to me at this point. I'm quite happy to go for a ride with them. They're very kind and the voice tells me in hushed tones that 'it will be fine'.

Half an hour later I'm in a cell ... no blanket or chair ... bare ... a plastic bench-bed. But I have the Power. It hits me – a flash of inspiration. I *know* how Terry Waite survived. I hear him say, 'Come on, girl, if I survived Beirut you can do this. God will keep you safe.' I am suddenly happy to be there.

I let my mind play games, let it journey and travel beyond the cell door. If I can communicate with anyone at a distance, I can survive anything.

'Do you know who this man is?' 'Is it ...?' I name a relative, long dead. It is actually the police surgeon. Mum and dad are there – they look confused and upset. 'I'm fine', I say, sprinkling water on the police officers, turning the lights on, the taps on, the lights on, the taps on. Why do they keep turning them off, don't they know that I *have* to turn them on ... energy ... it's giving me energy and power, and enabling the voice to be stronger. 'I can help you', I say. The police don't look too impressed. I smile knowingly – of course, they don't hear the voice. And then a lucid moment! They are discussing hospitals. I insist I want to be in Coventry near to where my parents live. (I'm not associating it with 'mental' wards or anything: I'm thinking 'general hospital'.) In my naïvety, I assume I'm to have a checkup; they must believe that I have power and they'll want to check it out!

The journey – it's cold and dark outside. As I am put into the police van, I am having second thoughts about this. The policeman on the right is okay, but the one on my left is evil the voice tells me. They must not change places ... or am I wrong? ... is it *left* that is good and right evil? Oh shit, what if I get it wrong? The Devil will get me, not God. Keep chanting. I think that I've got it sorted ... right is definitely good. Okay, so treat the Devil with contempt. 'No, don't spit, that's not very nice, is it?' says the policeman. But nobody understands that he is Evil. 'The Devil has a smiling face' says the voice repeatedly throughout the journey. We arrive at the hospital. The journey has been a nightmare. I remember sitting sideways-on, hurtling through Birmingham at what felt like breakneck speed. I've babbled, screamed, spat, chanted, shouted and kicked. The police seem glad to arrive. They drag me in through the doors, still kicking and screaming. The police officer on the right is apologising profusely for hurting my arm – Satan on the left doesn't give a damn. I'm covered in bruises.

And then it dawns on me ... this is where the party is. Of course, Patrick will be here, as will my friends and family. I wave the police officers goodbye; cheerily thank them and apologise for the trouble I've caused them. I'm surprised that I can no longer hear a voice, but assume that's because I've arrived at my destination. The job's done! I go with the doctors and nurses to get changed ... bit pissed off with their choice of party frock. 'Hey, hang on ...' Wham! The needle goes in. I'm helped into bed. I sleep and sleep, miss Sunday out completely and awaken Monday morning fairly fresh, alert and voice-free. I'm back to 'normal' (whatever that is) within a day or so and let out after five days. No medication needed; told this was a 'brief psychotic episode'. Back to my son in time for Christmas; telephone police; apologise profusely. The officer I speak to seems genuinely pleased I have recovered so quickly, tells me to have a good Christmas and put it all behind me.

RECOVERY AND BEYOND

One of my favourite quotes is R.D. Laing's (1967: 110), 'Madness need not be all breakdown. It may also be breakthrough', and over time I have believed this to be true for myself and others I have met or worked with in the psychiatric system. However, there were to be several more of these 'breakdowns' before finally breaking through, beyond the recovery journey to the place where I now am, a place of thriving.

On five more occasions over the years I was to experience the internal dialogues and, although I always believed they were messages and signs from another dimension, I never again heard them in quite the same way. Between the first experience and the second, I had fully converted to Christianity and so I subsequently held the conviction that I was hearing messages from God, the Holy Spirit or angels. My belief that this was so was strengthened by a meeting with Terry Waite, whose voice I had heard so clearly some years before. It felt like I had come full circle in my understanding, almost like déjà vu.

On another occasion, which led to me being compulsorily detained once again, I had 'communicated' with the voice of Spike Milligan, and visualised us at a party. Just one year later, I was actually picking him up at his home to drive him to Coventry to a charity function I had organised and felt once more an overwhelming sense of déjà vu.

Perhaps the most poignant episode of voices was just before Easter time in 2002, when once again I ended up compulsorily detained. For weeks, I had been getting up at the crack of dawn to drive to Corley, a village just outside Coventry. For no reason that I could think of, a spiritual voice in my head was telling me I needed to be there, to get involved with the village community in some way, that it was an important place for me. I started spending time at the local pub and got to know quite a few people, and before I knew what I was letting myself in for I had agreed to buy a horse, put my house on the market and was planning to move out to the village. At the same time, I was more and more listening to my spiritual guide, working hard, eating and sleeping little, and eventually I burned out. My family were concerned, called in the crisis team and, much against my will, I was once again in hospital.

During my stay, brief as always, thankfully, I was assigned a bed which faced out in the direction of Corley and I would watch, imagine myself out there and listen to a new voice, that of my father. We discussed which of us God was calling to Him first. I insisted it should be me, that my mum and brother needed him, he was just as insistent it should be him that was 'taken'. We 'discussed' much about life and dying, it felt that he was preparing me for his death, and the conversations were as real to me as any I'd ever had with him. They lasted for several days then disappeared, and I returned home within the week.

I spent a lot of time over the next few months going over to Corley with my parents and son. We would visit the stables; my son and I would take turns to ride our horse; we would go for meals together and I showed them the house I was hoping to buy. I learned much about my father that I had never known before – the most surprising thing being that he had actually lived in the village for a couple of years as a young boy, and the fields and lanes I rode along were the very ones he'd played in as a child. Looking back, it was very special spending such quality time together as a family in that place, though I made the decision not to move there after all. A year later, Easter 2003 – almost exactly year to the day of my going into hospital – my father died and, although it was a desperately sad period, I drew a lot of strength remembering the 'conversations' we'd had.

As I previously stated, I now feel at a place in my life where I am thriving, using my experiences in a positive way, currently working in partnership with my colleague and friend, Mike Smith, a former nurse, delivering training and consultancy on a variety of mental health issues.

There have been two main turning points in my recovery. The first was many years ago, when after a period of deep depression I happened to befriend some young homeless people and ended up setting up a local office for the Big Issue magazine. I found myself slowly starting to enjoy life again, to laugh and put my depression far behind me. Looking outwards, helping others and having a valued role in life, has been reported by many as being instrumental in their recovery. For me, it was an epiphany – that what I had experienced could be put to good use. Having a reason to get up in the morning, a purpose to the day, and mixing with a range of people – the vendors I supported and workers from the organisations I linked with – helped to build up my confidence. They all accepted me for who I was, and were not judgemental about my past.

Following on from running the 'Big Issue', I set up a support group in Coventry, 'Krysalis', for people with mental distress, and set about using my teaching experience to run training courses so that the members could go out and deliver user-led training to professionals in the area. This led on to me meeting many people working in the area of recovery – Marius Romme, Sandra Escher, Mike Smith, Ron Coleman, Rufus May, Mary Nettle, to name but a few. Learning from them, from a non-medical perspective, was of huge significance to my recovery: it helped me site my experiences into a context which I understood and could rationalise and, thus, work through.

A more recent turning point has been the publishing of my first book, *The THRIVE Approach to Wellness*, co-written with Mike and drawing on our joint expertise and experiences over the years. In the book we talk about moving beyond recovery to a place of thriving that is not just the place where you were before the distress but the place where you would have got to without the experience of ill health ever happening. Writing on the process of recovery has proven extremely therapeutic and profoundly liberating. It has helped me value my experiences and turned negatives into positives. Finding meaning and context within the 'madness' has proved helpful – although I did some things which appeared crazy to others I now have an understanding of what it symbolised in my life: a yearning and a searching for meaning, amongst other things. I do not believe there is any one way to recover; it is completely individual, though there is much common ground. Having hope for the future was crucial to me, as it is to many others. But perhaps just as importantly for me is the idea of emancipation and reclamation, freeing myself from the constraints of being regarded as a previously ill person, and choosing to regard and value myself and my experiences as unique.

Seeing my experiences as spiritual rather than illness has also been pivotal in my recovery. I do not believe myself to have ever been ill, simply distressed, in need, crying out for help – which forms the basis of how Mike and I now work with others. I have always rejected medication, other than where it has been forced on me in hospital (with very bad side effects) therefore I have had to rely on inner resources, natural resilience and lots of sheer hard work. I am often asked if I regret any of what has happened. Well, I probably regret some of the pain I have unwittingly caused others (though Paula very generously states that I gave her a much better understanding of the issues surrounding mental health and the true meaning of crisis!), but I look back on what I had – a very tenuous understanding of life, values and priorities, then I look at what I've gained in terms of true friendships, fulfilment, and a joy for living, and I feel truly blessed. My voices are ever with me – integrated and a part of me, as they were all along – but these days I would call them my intuition, my inner reasoning and my guardian angels.

MIEKE SIMONS

INTERVIEW WITH SANDRA ESCHER

If you don't mind, let's start with your childhood, would you like to tell me something about that, please?
I was born in the middle of World War II, as the eldest of four children. I was very much wanted. My father adored me. My mother was more like the archetype of a good woman. She always treated us really well. She was a very strong woman too. The younger sister who came directly after me was born at the end of the war right in the middle of all the warfare. Breda was liberated at that time. That battle took place near our house. Apparently it was all very chaotic. My mother told me later that I walked around feeling distraught. I felt excluded by my mother. I spent most of my time with my dad. I am most like him too. Since I was a child that never laughed, she took me to a doctor when I was 2 years old.

My father became ill when I was 6. As I child I never really noticed what was wrong with him. He decompensated, as they call it. He had married late in the middle of the war. My parents had four children in five years and my father found that difficult. Furthermore, he had been spoilt rotten by his mother and my mother could not keep that going at the same rate. Initially my father was admitted to a couple of local district general hospitals. He was certified mentally ill when I was 9 and left for good to a psychiatric institution. I would only see him there when we visited him during the holidays. There was always some anxiety then since every time we had to wait and see whether he was OK or not. I have not suffered a great deal because of my father's illness. I felt relatively safe with my mother. Since she started letting out rooms, we were pretty comfortably off. When I was 12, I went to boarding school. That was the best solution for my mother, since I would get a good education there. My opinion on this solution was not asked.

When I compare myself to other people, I enjoyed an easy and happy childhood. My first threatening problem was when I lost my job. I was 39 at the time. I enjoyed my job and I had put my heart into it. The problem arose because I got into an argument with a colleague who had worked there longer than I had and who did not feel like clearing up the argument. My then husband worked in the same hospital and did not back me up at all. I started to reproach him over this. A distance developed between us. I thought it was really unfair what was happening. Moreover, it was the first time that I had been rejected. I just stared into a black hole in front of me, since at the time there were no teaching jobs any more. I started therapy. All my anger and sadness came out and I flipped. I saw all kinds of delusions and became very frightened too. In hindsight I have to admit that I was behaving very weird at that time.

My husband got fed up and got colleagues involved. He took me to the competition (a different psychiatric hospital from the one they both worked at). It was decided I would be admitted. On the day of my admission, my mother was diagnosed with cancer. She passed away three months later, but by then I had already been discharged from hospital. That was what my life was like when I lost my job: my husband was not on my side and my mother had passed away. After losing my job, I moved out. I wanted a divorce and that was mainly my decision. Since I was still pretty depressed, that process was not making much progress and somehow I had this idea that things may get better between me and my husband. We were also still seeing each other. One Wednesday afternoon, I visited my former house for the children, to do their laundry and look after them. I saw all kinds of signs which made me think that something was not quite right. I confronted him with it and it turned out that he had a lady, as he called her. That was the final straw for me, whereas I had hoped that things would turn out for the better in the end. I was very angry, very disappointed, very jealous mainly, since I had been rejected once more.

That happened in December (1984), I was 42 years old. Following that this voices business gradually started. It was a gradual thing. I was very busy in my head. My mother occupied my mind and I kept on talking to her a lot too. A number of voices emerged around me. About five of them I think. I was constantly talking to them and then you lose your sense of reality. I became chaotic too and confused and tried to look for support from my family. The voices also began giving me orders which I executed which led to an even bigger chaos. People around me thought that I needed to be admitted and this happened. I was readmitted to Santpoort. I began to walk around in circles outside a lot in order to be able to talk and talk. I had promised myself not to talk about the voices in this clinic. However, after three weeks when I felt safe again, I absolutely wanted to know what it was all about. How it had all started? I thought the psychiatrists would know, but during their studies they were not taught about dealing with voice hearing. They feel pretty insecure about that, they basically do not really know what advice they should give you.

RECOVERY

During the aftercare I met a psychiatrist who claimed that he knew that hearing voices in your head existed. So he did not tell me: 'You're crazy', but 'I don't know anything about it' and 'I don't know how to teach you how to deal with this.' I did not mind that so much as I had plenty to take care of anyway: my divorce, getting my children and my house back. I needed a great deal of energy to manage reality and this psychiatrist was particularly good at that; managing reality. I also noticed that it was very important to occupy myself with these kinds of things. So I had come across a psychiatrist who supported me with a sense of reality and that was exactly what I needed at that time during that year. From that moment onwards, things started to fall into place again. Based on my frustration regarding the voices, I decided to do my own research. I started reading about it and discovered that far more was known about it. At that time I came into contact with Pieter Langendijk, a psychologist (and complementary therapist) who was married to someone who heard voices and who comforted me by telling me that it was not something odd at all. It was not madness at all. You can deal with the voices, if indeed you start a dialogue with them, talk to them and try to keep them in a positive mood. If you are positive you attract this positivity, if you are negative you attract this negativity and then you will get negative comments too. I learnt that at the end of the day it was my own responsibility whether or not I executed the orders and accepted the resultant consequences. It is always your own will that is above everything else. Your environment can support you in this, like, for example, 'Mum, look what you are doing now' or 'Mum, look what you got yourself into this time.' Fortunately my daughter is very good at that. Intuitively she feels whether I am doing the wrong thing or involving myself in a wrong relationship. I learnt how to deal with the voices through myself and my daughter.

After hearing voices for about three years, quieter 'normal' times dawned until the point that I wanted to buy a house, since we finally managed to divide our assets after six years. It turned out I still was not able to cope with stress well enough. The moment I moved into the new house with all my worldly belongings, a hellish cacophony erupted in my head. I recognised the symptoms and decided to remain calm and to clearly differentiate what was real and what had a cosmic impact on me. After not having slept for about ten nights, I decided that they were not going to drive me crazy and I started swearing at the demons and I told them to leave my head and my house. Just like 'them' I became possessed. By shouting I decided that I wanted to remain in control of my house and my head. It worked this time. I was able to escape the real madness and the craziness and that gave me new strength and courage to go on and to endure and face up to this anxiety and insecurity brought about by this transitional period.

SUMMARY

To summarise my story: I start hearing voices when I am in a situation which threatens my existence like my divorce and the purchase of my house six years later. The first time it confused me so much that there was nothing I could do with it. The second time I was indeed confused, but I was clearly able to cope with it in a better way. I was able to set limits to the impact of the voices. On both occasions, my voices presented a polarity: both the opportunity to escape from the orders, which made me none the wiser, as well as help in analysing my problem. The voices verbalise my emotional battle between tackling my problem and running away from it.

During the intermittent period I met Romme and Escher, I told my story at the First World Voice-Hearing conference in the Netherlands in 1987, I participated in the foundation of the 'Weerklank' ('Resonance') Association, played a active role in it and had met a great deal of voice hearers which made me feel more self-confident about hearing voices. A highlight in my recovery was that as the chairwoman of 'Weerklank', I was able to tell my story at the hospital where I had been admitted in the past.

For many years Mieke Simons was the chairwoman of the board of directors of the 'Weerklank' Association – the Dutch network for promoting the interests of voice hearers. She also found a part-time teaching job. She is retired now and spends a great deal of time with her grandchildren.

MIEN SONNEMANS

WITH MARIUS ROMME

Mien Sonnemans is 60 and married to a very supportive husband. She has one son, two daughters and several grandchildren. When she was seven years old she started hearing voices, just before her first Holy Communion. That was when the sexual abuse by an assistant priest started.

As a child I wasn't confused by the voices, to me it was normal. I never talked about them when I was a child. I wasn't afraid of them. I often did what they told me to do. I had two nasty and one good voice. The nasty voices pushed me to destructive acts, kicking against things or hurting myself. The positive voice helped me now and then. One nasty voice told me I was a child of the devil and good for nothing. The other nasty voice talked about the same things, again saying, 'You are good for nothing, you are not able to do anything, be glad with the crumbs that are left.' If I asked them why they acted in such an ugly way they said, 'because you are ugly'. These voices remained dominant until I was 30 years old. Afterwards, I was hardly bothered by them anymore because I had decided that I should put my children first. But the abuse history still haunted me and therefore I became depressed. At a certain moment I started to seek help. I had treatment for a while at the community mental health centre, but I only got medication. That didn't help and I just suffered from side effects. My therapist didn't tell me anything more than 'swallow your medication and keep your mouth shut. Keep the lid on the cesspool.' Around my 50th birthday I collapsed, all my energy was wasted. I started to think more about suicide. I wrote a letter to the therapist at the CMHC (Community Mental Heath Centre). I asked her to help me to step out of my life in a decent manner. This was when the alarm bells at the centre started to ring.

We had been talking together, three staff members and me, and that discussion made clear I wanted different treatment. I took a hard line (I even hit the table with my fist). My CPN told me she had read about a hospital, a psychotherapy clinic run as a therapeutic community. I started therapy and the abuse history was uncovered. I didn't talk about my voices during the first admission. I went there simply to stay alive. Nevertheless, the voices returned fiercely after years of absence. I started to recognise one of them as the perpetrator of the abuse and I became extremely anxious. The voice of my mother I got for free. The voice of my mother I found especially confusing.

RECOVERY

It wasn't until my second admission that I spoke about my hearing voices and that one of them especially was very aggressive. Until then I hadn't talked about the voices with anybody. I didn't get any special therapy for the voices in the psychotherapeutic hospital, although they did account for it in their general therapeutic approach. Because I got more insight into myself I began to understand my voice-hearing experience better.

In my case it originated in the traumatic experiences of my childhood. From the moment I understood that, I could place it and work on it. The most benefit I had, and still have, is in taking for granted that, in some way, I create those voices myself. It relates to how I look at myself. For years I had lived with the conviction that it was all my own fault, that I was deemed a devil's child from birth on. This conviction I had to turn around. By working from my own reasoning and, consequently, saying the opposite to myself, I did gradually succeed in turning the conviction around. It sounds simple but is hard work and proceeds only step by step. I call it the 'Cees-method', Cees being the first name of my therapist. Sometimes I don't succeed and then I use what I call the 'Tiny-method'. Tiny is the psychologist from the CMHC and this method is about communicating with the voices, asking them what they want and answering them; for example, telling them that I am not a child anymore and can do what I want – that *I* determine what I do and not them. Sometimes this helps but when it doesn't I become very angry and figuratively kick them out of the door – the Cees-method again.

I have accepted that they are there and found a way to cope with them. It is something that belongs to me. I can't avoid them and I am not panicked by them anymore. I absolutely don't feel ashamed of them anymore. I can even talk with my family about them. When I told my husband and children, their first reaction was: 'Is it very awkward?' and 'Now we understand you better, so many pieces of the puzzle have fallen into place.' I didn't have to keep silent about it anymore. My children accepted it completely. My husband is very supportive, even if he doesn't understand. I don't go deeply into it anymore. If the rest of the family understands, it's no longer so important. For a while I felt the urge to let everybody know; I don't have that any more. There are people who are prepared to listen to me, that is enough. I no longer need to tell everybody. Now I can see that my brothers and sisters didn't reject me, I don't panic every time and that gives me peace and space. The greatest support I received was from my therapist in the psychotherapeutic hospital. He was the first one I told about it and he immediately took me seriously. He showed me the right way to cope with the voices, not to obey them but to neglect them. I must confess now that I kept silent about it for forty-nine years. It was him who taught me I wasn't mad, that the voices related to my past and that I shouldn't go along with what they said and expected from me. I had to neglect them and show them the door. After I had talked about my voices with the therapist at the psychotherapeutic hospital I spoke to the psychologist at the CMHC and she also took it seriously from the start. It confused me, though, when she advised me to discuss with the voices. Later on in my process I learned when it was good to send the voices away and when it was good to discuss with them.

It helped me very much to realise that the hearing of voices is a reasonably normal phenomenon, that you can and may talk about it, that the voices express what happens within me. It also helped me to accept my voices and my past and the relationship between the two. I can now express myself much better. I am very glad I have succeeded so far, although I still encounter certain things. Sometimes I am confronted with triggers. You can't eradicate all damage. For a long time I was stuck in the victim role. Because of everything that happened in my childhood I didn't think it was worth working on myself. I acted in the way I had been told: 'You can't do anything, you will never be anything.'

To recover you must regain yourself; for that I had to release myself from everything that was being said in my head. Trusting oneself is a learning process. Gradually, I learned to fight for myself and for that I needed much support and acknowledgement. I got this in the self-help group I joined. There, I gained self-esteem. I started to really talk about my voices. Before, I had tended to isolate myself and was very lonely. In the group I learned how to talk about voices when I was outside the group and that reduced my isolation. I no longer became afraid and when I wasn't afraid I didn't see shadows and devils anymore. The voluntary work made me more self-confident too. I didn't have those dips anymore. For my recovery three things were important; finding good therapy, telling my family about my past and doing voluntary work, even though my husband was opposed to it. Together with some other women I established the foundation 'Willpower' for women's assistance. The three of us are the daily board. I recognised that when emotions come up I can stay level-headed and give solid advice. I can slow them down if necessary. Not convert everything into action.

To be clear, I hear three voices and recognise them. The aggressive voice is from the assistant priest, although he is sometimes nice. The second voice is from my mother and she is always angry. I find this the most difficult voice to cope with. The third voice is from Cees, the psychotherapist from the hospital. He is a good voice and a kind of guide. I have heard this voice for three years. I can cope with the voices now. I can function in a group and I can cuddle my grandchildren without a voice telling me that I should do something to them.

ODI OQUOSA

INTERVIEW WITH JACQUI DILLON

Odi Oquosa is 37 years old and was born in Nigeria. In 2000 he was tortured for three days by officially endorsed armed vigilante groups, commonly known as the 'Bakassi Boys'. He still bears visible injuries on his body. These groups are responsible for the execution of hundreds of people and for the torture, 'disappearance' and unlawful detention of scores of citizens. The international human rights organisation, Amnesty International, assisted Odi in seeking political asylum in the UK. He now lives in Brighton. He is a shaman, a community artist and a healer. Odi facilitates workshops that encourage people to heal themselves through non-medical treatments like, art, poetry, dance and music.

I was born a warrior prince. My mother and father made my body but the spirits made my thoughts. Since I was a child I was captured by the spirits of my ancestors. I heard the voices from history that told stories of colonisation and slavery. I am connected to the history of what has happened and what continues to happen to my people. I owe my ancestors respect and obedience. When they call, I must follow.

I started travelling the world when I was 18. In 1990, when I was 25 and a successful textile designer living in Switzerland, I began having unusual experiences. I would have premonitions of things that were going to happen, accidents and things like that. The voices of the ancestors would tell me these things that would protect me and help me to protect other people. These things can frighten you and take you into another world; they can make you mad if you are not ready. This was my ancestors preparing me to take responsibility. They told me that I must return home to Nigeria to become a shaman.

So I returned home to Nigeria. I went to the sea and put my hands to the earth and that is when I got communication from the ancestors and gained knowledge. I began to see the past conflicting with the present. If you do not deal with the past it will come back again and you will have to deal with it in the present. Our past hasn't been understood and the ancestors chose me because I am part of them. At that time the 'Bakassi Boys' were killing people, burning down houses and bringing fear. I decided to confront them by going on radio and television and speaking out. I told the police but they could do nothing. I finally went to meet with the 'Bakassi Boys'. On my third meeting they abducted me, telling me they wanted to kill me. They tortured me – my body is full of marks. I was strapped down, beaten with machetes and cut all over.

My family intervened and they released me. After that I started having panic attacks and nightmares. I'd see people chasing me with machetes, even in my dreams. My voices were telling me I needed to go through these experiences to understand shamanism. I had to be wounded to understand about pain. I started painting and writing stuff about my experiences. But then the 'Bakassi Boys' came to my office and burned down the whole place. I lost all my work. It was hell.

I knew then that I had to escape from Nigeria and so with the help of Amnesty International I came to England in 2001. I brought a lot of evidence with me about what these vigilantes had been doing to people. I was living in London but the chaos of the city made my panic attacks worse and all I could hear were negative voices. I feared that people were following me and that they wanted to kill me. It was a very bad time. So I went to Brighton to be near the sea. I wanted to be close to nature and the elements so that I could heal myself.

Because of the problems I was having, my GP arranged for a psychiatrist and a social worker to come to my home. I had to talk to the doctors, who sent me to a psychiatric ward. They saw me as a mad person, who was delusional, as I was still talking with my voices. They diagnosed me with schizophrenia. They told me that I needed medication and I said, 'But I am the doctor, not you!' They asked to meet with some of my family and friends, so they came down and they said, 'Yes, this is our culture', so they stopped pestering me to take medication. They began to understand me by reading my poems and looking at my paintings and sculptures. They began to see that I wasn't mad – I was a person.

My voices helped me to combat the panic attacks and flashbacks. As the panic attacks continued, I started getting angry at my voices and at myself. Then one day my voices told me, 'You have to fight. You are a warrior'. So I brought out an old tribal sword, a double edged sword and I hung it up in my flat. The next time I had a panic attack I saw the machete men but they ran away. It was a symbolic event but it was a turning point. I haven't had any panic attacks or flashbacks since that time. Now I am fearless again.

I now help others who have had similar problems to me. The hospital in Brighton now involves me and I use my knowledge to offer one-to-one support and give people things that the system cannot give to them. I use natural things like stones and wood to help me connect to people that the system considers seriously mentally ill. I help them to find themselves. I also run workshops for professionals to share my knowledge as a shaman, an artist and a healer.

OLGA RUNCIMAN

THE VOICES OF ME!

It was asked of me, and I subsequently felt inspired to contribute to an anthology about me and my voices; two things which are so separate and yet so together. How did I survive them, and yet how could I not? I needed them as much as they needed me and, together, we created me, a fragmented child, who became a fragmented adult, who finally became whole, became me, became Olga.

I heard my first voice as a very young child, perhaps around 4 or 5, I don't recall. I do remember however the first time I heard him. I was sitting playing alone inside our house and he called my name very loudly. He had a deep voice which almost had an echo to it and it seemed to come from above and around. I didn't recognise the voice and was immediately curious as to who this strange person was calling my name, and I started to search for him in the house. I searched everywhere, and every time he called my name I would shout back 'Yes I am here!' or something to that effect. I didn't find him, and I became increasingly frustrated and distraught, and in the end I became very angry at his ability to hide himself so well that he was impossible to find.

Over the next period of time he kept appearing as just a voice and, very quickly, I accepted that he was invisible, that he was good and that he was there to help me. I also soon realised that he had the ability, in my then small world, to predict happenings and situations which I could then avoid or cope with, with his help. As time passed, he became my comforter and my guide in this labyrinth of emotional turmoil which was my home, and he came to play a big role in surviving those early years of my life. I called him God.[1]

My second voice, who has perhaps always been there, is a small child, a little girl, *my* little girl. Always with her back to me, always alone – so very, very alone. Dressed mostly in red, she never talks, only screams, and even then not that often. Raising her head, she can scream out loud – the agonising pain of utter abandonment – yet she never has and never will be heard.

---

1. God came as a 'helper voice', when my life as a child was at times very difficult, and he was there until I lost faith in religion and therefore him, and I threw him out. ... continued ...

Sometimes, she lets out a few shuddering sobs. Otherwise, she sits there cross-legged; her back to me, huddled over some secret activity which only she knows. I know she is a part of me, a secret part, and I do so want to unlock that secret, yet I don't know how to reach her; she sits there so close I can almost touch her, yet she is so far away I might as well be on another planet where a lifetime of travel will not bring me closer. She is my enigma, the big question in the tapestry of my life, my why, why … this?

My third and fourth voice came later, much later; they came when I threw out God. Why did I throw out God? I threw out God and they came in, sneaking in like thieves in the night, stealing my soul, filling my world with blackness and hatred. A seeping black pool of hatred and destruction, causing me to burn my tongue and cut my arms – only that, again, was later, much later. They were my failures, my guilt, the living proof of how spectacularly I had failed; never good, always bad, a constant reminder of my dirt, the dirty little girl who became the dirty filthy me. Slowly – or perhaps it was in reality quite quickly – they poisoned me; black tendrils stretching out, moving in, going deeper and deeper, and then … they were stopped. They were stopped by the very thing they themselves were: failure. By being my failings, they themselves were ultimately doomed, doomed to fail in their mission: a complete poisoning of all of me. For, somehow, a fragment or fragments of me remained intact, were immune to the poison; remained clean, serene, strong and powerful and wouldn't let the poison in.

They have been my constant companions, always there but not always present. Sometimes they fill my head, taking over my tongue, saying words I do not recognise – recognition in the sense that that is not me, it is a stranger borrowing my mouth, my tongue, saying terrible things which hurt, cutting like a knife into the soft part of me. Or worse, spreading out, hurting those whom I hold so dear, which in turn hurts me again and again, as the pain reverberates and comes back to me like waves. Other times, their blackness is far, far away, covered by layers of calmness, strength, love and happiness, trapping them so their black tendrils cannot escape. On those occasions they have no control, they are themselves controlled by me, a united me, and their power is reduced to nothing. So how is it possible that they can still sometimes spew out black tendrils? I like to think they are an echo, sometimes

---

… continued … That opened the door wide to the two poison voices and the group. They became very dominant when I went to my second boarding school at around 10 where I was exposed to massive bullying by the other girls, but the worst was by the teachers. I was also sexually abused by one of the teachers there. The headmistress of whom all were afraid including many of the teachers, acquired in my eyes tremendous power and she, though not a priest, would hold many school church services. God ceased to be of any help as nothing I did or said made any difference and the headmistress, by pretending to be a priest, and God not striking her down for blasphemy, made her more powerful than he and I lost my faith completely.

a loud echo but just that, an echo, nothing more. Yet I know they are my past impinging on my present, distorting and trying to poison, always poison.

Then there's the joker; he's a latecomer, arriving long after all the others have been here for what seems like an eternity. He's actually quite wise in his funny sort of way and he's also the finisher, the ender of poison. I know, when he comes, summarising the whole episode in his joking jokes sort of way, that he is the bringer of peace, and I welcome him. I know also that, for the outside world, he is the most scary. He makes me laugh and the outside world interprets, they don't understand, and hearing my laughter their interpretation moves in, 'She is insane,' they say, 'lock her away.' I like his jokes. By joking, he disperses the black tendrils, making them dissolve, withdraw and neutralises their poison. His ironic but oh so true jokes go straight to the centre, drawing little blood in his precise interpretation of reality, my reality. And when I understand his message – because I don't always – he has used few words, where I would probably have had to write a whole chapter to see that light. More often than not, he makes me see the absurdity of this whole episode, how completely small and insignificant it is when measured within the perspective of the rich tapestry that is my life. That episode he highlighted was but a speck, which for a short while was allowed to fill and open the door to the black tendrils of poison. He shuts that door.[2]

Finally ... almost, we have the mumblers, the murmurers, never saying anything clearly, always just outside the clarity of words. They are a group of an indeterminate size, sometimes huge and threatening, other times far away, like storm clouds gathering at the edge of the horizon. They are the warners, warning of dark times approaching. Their approach can be at times so subtle that suddenly they are there like a flash storm catching you unawares; at other times their murmuring is like a far distant thunderstorm; rumbling, getting ever closer, warning of the impending storm. Their mumblings are confusing, their message unclear, but they are always there at times of weariness or mental exhaustion, confusing me, distorting the meaning and the words of the external world. Other voices start to include dark and sinister messages and motives, hidden motives, making those people shadowy and threatening, just like those storm clouds gathering. Words of kindness twist and become

---

2. He comes when something triggers me and the poison voices flair up. He puts things in perspective; I suppose he in a way represents reason. If I am triggered by someone doing something to me and I go into this black space, he can put that actual episode with that person in perspective, and he does that often by joking and making me laugh, and humour is a great thing for me. I also find him quite clever because he can summarise that situation in quite an analytical manner that makes sense and deflates the power of the episode. Once that happens the poison voices disappear and I am back to me again.

cruel and harsh, echoing the past where things were never as they seemed. Why should others be kind now – when I am big, strong and oh so grown up – yet cruel, using and abusing me when I was a little girl? Shouldn't it be the other way round? Shouldn't it be not at all – do you see now? How they can confuse?

Last, but really the beginning, God came back, only now he is not God, at least not in name. He is the good one, the good voice – and, with his return, everything changed; the balance of power, the balance of control. With him I began the journey of union, uniting the fragments, joining each piece of me to me, to finally become whole, become me, become Olga.

MY VOICE, THE VOICE OF ME (RECOVERY)

Becoming me, becoming Olga, was a journey, a hard journey but also a journey of joy and ending in love. Journeys are strange things, you think you are going in one direction but suddenly you are on a different road in a different country; people say strange things to you which are difficult or maybe even impossible to understand.

On this journey to becoming whole, I passed through a land which was so well known [psychiatry], yet being on the other side it became alien. The language I used to speak in this country ceased to exist; I understood their empty words but my words were seen as insanity. I was a schizophrenic they said: 'Please remember that, oh, and while we are at it, remember to stop thinking there is a cure, you are a chronic, a chronic schizophrenic, a biological defect with an incurable disease.' I, too, when I had been on the other, other side, studied the books and learned the biology, had been told, and believed, that this was a chronic disease. But now it was me, and I couldn't believe it.

In the beginning I told them my troubles but nobody listened, just wrote them down. Why they wrote, I don't know; it was not relevant and played no role. What was important was teaching me my place in the biological scheme of a medical model. Chemistry of the brain was out of sorts due to genetics, so chemicals to fix my defect was the order of the day. Orap, Cisordinol, Risperdal, Leponex were but a few of the ones that I tried on this ten-year journey. I grew big and fat, apathetic and stiff and, as for my brain, well, it ceased to connect; disjointed and trapped, it filled with wool, creating a distance between me and my life. 'It will help with your voices, which are just a symptom of this serious illness; they are not real, don't you believe it', they said again and again. My feelings were blunted, my emotions were grey, the colour was gone and all I had left was emptiness, endless meaningless emptiness which filled me with despair. That I could feel. Time stretched out, slowed – or probably it was, in reality, me, who ground slowly to a halt. I would sit in a chair and think 'What should I do today?' and, suddenly, today was dark, gone, night had arrived. Another meaningless, purposeless day had passed. Thank God for the pills, at least I had slept most of *that* day away ... again.

I kept asking them, 'Are you sure there isn't a mistake? Surely it's not possible my life will be like this for the rest of time – my time?' I stopped asking when it was no longer I who heard the words of hopelessness. I drove them insane ha! ha! by asking and asking, surely there were exceptions to this horrible rule. But no, neither they nor I had ever heard of recovery; that many before me had recovered and that, *yes, it was possible!* The silence on recovery in the system was deathly and filled the wards and corridors with hopelessness, not just for me but for us all, staff and 'schizophrenics' alike. And then the hopelessness spread. After a year (or was it two), my family was informed; all of us together. I had asked again 'Surely, surely, this is not true?', and now it became imperative that reality was upheld. I had to accept, once and for all, that this was my life and that I must acknowledge it. What better way then, than before witnesses, the witnesses of my past. 'Olga is seriously ill and will never recover,' they said, 'she is too fragile and requires help the rest of her days; she will never work and must of course take medication the rest of her life.' I wanted the ground to open and swallow me alive but, instead, my voice joined the deathly silence of the system, never again to ask, 'Surely, surely this cannot true?' The voices of me, though, were not quieted; they did not go, ever, no matter what little round or long red or green pill I took to silence them ... or was it me?

The staff were sweet and kind and they did their best, they just didn't know better and neither did I. I did, after all, once belong to the other, other side, so I know. Diagnosis and prognosis ruled the day, so meaning and understanding got lost on the way. They are the experts, they've been approved, they must perform and choose genetics as, here, they can rationalise, justify why they cannot possibly, possibly be one of us. The insidious fear that's lurking; that maybe, perhaps, they are not so different after all, is 'experted' (or is it exported?) away, but certainly not faced.

So how did I recover?
By looking death in the eye. In my preparations for meeting death, I wrote a lie; a lie that shone out of the paper and seared my eyes, and I knew, even though I did not believe this strange four-worded sentence, I could not leave this earthly world on a lie. I wrote 'I have tried everything' – but I hadn't. I had not done it my way, so busy was I listening to others – the so-called 'experts' – experts who, in reality, are as much in the dark about suffering of

the mind as the sufferers themselves. So I prepared a plan, a concrete plan, which, in the beginning, could be followed step by step and where belief in the plan was an irrelevant companion.

I was conventional, or so I thought; apparently, in reality, I wasn't really. I chose therapy with a therapist I had known from before, the difference this time was that I had nothing to lose, so no holds were barred and all could be told. 'But therapy is not good for a schizophrenic like you,' they said, 'it would unearth too much and make you more ill. Settle down, make a scarf instead, that will help.' I chose therapy anyway. My therapist could see a difference in me – that I was serious – and it filled her with hope, my hope, hope that began to move back into me giving me strength and light – but, most important, it was the start of my journey back to the living.

Medication: now that was a tricky one. For years I was told, and truly believed, that I would feel so much worse if I stopped my little white pill (or was it red? ... there were so many they confused my head). But now, with death staring me in my face ... who cared ... it would just give me more reason to die if I felt more pain. So they said 'No, don't stop', but I did it anyway – in secret. And, little by little, the woolliness receded, my head became clearer, my feelings returned. I felt the pain, the anguish of my new understanding, but I also felt joy and a zest for life – they had lied, I didn't feel worse, I felt alive. The colour returned and, here too, my journey began. I had grown fat with these pills of mine; I'd never been that, so a diet was in order in this new-found cure. I started with Weightwatchers; I just had to mind my points, it was irrelevant on what and that I could follow. I followed my points and the weight got lost, I began to move, my energy was back. And then one day I had to shop. My clothes were too big and I needed new ones, but now, suddenly, I could shop in a regular store for regular people with regular sizes. That put a smile on my face, because now I could dress for this journey of mine.[3]

I had had a dream, once. I was going to be the studier of stars, the first woman in space and that required exams, not permissible at this school of mine. That is, until physics was suddenly allowed, private tuition no less, by a teacher who had said that he could see something special in this young child ... only physics became physic*al* and the dream died.

However, with this new found plan, I wanted to learn and stimulate my mind so I could at least go out with a (big) bang. So the dream was revived: a course was found to study the stars, the planets and the beginning of

---

3. Going on a diet, self-image, how one looks, is important for many, also for me. I had become fat, formless and inert. To actively take care of myself physically by losing weight, fixing my hair, makeup, clothes and going out into the world with my head up is empowering on many levels.

existence; and to my surprise I found my reason, a purpose for being. I found that there's more to life than death, that there is something bigger, greater and more meaningful, and that life is no accident! So amazed was I at the grandness of the cosmic universe that I felt a transformation occur within myself, and with that transformation my true journey began. My voice from my childhood returned and God came back – only now he is not God, at least not in name. He is the good one, the good voice. And with his return everything changed, the balance of power, the balance of control. With him I began the journey of union, uniting the fragments, joining each piece of me, to me, to finally become whole, become me, become Olga.

Addendum

When I became a client of psychiatry I lost everything job, studies (I was back at university going to become a psychologist), friends not to mention my self-respect, self-worth, hope and dreams. When I got my life back I thought it was only temporary as I had been taught and told that schizophrenia was chronic and incurable.

A friend of mine persuaded me to go to a conference and there I met Jørn, who was talking about recovery, and he changed my life. While Jørn and I were talking, the first time I met him, he asked at one point why was I 'so interested in recovery' and I said, 'Because I think I am one of them.' He looked at me and said very spontaneously 'do you want to work for me' and I equally spontaneously said 'Yes'. That's how I ended working as a recovery coach at the castle (Slotsvænget) and he also introduced me to the Danish Voice Hearing Network which was just about to hold it's first-ever general meeting and become an established network of which today I am the chairperson.

PATSY HAGE

MARIUS ROMME

Patsy Hage is considered to be the figure-head of the 'accepting voices movement' by many voice hearers. She was the start. Her perseverance made me think differently about hearing voices. By publicly talking to me on a TV show about her experiences and the problems she encountered in traditional psychiatry, she started something of which she was personally unaware. Patsy is remarkable in a number of ways. She is one of the few people who in her behaviour continues along the same course, if she considers the arguments reasonable, like talking publicly on TV about her experiences with voices at a time when nobody else did. She is also a person who would never voluntarily seek publicity. After the first World Congress for Voice Hearers in Utrecht in 1987 she distanced herself from the voice-hearing movement. That is why so little is known about Patsy. However, Patsy and her story cannot be omitted from this book.

Patsy was the first person in whom I accepted voices as reality. This possibly also means that she herself has not benefited from this approach as much as the many others in this book. Patsy and I still had to discover all kinds of things. Our research was yet to begin. At that point, we did not know that it was related to threatening incidents.

This story consists of two parts:

1. A brief history of her voice hearing, as she explains to Sandra in an interview in 1998, taped on video for training purposes. By then, she had not been occupied with her voices for a long time, but in this interview she tells Sandra about possible links with her life history.

2. Her recovery story that I described on the basis of my recollection of our conversations. After her marriage, when she felt safe and accepted, Patsy wasn't bothered any more by her voices. At that time she visited us to tell us that in hindsight she had the idea that she herself had created the voices in her head.

A SHORT HISTORY OF PATSY'S EXPERIENCE WITH VOICES

I was 8 year's old when I started hearing voices for the first time. I was in the attic with my brother. We were 'acting'. I had a scarf wrapped around my head and a candle in my hand. The scarf caught fire and I screamed for my mother and whilst on fire I ran down the stairs. I thought I was going to die. I was admitted to hospital with the most terrible burns and that is where I started hearing voices for the first time. Initially the voices were friendly and I talked to them, for example, at the dinner table when my parents were arguing. I could not cope with that. I have never been able to deal with aggression.

When I was 16 years old I ran away from home and I was put into foster-care. I had hoped to get rid of the voices. I believed that the voices were linked to the bad atmosphere at home. If I were to be away from that, they would disappear, but instead they became very aggressive at that time and they dominated me, particularly by refusing me all kinds of things. When I was 18 my father passed away and I went back to live at home again. I started my studies in Nijmegen and the voices were so loud there that I could not concentrate at all on my studies. I failed. I went back home and did a dog-grooming course and I worked in this profession for a while in the garage of my parents. Subsequently I found myself a little house of my own in a pretty unsafe part of town and I was very scared. I more or less locked myself in with the protection of two dogs. I did not go out at all any more as the voices would not let me. At that time, a friend of my mum's referred me to Marius Romme.

RECOVERY, AS RECALLED BY MARIUS ROMME AND CONFIRMED BY PATSY

In the case of Patsy we see a partial recovery. She visited me in 1984. Six months after the voice-hearing congress at the beginning of 1987, she got married. That is when she wasn't bothered anymore by her voices. She raised two children and she lived an independent life with her husband and children. Her issue with aggression has not been resolved. Although she really knows what she wants, she can get insecure very quickly. I will recall what I remember of her therapy here.

From 1984 onwards until her marriage in the second part of 1987, I had regular conversations with her, initially on a weekly, but later on a fortnightly basis. When I met her for the first time, she had some rather noticeable scars on her face and it was apparent what had happened to her. She found it difficult to talk about this, as she was ashamed of it and it formed a barrier in her contact with others. I advised her to visit a beautician in order to learn how to conceal her scars with make-up. This handicap was avoidable and only aggravated her insecurity. She followed my advice and this had a good effect.

She had been referred to me and the referral letter mentioned the possibility of her problem being linked to her difficult father. Since, at that time, I would never have associated problems such as a burnt face, a difficult father and voice hearing with each other, this link was, therefore, never forged and instead we started talking about her then current problems such as housing and the voices. As a psychiatrist I discussed the voices in terms of a symptom of a disease. She was not satisfied with this as my way of talking about voices did not help her. She was impeded by the voices and wanted to know how that could be changed. Medication had not really helped her. The medication made the distance to the voices slightly greater, but at the same time, limited her too, since when she took her medication she could not concentrate well on reading, something she enjoyed doing. Therefore I reduced her medication and taught her to self-regulate it by just taking a little bit more for a few days when she was impeded more than usual. However, Patsy wanted me to accept her voices and to talk about how much they bothered her and particularly to give credence to the reality of the voices. It took her a year to convince me that the voices problem is not the potential disease, but it was the bother that it caused her. At that time she could not talk about the voices in detail either, the voices did not allow her to do so.

Since Patsy could not talk about them, we decided that she would write down her experiences with the voices at home and she would bring her notebook with her so that I could read it and together we could think of the things she could do. From our conversations it became apparent that twice a year she was bothered even more by the voices, sometime in May and sometime in November. It turned out that her original burns accident had happened in November and that her father had passed away in May. At that time I had no idea that the burns accident through the accompanying mortal fear could be linked to hearing voices. Her father's death had been traumatic for her for several reasons. At that time I did not have a clue that voices are often linked to unpleasant experiences, which can also be the reason for their varying intensity. For Patsy these were both the threatening experience of the burns accident as well as the threatening feeling of aggression.

Since Patsy felt very unsafe in her own home and she more or less hibernated in there together with her two German Shepherds, I encouraged her to look for another place. That happened, but she did not feel safe there either. An aunt of hers was able to move in for while which helped. Later, with the help of her mum, she was able to buy a house in a newly developed part of town, not far from her mother. There she felt safe. The people who lived there fitted in with her social experience and it was not far from her mother. The importance of safety is not new in the field of social psychiatry, but that it has a direct impact on the voice hearing was new to us.

During the time that an aunt lived with Patsy, this aunt was also an example how to live a sensible life and in our conversations that also led to us discussing how one should deal with voices. We would find out in which ways one could deal with voices. It turned out that one way of dealing with the voices was to say to them: 'Come back tonight, I'll have time for you then, but not now.' This worked quite well for Patsy and also gave her a feeling of control and more freedom of movement during the day. In those days, we did not know that you could learn to live with voices and in order to achieve that there were a number of practical ways which people could make up themselves too.

Whilst searching, we realised that there seemed to be another way of dealing with voices too, 'anticipating when the voices appear and reviewing how you can deal with these situations in a different way'. Patsy had a new boyfriend again at that time and when they went out, the voices made her go home at 11pm, but that was too early for her boyfriend. If, before they went out, they agreed what time they would go home again and if they stuck to that, the voices would not appear. In our conversations it became apparent that 11pm had always been the time her mother had told her to be home.

During the period that Patsy went out with this boyfriend, she became pregnant by him, but she did not want to marry him, as the voices were rather critical of him and she had not told him that she was hearing voices – that was a bad omen, as such a secret gets in the way of a deeper relationship. Patsy wanted to keep the baby. However, soon she became very insecure and thought she was not pregnant, but that the voices were changing her body and that they would destroy her by destroying her body. This was not a minor problem. At that time, we both agreed on saying: 'You think that the voices will destroy you and I think that you are pregnant. Neither of us knows who is right, but perhaps you want to give me the benefit of the doubt and wait with me for nine months. If you are not having a baby then, I will assist you with suicide and in the meantime I will have you examined by a neurologist every month in order to ensure that the voices are not harming your health.' That is what we did and fortunately a baby was born then.

After the birth of Patsy's eldest son, she moved in with her mum again for a while and following that she moved back to her own home not far from her mother. In the meantime, she had convinced me about the authenticity of her voices and I checked that by asking Patsy to talk to other voice hearers about the voices. In these conversations, it struck me how real these conversations were and how well they understood one another. We repeated this a few times and that is when Patsy told me that she liked knowing that there were other people who heard voices too, but that it did not offer her enough of a solution for her problem with the voices. This was then the trigger to look, together with Sandra Escher, for people who hear voices and who had found a solution to their problem. Therefore, we felt that TV would be the best option as TV reaches every living room. At that point we found a TV talk show ('Sonja op Maandag' by the AVRO) willing to make a programme around voice hearing. However, Patsy had to personally tell her own story. As I mentioned before, Patsy is very consistent and although she found it very scary, she did not feel there was another option for her either. After all, this was a possibility to get closer to a solution for her problem. Sandra, together with Patsy, prepared her story with the TV talk show presenter and carefully discussed the questions that would be asked. In order to create a news item which would serve as the reason for making a talk show about voice hearing, Sandra made up that we were to hold a first voice hearers' conference. There were 700 responses by telephone to the TV programme, of which 550 heard voices and 450 supplied their address details. In conjunction with Patsy, we developed the questions for a survey, which would serve as a contact tool. Some months later, in February 1987, the first congress took place and a network for voice hearers 'de Stichting Weerklank' ('The Resonance Association') was created. The voices movement was born. Together with her mum and her new boyfriend Patsy visited the congress, the secrets had been unveiled. Six months later Patsy got married and our contact reduced to once or twice a year based on mutual interest.

Not long after Patsy got married, she and her husband visited me and she told me that, in hindsight, she had the idea that she had personally created the voices in her head. Together we believed that the acquired safety had been important in making the voices redundant.

For the purpose of this book, I have classified Patsy with the voice hearers who have partially recovered, since Patsy did indeed realise that her voices were strongly linked to her inability to express aggression, but that she had never really learnt how to express this. The safety aspect and not being able to express aggression well, as well as blaming herself for things probably also form the reason that the voices returned sixteen years later. At that time, at her request, she divorced her husband. She started to suffer from the voices again, but she did recognise that the voices were a reflection of her own feelings. However, as a result of her depressive moods, she finds it difficult to distance herself from her self-accusations of being a bad mother. She is not overwhelmed, but she is bothered by the voices. Sixteen years without voices and being able to function well in a family with two children was enough of a reason for me to include her story in this book. For Patsy, voices are a mirror of the soul too, i.e., they reflect her mood.

PEGGY DAVIES

WITH PHIL THOMAS

My name is Peg; I am 64 years old, retired, and living with my friend Sheila in Wales, by the sea. My main activities are of an outdoor nature now: I enjoy walking, bird watching and my Church.

My voices have been with me since my early twenties. They seem to be at their most intensive when I am under pressure and can be of a destructive nature. The voices are in my head, although I am aware of external influences such as a 'little devil' on my shoulder, whispering in my ear. The voices became my constant companions. Although destructive, they were my friends and I did my best to obey them. For example: I should break into a church and remove the sacrament from the tabernacle as the voices told me, I could then cope with my life – one step better than committing suicide, which I had attempted on a previous occasion.

My first experience with psychiatric help purely, suppressed my state of mind and controlled my activities. Then, some years later, as a result of eight years with severe cramp and headaches, I attended a pain clinic. Here I met a doctor who encouraged me to be more open, to talk to her and to Sheila, my friend, of things I had repressed for many years, for example, my adoption and my schizophrenia. I did not talk about the voices as they did not want me to. The plague of ringing headaches disappeared! But the voices did not.

Seven years ago I met Dr Phil Thomas and was relieved to meet someone who was really interested in voice hearing. No one before had wanted to know, in spite of being admitted to hospital for ten weeks, out of control of myself and others. My voices were not at all pleased to be discussed and told me on one occasion, in Phil's presence, to 'shut up and get out', but I did not tell him at that time. Phil had me admitted to Dyll y Cas for two weeks and, with intensive therapy, I found I could be open and discuss my voices; in fact a new one appeared and took over, thus enabling me to cope with the destructive ones. As a result of Phil's work and Sheila's support, I coped very well, handling the voices and enjoying a more positive and free way of life. Previously, I had been repressed and introverted, preferring to stay indoors if I could. It was suggested I no longer needed depot injections and I was weaned off them. Sadly, it did not work for me and I now have a small daily dose of Olanzapine. The voices are back under my control and I scarcely hear them.

Sheila and I have just returned from an expedition to the Antarctic and I thoroughly enjoyed it. I really wanted to participate in all the activities available; something I couldn't have done in the past, I was too afraid. At home, I can now drive the car, just locally, having been too apprehensive for years. I now feel alert and independent, although I do realise the continued support of a friend and a good psychiatrist has everything to do with it.

PETER BULLIMORE

WITH SANDRA ESCHER AND MARIUS ROMME

From the age of 5 to 13 I had a tormentor. You would call this woman an abuser, I call her a tormentor because she not only abused my body she tormented my mind as well. She was a babysitter who used to look after me on Friday nights. At first things were alright, but then she used to put on a television programme called 'Appointment with Fear'. I'd say I didn't want to watch it as it frightened me but she would say, 'You must watch it'; then she would then turn out the lights and we would have to watch it in the dark. Abusers are very clever. She would keep giving me drinks and after a while I would say, 'I want to go to the toilet', and she would say, 'You can go but you are not to put the lights on'. I would be too frightened to go upstairs in the dark and would wet myself. When my parents returned the lights would be on and the television turned off and she would tell them: 'I told him to go to the toilet, but he took no notice.' She was the adult and so they had no reason to disbelieve her. I felt that they would believe everything she said. When you are really frightened of someone they can do anything to you. Once she had gained this power she could do anything she wanted. The abuse was sexual, physical and, some of it, downright disgusting. On occasions, she would bring a friend along to join in. It even got to the point where she would tie a silk scarf around my neck and hang me from the banister. As my eyes rolled she would let me down.

In a sense, you could say the paranoia came first because when I was going through the period of abuse it started to affect my behaviour. I became socially isolated; I wouldn't go out in the school holidays as I felt everyone knew what was going on but no one wanted to help me. They would be laughing about me and making fun of me. My mother told me one day, 'You can't stay in all the time. You must go out', so I would go to a local park where there was a small putting green, and I would get one golf club and two golf balls and I would play golf against something I could hear. I played against a voice. It had no identity or gender; it was just one voice. I think I was about 8.

At first, it was reassuring but, as I got older, the voice took a sinister turn: it told me to hurt others. I think the reason was, because I was getting older, my body was starting to respond to the abuse. I hated the thought of it but found some of the feelings pleasurable. This really confused my mind. My behaviour got out of control and I stopped trusting anyone. I was starting to be seen as dysfunctional. I was playing football with a friend of mine and the voices told me to hit him. It was like my head would explode. I did hit him but couldn't explain why. So then I got hit by my mother.

The lowest point of the abuse came just before my 13th birthday. It was midweek and this woman came round and asked my mother where I was. She told my mother she would go upstairs to help me with my home work but she came in the bedroom and had full sex with me on the bed. I thought, 'What if she's pregnant. I'll get the blame. I get blamed for everything else.' Fortunately she wasn't pregnant, but this gave me the courage to tell my parents that I didn't want her coming round on Fridays anymore. As I could look after myself, they agreed. The abused stopped and I became voice free. I was still fearful of the world and didn't trust anyone, but from 13 to 17 I lived a so-called 'normal' life. I had started work but had never spoken about the abuse.

I met a young woman and fell in love. She was my first love. We went out for a while and she then became pregnant. At this time I was working for a steel firm and there was a recession. I lost my job, my wife then became pregnant again. We now had three children and limited income and the stress was unbearable. The house was going to be repossessed and the bills were mounting up. I eventually found work manufacturing fire surrounds but I was working seven days a week and not making any impression on the debts we had accumulated. I started to feel the world was against me and the voices returned. I was walking home one Friday night with my wages in my pocket and I heard a really loud dominant voice say, 'You are Mickey McAvoy, you are worth millions now.' Mickey McAvoy had robbed a gold bullion security depot years before and I foolishly believed it, so I walked into the nearest bar and bought everyone a drink, thinking I had millions. My wife went mad when I went home with no money and I couldn't explain why I had done it.

Things ebbed and flowed for a while with voices and paranoia. I was then approached by a friend of mine who asked if I would kick-start a business making fire surrounds. He would put up the money if I put in the knowledge. In the first year we turned over one million pounds.

With this came a lot of stress and pressure as we were working eighteen hours a day, seven days a week. Then my wife, unknown to her, became my tormentor. She loved the flash lifestyle with plenty of money but would complain that I was never at home with her and the children. She would ring me when I was working late and start shouting down the phone. I started to feel that a woman was abusing my mind again and with this and pressure of work my life started to spiral out of control.

During this same time there had been a problem at work, a man was shouting down the phone and I told him to 'Fuck off'. My business partner said, 'You can't speak to people like that in business', so I hit him over the head with the telephone and drove home. I stayed there for three weeks. I didn't eat, wash or shave. I sat in a chair, locked in a world of voices, paranoia and depression. Eventually, the doctor came and admitted me to the local psychiatric unit. My wife eventually threw me out of our home as she said she'd had enough. She had found me a flat to go to but never told me it was unfurnished. So I moved back in with my parents til the flat was sorted out. I spent hours walking the streets feeling intimidated by buildings and people. Buildings used to laugh at me.

Over the next years I had many admissions, often on section. I didn't find them helpful as I was taking a combination of many drugs a day. It was like all the system wanted me dead. At this time I was told about a hearing voices group; I went along and it was an amazing experience; I could at last take off the mask I had worn for years; at last I belonged somewhere, meeting people with similar experiences. I then foolishly stopped going. I decided I would evaluate my own life. I used to employ nine people and I hadn't seen any of them since my breakdown. I was starting to think: 'Perhaps they were my disciples and they all betrayed me. Maybe I stopped the voices group because my paranoia was more up-front than my voices.

After one of my last times in hospital, I spent a lot of time doing nothing; my divorce had come through and I felt some pressure had been taken off me. I then met a woman who was younger than me. I was warned not to go out with her as she had a violent past but I thought, 'I've been on my own for a while, in for a penny in for a pound.' At first, things were fine, then, one Friday night, she got really drunk and for no reason smashed a vase into my face and carved my body up like a chess board. I needed fourteen stitches. Me and women don't seem to mix on Friday nights. This went to Crown court and there, for the first time in a long time, I was told that I was right. This was actually the start of my recovery.

PETER'S RECOVERY STORY

It was actually after I had won this court case because someone had slashed my face. I came out of the court and a very good worker called Sally Bramley, who had come with me, asked me how I felt and I said, 'Fine'. She asked me if I had any voices or felt paranoid. When I said no, she said, 'You've just turned the corner in your life, you must build on it. You need to do something.' We went across the road to this pub and all the time she was saying, 'The other hearing voices group is shutting down and I want you to start one.' At first, I was just finding objections but I got a lot of support from Sally; she pushed me to start this group and convinced me I could do it. She kept pushing me and pushing me. Perhaps I needed that push.

I suppose I had become a victim of authority. It had always played a big role in my life and I thought of that babysitter as authority. I have been in trouble with the police who were authority, and the psychiatrist was authority; so I began to think, 'Don't start going against what you can't beat.' I told this to the hearing voices group, to people from the network who came to do a workshop. I spoke to one of the trainers, saying, 'I like the way you work with voices, but yours have identities, mine are all demons. They just sound *horrific,* strange tongues and everything.' He said, 'You have to address the demons of your past.' That was all he said. And when I looked at my life, the demon of my past was my abuser. I still used to see her regularly in Sheffield walking on the street. When I saw that girl I would run away in real fear. Then, one day, I decided I would listen to what this guy had said to me. I would not run away. When I saw her down the street my first idea was to run. My heart was beating but I kept eye contact, I kept walking closer to her. She turned her eyes and looked the other way and I then felt I had altered the balance of power. I didn't have to fear her anymore. It was actually meaningless. It meant nothing. OK, this woman was a tragedy, but so what? I was letting have her power with all the resulting problems: voices and paranoia.

I went home (I lived on my own at that time) and locked myself away for two weeks. I just started to listen to the voices. I used to let them say what they wanted. I could hear the content now. The more I listened – I listened for hours each day – the more I realised there was one dominant voice. Although they were speaking strange tongues, speaking like demons and devils, I realised that there was one voice louder and more critical than the others. I identified the dominant voice and I actually decided I was going to make that voice my abuser. The reason for this was that I was kind of strong in my own mind to do it, and she had destroyed my life enough. The dominant voice was actually an abuser, so I made it her. The tone did not really change but I realised it was actually her and I could start to challenge her. And once I had diminished the fear, I realised the voices could not hurt me and I could actually control my life. It took a lot of time. I got off medication, went back onto it again, and have had hospital admissions from that, but once I diminished the fear, I found a starting point from where I could begin to move, where I had something to recover for. I actually could have a life, even without the voices around. I did not know what that life was but I wanted something. I did not want to be walking about shuffling my feet, stiff with medication. I wanted to function in society. I think I just wanted to do what everybody does: go to the pub, speak to people and not be questioned: 'Why are you walking funny?' I wanted to have a relationship with my kids again.

So I set up a group on support and education. We were getting guest speakers in with different ideas. I read the book *Accepting Voices* and a lot of things related to my life. When I kind of challenged the dominant voices I needed some more focus in life so I contacted the Hearing Voices Network in Manchester. They invited me over to meet them and then I just felt this is what my life needed to be. I have come through a hell of a lot so I like to put something back. I got involved with more training and started doing some writing. I found a purpose again. I had been in business; I had earned a lot of money in business, but it put me in the psychiatric system. So it is not about money now, it's about change. And if you want to change you need to do something. That is the main thing: seeing that people can recover.

Recovery is a very individual thing. You have to define it for yourself. Look at what you are, look for a purpose in life again, because then you can start to move forwards.

I started the paranoia group two years ago. It came about when a psychiatric nurse rang me and said: 'I have this young man who's doing nothing with his life. He just stops in bed, goes to the pub, has a curry and goes back to bed. Can you help him in some way?' I said, 'If you tell him to ring me I'll see what he wants.' He lived quite far from my office, so when he rang saying, 'Can I come to see you?' the easiest option would have been to say, 'I'll come and see you.' But instead, I said, 'You'll have to come and see me.' That was the first step on his journey to recovery – just getting there. He turned up looking very scruffy and I asked him what he wanted to do. He'd trained as a social worker and worked in drug rehab and he said, 'I've got quite good group skills. I used to do a lot of groups and I'm really interested in paranoia. Do you think we could set up a paranoia group.' I said we could try, because there wasn't anything at the moment, and we could finance it from the hearing voices group. So we booked a room, we made a flyer on the computer, photocopied it and sent it everywhere: voluntary, alcohol and drug rehabs, etc. People came up to us and said: 'What's this paranoia group you're starting?' I said, 'It's exactly what it says.' Then they said, 'You've got no chance – people will be too paranoid to come.'

We just booked a room in this old school. We set it for 12.30 on a Tuesday and thirteen people turned up. Fantastic. For example, a worker from Sheffield Mind took a flyer up to his house from the paranoia group. He actually left his home that day, got on a bus and came to the group. I asked, 'Why have you come? ' He said, 'Because I thought it was only me, that I was the only one who suffered with paranoia.' This man wanted to meet others. Two years later his recovery has been fantastic. There is another woman who was in the police force. She saw some police officers beating someone up in a cell. She threatened to report them. They said, 'If you report us we'll make your life a misery.' She did report them and they did make her life a misery. They really bullied her for as long as she was in the police force. She actually had to leave the force. She has a massive paranoia about the police because they said, 'If you breathe another word we'll get you.' So you can see that her paranoia is real. It really took over her life. She is now doing an advocacy course. There were also two women who turned up because their husbands had said they were paranoid. We kind of built up a paranoia network from there. The paranoia group became a success and, now, I am travelling the world delivering training on hearing voices and paranoia to professionals and I also do individual consultancy work, usually with people who have been told by the system that they cannot recover.

PETER REYNOLDS

WITH JACQUI DILLON

Peter is 52 years old and married with two children and four grandchildren. He is currently working as a mental health advocate and is involved in other mental health related work: an advisory group, research, etc. Peter enjoys music, fishing, personal development, cooking and eating, football and spending time with his grandchildren. He also attends a Hearing Voices group.

I hear voices behind me and I also hear them in my ears. They are inside and outside of me. When I was psychotic, I believed that I was being talked to by aliens. I had a conspiracy theory that everybody was against me and taping me, that I was on cameras in the house and that my phone was being bugged. I hear voices but I am not psychotic anymore and it doesn't have the same power over me as it used to. Now, I feel that my voices come from me. They are clouded memories of things that have gone on in my past.

I hear six voices: I have *Socrates*, and he comes along when he fancies. I can't conjure him up but when he comes, he talks of philosophy and psychology and medicine, all sorts of brilliant things. On the bad side, one is *my father*. It is not his voice but it is what he would say. He ridicules me and makes fun of me, just generally taking the piss out of me like my father did. His voice tells me that he never did anything to upset me, which just isn't true. I have the *blasphemer* and he just swears all the time, along with *profanities*, another voice that curses me. There is another one called *dangerous*. He tells me to walk in front of buses and cars all the time; makes me see how close I can get to the railway line on the tube. He's a bastard. He wants me dead, very much like my father did when I was younger. One of the voices is *the man that my mother had an affair with*. He talks to me about my mother sometimes. What he says is crude and horrible. That is the time when I will take medication because he is so destructive and he hurts me so much.

It didn't start off with voices; it started with noises when I was about 9 years old. I could hear whistling noises coming from behind me. They would go up to a peak and then go rapidly down. They had always been in the background as noises I could hear – schoolyards in my head, children shouting and screaming. I think the voices were provoked by my mum and dad's relationship. My mother and father were always accusing each other of sleeping with other people; my father hit me once and said, 'I don't know if you are even fucking mine' – so if that isn't stress for a child then I don't know what is. My mother and father were permanently arguing as I hit my teens and I was trying to deal with puberty as well. A lot was said about sex. Shouting and screaming: 'You took him up your Nan's and fucked him on the settee', and it left me with a sexual problem. I started self-harming; I'd pour surgical spirits and bleach on my genitals; I thought I was diseased; I wouldn't eat or drink in the house as I believed I was being poisoned.

When I was 13, my mum died, so the family disintegrated. Not long after, my father came to me and said, 'I got married and this is your new mum.' This was six months after my mum died. I said, 'She isn't my mother and you are no father to me, I'm moving out.' I had all these unresolved problems, and then I was seduced by my sister-in-law. This happened before I had my children, when I was a teenager, from age 13 onwards. That went on for two years and then I just said, 'I am not doing it anymore, you can tell him if you like', because she would threaten me, 'If you don't continue doing it then I'm going to tell your brother.' She said, 'But you enjoyed it', and there was a part of me that did enjoy it. I was a 13-year-old boy being initiated into sex by an older woman but it was my brother's wife, so it was all very confusing. I was so screwed-up by all that had gone on and I didn't know if I was really my dad's son. I questioned many things about myself but I didn't deal with this until much later on.

Then I met Linda, my wife; I moved to the East End and the stress continued. Firstly, when my son was born and then when my daughter was born. They were really stressful times. I was only 17 when I became a dad. I knew nothing at that age and I had a kid dropped in my lap who I adored and loved, but I just didn't know how to be a father because I'd never had a role model. The voices started the day my daughter was born. I felt like the responsibility was too much for me to handle. I'd go on walking trips for five or six days and come home filthy like a tramp, eat something and get in the bath, go to bed and just sleep. Then a couple of days later I would be off again because I felt like my whole house was alien to me. Everybody wanted something from me, especially when the voices started. In the end I had a physical breakdown caused by mental ill-health.

I first sought help in 1974. I was suffering with delusional depression. I started to self-medicate with alcohol, which led to depression and some psychotic state that I was in. I was on a whole range of drugs at that time and I was in hospital for some months. I was out after about six months but then I relapsed with full-blown voices. They diagnosed me with reactive depression with psychotic episodes. I was having terrible side effects from all the medication. I then got involved with cocaine. I was taking about a gram a day just to get rid of the voices. It worked very well until I tried to stop taking it and realised I was addicted. I spent all my money on it. So then I had to be rehabilitated for that – cocaine and alcohol abuse. I had a lot of hospital admissions: I have been in hospital twenty-five times in the past thirty years, so that's nearly once a year. The longest time I stayed in was two years and four months, mostly in the Intensive Therapy Unit before I was put on one of the wards. I really don't know how people get well in there, I really don't. When you are in hospital you don't have problems because you aren't dealing with them, but as soon as you are discharged, all the shit comes back up again.

They were never interested in the voices; they'd just say, 'Well, what do you think it is? How can you explain it?' They were looking for some insight in me. All the time I was asking: 'What is it, what is it? Tell me'; I wanted to do something about it. I then got diagnosed with bipolar schizoid-affective disorder. I was put on medication for the next fifteen years, but it never got rid of my voices. They left it to drugs to deal with me. I wasn't in any kind of therapy. The last diagnosis I got was paranoid schizophrenia. So I've had the full book – reactive depression; anxiety; agoraphobia; manic depression, schizoid-affective disorder and then, finally, paranoid schizophrenia.

When I first went to the Hearing Voices Group, I was very depressed, very down, almost suicidal, and I didn't speak for about three months. I didn't know if it was safe to talk about my voices because whenever I had spoken before, especially to the medical team, I'd be hit with another drug, so it made me reluctant to tell them what was going on. I discovered that most people had similar problems to me and it was a relief to find out that I wasn't the only one. Everyone seemed to be suffering alone until they came to the group. We exchanged coping strategies, ideas, advice; just being a part of a group helped me a lot. It showed me that there were a lot of people going through similar problems to me and I could relate to that because they were ordinary people with ordinary problems. To be a voice hearer is a lonely thing sometimes and there was a network there for me to engage with. I've done a lot of work on myself but only with the help of the voices group. In the group people say, 'Oh, when I was struggling with that, I did this', and you say, 'Wow, that's a good idea!' We don't dish out drugs, we just listen to people. In the group I spent time talking about my guilt in relation to what had happened between me and my sister-in-law. It's only this year that I dealt with it and it happened thirty-seven years ago. Part of me did enjoy it and part of me wished that it had never happened. In the group I was made to feel that it was OK to enjoy a part of it and that it was wrong to feel guilty about all of it.

It's thirty-two years now that I have been hearing voices. I've learned a lot about myself and about other people. I haven't been back to hospital for nearly six years. I now have insight into my voices, gained through the voices group. I cope very well with them now; I challenge them more than I used to because I have gained confidence and self-esteem; I don't do everything they say. I like it when they get nervous and frightened. I get an internal dialogue going and I question what they ask of me. I say, 'What do you want from me?' Sometimes, challenging the voices makes them have a knee-jerk reaction. When they say, 'Kill yourself you bastard, you are no good', I know that I am better than that now. That was a big change – knowing that I am better than the things they tell me to do. They've changed in many ways; they've changed in content. I still get the blasphemer, but not that often now. I must be doing something good because it's shut up. Socrates I love. My father I don't like, because it's always criticism. The way I deal with it now is that I think of something that I've done for someone else and if I can understand where they are coming from it helps me a lot, feeling connected to people. If my voices try and manipulate me now I just think, 'What can I do to stop them?' I give them space but I won't engage with them and they get bored and piss off. I learned all this at the Hearing Voices Group. When I talk to someone now and they say that their voices are bad, I say, 'Well, what is that about? What is happening?' You do find a reason if you look long enough and hard enough. I've got a network of friends now, they are all voice hearers and we ring each other up when we've got problems and help each other out.

After about two years of attending the group I got involved more in its facilitation and I really grew from that and went on to do bigger and better things. I am now an advocate three days a week; I facilitate the Hearing Voices Group when the facilitators are away. After all, I've had it first hand for over 30 years, so I have a lot of relevant experience. I don't class myself as a schizophrenic – I class myself as a voice hearer.

RINY SELDER

WITH MARIUS ROMME

Riny Selder turned 51 in 2006. She is divorced and has a daughter. She is actively involved in women's support. Together with Flore Brummans and Mien Sonnemans she founded the 'Wilskracht' ('Willpower') Association for women who cannot get psychiatric help. With the help of subsidies they purchased a caravan. It is in this caravan that these women can stay the night without other people knowing of their whereabouts: it is a kind of runaway refuge. Furthermore, the association organises self help groups, for example, a group for voice hearers, as well as social events such as parties, Christmas festivities and holidays.

Similar to Mien Sonnemans and Flore Brummans, Riny's voice hearing is linked to sexual abuse. However, she hears a positive voice. Riny Selder was sexually abused by her brother between the ages of 6 and 13. At the time when the sexual abuse started, Riny's grandma passed away. At that time she started hearing the positive voice of her grandma. She had, in fact, a better relationship with her grandma than her mother. The voice tried to comfort her and assured her that everything would be alright. She told her mother once that she had heard grandma and her mother was livid and said: 'You're crazy and I'm going to have you locked up if you don't stop. You should not mock grandma's death.'

After that Riny never talked about it again, until she told her GP when she was 36. Her GP was very sympathetic and referred her to the regional institute for community mental health (RIAGG). They did help her come to terms with her incest experience, but less attention was paid to the voice. Since she refused medication, Riny was declared 'finished with treatment' after twelve and a half years. They did refer her, however, to a self-help group. She is still actively involved in this. The self help group has helped her as the voices were accepted and she could talk about them in an accepting atmosphere, without being declared crazy.

Riny has only ever heard one voice and that was a positive voice. Since people told her she was crazy, she always thought of herself as different, instead of benefiting from this positive influence. As a result, Riny suffered unnecessarily for many years.

How did you deal with the voice? Did you recognise phases of confusion, better understanding or stability?

As a child I was not confused by the voice. A child does not separate fantasy and reality from each other. Around the age of 15, I started to realise that hearing voices was not normal. My voice was not negative, but a watchful eye over me. I once stood on the Maas Bridge and then I heard a voice telling me not to jump. The voice always tried to get me out of my sombre mood. Initially, around the age of 15 I was sometimes frightened. I would then give in to the voice by withdrawing, in a corner, that's when I felt safe. For me, that was a way of dealing with it. I would often put on some music too. Music helps, it releases my emotions. I feel better then. Later I started to wonder how I needed to learn to deal with the tension (in my body). I started body relaxation. I gradually changed the relationship with the voice too and started to get more of the positive side out of it. Stability only occurred when the general problems were dealt with.

RINY: MY RECOVERY

I have very positive treatment experiences. In 1991 I visited the regional institute for community mental health (RIAGG) for the first time; my therapist was a gem. She really had to drag things out of me. It was six months before I really started talking. Initially we worked on the traumas, the voices were discussed and according to her there was a relationship between the voices and the traumas. To be honest, I have to admit that it was a complete therapy package. First coming to terms with the incest, the voice hearing followed later and after that borderline. The only thing I was frequently told during this initial treatment period was that I would do better if I were to take medication and have myself admitted. I did not consent to this and I endured everything fully awake. This meant that the first thing that broke down was my relationship as the pressure that was put on it became stronger and stronger.

It was then that I really felt that I never received real love at home and that I was not really able to give either. It all got too much for me, expressing 'these feelings' to my ex. Everything I did, I tried to do it like a robot, not showing emotions and definitely not getting intimate, I had lost all respect for myself and did not really know who I was. It was not until later that I started to realise that I was only a human being of flesh and blood and that I was allowed to have my feelings and desires and that I was Riny. However, I had difficulty with that too. The voice, of my grandma, guided me, encouraged me and at that point I wanted to prove myself in all kinds of ways.

For many years, I escaped into my work, increasingly fanatical and increasingly aggressive. Until I reached breaking point. The suicide attempt of my daughter. At that point I did everything to recover and I followed both individual and group therapies in order to get better. Or for want of a better word: learning to deal with it. After twelve and a half years I was finished with treatment with the regional institute for community mental health (RIAGG) and I have now found my niche with the self help groups of Time out. However, occasionally my grandma calls in with her voice and she says: 'Child I am proud of you and I knew you would do it, keep the peace within you.'

Who have contributed most to your recovery?
I owe a lot to my GP, who was there for me day and night. Two very good girlfriends supported me in my search for treatment. I owe a great deal to a therapist at the regional institute for community mental health (RIAGG) she taught me how to talk about it and I started to realise things. Her successor stimulated me enormously to keep going too. The Time Out Association respected and stimulated me. In my case, it took a long time before I had truly accepted my traumatic experiences. I underwent a lot of therapy at RIAGG. That helped me. Following that I started to keep myself busy with voluntary work which gave me more self-esteem. I took more self-initiative and empowered myself as a result. Now I experience that people who have not seen me for a number of years, they don't recognise me any more, in a positive way, that is.

I have only ever had a positive voice, but I still could not cope with it. In the voice-hearing group I experienced the importance of others accepting that you are hearing voices. The voice-hearing group gave me more self-confidence. Others see that you have grown, I kept myself to myself very much, now I am a blossoming flower.

ROBERT HUISMAN

WITH SANDRA ESCHER

Robert could be followed for many years since he took part in the pilot study of the research with children in 1993, followed by the actual study between 1996 and 1999 and finally the follow-up study in 1999, all in all from the ages of 15 to 22.

The first time we met Robert, we were looking for children hearing voices for a congress which was held at Artis Zoo in Amsterdam in 1993. Robert is 15 years old at the time. Robert has been hearing voices from the age of 7. It started with three voices. The death of Claudia was the trigger. Claudia was 4 years old and a classmate of his brother. Her death had a great impact on him. He became very insecure, came home crying to his mum and for a long time he would take a rose to Claudia's mother every single day.

From the age of 4 onwards, Robert was occupied with death. Aged 7 he started hearing voices. They had moved to a house where someone had hanged himself and subsequently he was confronted with Claudia's death. It started with three voices, the voice of granddad. Granddad is a wise voice. He had had a good relationship with his granddad and played lots of games with him. Granddad died after hanging himself. Robert was 4 years old at that time. He also heard a voice of a man and a woman who were about 40 years old.

Granddad's voice is positive, the others negative. For example, when Robert is out cycling and thinking about braking, the negative voice says: 'Cycle on' and granddad's voice says in return 'Stop'. When Robert cycled on he got involved in an accident. The negative voice also interfered at school during a test: 'Why don't you just stop?' The negative ones also threatened, if he did not obey their orders an accident would happen, for example, 'that his mother would die'. The voices usually talk to each other about Robert.

The voices offered advice, helped find solutions for problems (granddad), but also criticised, refused him things, made him angrier, talked at the same time as his conversations and interrupted pleasant activities. Robert does not enjoy the voices. He is scared of them. At the age of 6 i.e., before he heard voices, he visited a child psychologist once because of his mortal fears. When he was 12 Robert also had a conversation with a child psychiatrist, who blamed it on insecurity and who did not want to turn it into an illness. During our conversation, we confirm this thought, all the more because

Robert had been confronted with death in such a dreadful way. His mother strongly supports Robert. His father finds him a bit of a softie, not an unbelievable response.

Sandra Escher meets him again three years later, this time for the first interview of the children's study. He is 18 at that time and occasionally still hears a voice in his head and he thinks that it is someone else. He can have a dialogue with the voices then. He is not scared of them any more and he can pack them off. He can refuse orders. Robert can call up the voices and cut himself off from them. In his daily life, everyone knows about his voices and Robert talks about them when needed and that is not very often any more now. It's been two years now that he has felt that he is in control of the voices. That happened after he had to retake a year at school and suddenly he knew what he wanted: to earn money. He started army training. He did not like school.

At the final interview, another three years later, Robert has grown into a great big fellow who exudes self-confidence. He graduated from the marines. That involved serious physical and mental exertion. He started hearing voices again for a short while, but that ebbed away. His mother is as 'proud as a peacock' of him. He is doing very well. A lot has changed compared to the first meeting when he was fifteen. Robert has moved in with his girlfriend. During the last three months he went to Bosnia as a professional serviceman. Right in front of his eyes, someone of the mine disposal service stepped on a tank mine. There was blood everywhere. At that point, he had expected to hear voices again, but that did not happen. He believes that the absence of the voices is related to his own decision that he does not want them any more.

Robert has been pretty scared of the voices. As a result of his profession, he has learnt to cope with fear differently. 'The fear disappears quicker than you think', he says. At work he needs to concentrate and cannot afford the distraction of the voices. Nobody at work knows about it. He is concerned that if anybody found out, he would be fired. Robert believes that his voice hearing is related with a good guide, with a spirit and with a special gift.

At the follow-up research, Robert still assumes that the death of Claudia, the 4-year-old local girl, was the trigger to the voice hearing, but that he had already been preoccupied with death a great deal anyway. For a long time he remained insecure and did not really know what to do with his life. At a certain point, he realised that the voices threatened, but never delivered the goods and that is when he lost his fear of them. Robert claims that learning to talk about his emotions has been a lasting support against the voices. From the moment he chose for the marines, he got direction in life. He has not been hearing any voices for the last two years.

Over the last twelve months, Robert has been confronted with a number of things. His other granddad passed away, his relationship ended and he moved. At none of these events did he hear a voice. He sees hearing voices as a gift. Mother believes that if we had not visited them in 1993 and had not made hearing voices more acceptable, without calling it an illness, for the family, particularly his dad, things could have looked totally different for Robert now.

RON COLEMAN

MARIUS ROMME AND SANDRA ESCHER

We (Marius and Sandra) would have liked to have started these 50 stories with Ron Coleman, because to many people Ron is very special. We have known Ron since 1991, and seen him change in a way that most people who meet him today find hard to believe.

We met Ron when we gave our first presentation about the accepting voices approach in Manchester. After our presentation there followed three voice hearers, all members of the first self-help group, who each told of their experiences. Ron was one of them. He had prepared a written speech and hardly looked up from the paper. He looked slightly paranoid, locked up within himself, and had a poverty of movement. Ron's physiognomy was exactly as one tends to see in psychiatry of a person diagnosed with schizophrenia; a diagnosis given to him by Dr Alec Jenner, Professor and Head of Department of Psychiatry at the University of Sheffield.

We kept in contact with Ron, and over the years have seen him gradually grow out of his withdrawn situation of neglect and dysfunction, and overcome his anxieties. One example of many is from the time when the accepting voice approach was first on the move, and we were invited along with Ron and Phil Thomas, to give presentations in America. Since we were coming from different countries we agreed to meet at Chicago airport. Ron arrived dressed in his Scottish kilt. His reasoning was: 'If the plane crashed then I'd be recognised'! By then he had already set out to become the businessman he is today; he was carrying a very old and heavy trunk, tied up with a colourful rope because it was difficult to close, and containing books about the accepting voices approach which he intended to sell.

It took him three to four years to recover from the social drawbacks as a consequence of the psychiatric illness concept. People encountering Ron today find it hard to believe that this man, with his fabulous way of presenting and discussing his experience and ideas, was once diagnosed schizophrenic and presented all the behaviour that is generally associated with this diagnosis. When confronted with Ron's 1991 diagnosis people often say: '... but he must have been wrongly diagnosed.' Whilst we do not want to debate diagnosis, the experience of people like Ron provides evidence that voice hearers, regardless of how psychiatry may see them, can change considerably if given the chance. We doubt that anyone in the Manchester audience, when

Ron first told of his experiences, could have predicted his development. Ron himself saw his opportunities, and took them.

Ron developed as a hard-working, inspiring speaker, who has a talent for convincing people of the necessity for a different approach to mental illness. Over time he has built up a business and promoted the experienced-based movement all over the world. With his thriving business, in which his wife Karen also participates, he provides his family with a good life. Ron has become a family man. With Karen he has a large family of seven children. Ron is also very much appreciated due to his remarkable capabilities in helping voice hearers, presenting his knowledge and, not least, for his ability to relate emotionally to people.

Ron has published a lot about his own recovery process. We have composed this story from two books; firstly from an interview with Sandra Escher for the second Dutch edition of *Accepting Voices* (Romme & Escher, 1999) and, secondly, from Ron's story of recovery in his book *Recovery: An Alien Concept* self-published by Handsell in 1999. He now resides in the Isle of Lewis, Scotland.

The following story by Ron is taken from a translation of the Dutch second edition of *Accepting Voices* (Romme and Escher, 1999). He says: 'In the book of Romme and Escher *Accepting Voices* three phases have been described. These phases are experienced by voice hearers while learning to cope with their voices. The first is called the startling phase, because the onset of hearing voices is often quite sudden, startling and anxiety provoking. This first phase can be long-lasting, taking much time because the voice hearer often receives no help to move to the next phase, the organisational phase, where the voice hearer is motivated to gather proper information about hearing voices, and starts to change his relationship with his voices.

'I had been in the startling phase for eight years. I received many different kinds of medication; Clozaril, Methotrimeprazine, Lithium, Procyclidine and Clomipramine. The voices kept coming and the response from the psychiatrist was to increase the dose or change the kind of medication. No matter what was done the voices persisted and they were called 'residual symptoms'. I did not agree with this. This was not some 'left-over', these were real voices.

'My life was just a mess, a total mess. I had nothing anymore, and wasn't interested in anything anymore. I stayed in bed for about twenty hours a day. I did not want to talk to anybody. I was only interested in what was happening in my head.

'In the self-help hearing voices group I met Helen Heap and Anne Walton. They helped me to enter my organisation phase, where I started to organise my life again. They told me that I had to start thinking about my voices in a different way. I started to do that and probably gave Helen and Ann a very hard time. After about two years I decided to change my opinion. One morning I woke up and thought: 'This is enough. I do not want to take medicine anymore.' From that moment on I stopped. The next three weeks were like living in hell. After that I started to explore my voices. I decided where my voices came from. The voices were there because, as a small child I was physically and emotionally ill-treated by my father. The voices were also there because when I was 11 years old I was sexually abused by a Roman Catholic priest. I could tell nobody because I thought that he, the priest, stood between God and men. I had the idea that it was my fault because he said I had provoked his behaviour, I was leading him into sin and that I was evil. Around that time my relationship with my father changed. He had sorted out his own problems and he started to support me. At school I took a special position. At school I was not punished anymore, because sports were valued very highly. I played rugby very well. That is the reason that at that time I did not become ill.

'The voices were there because when I was 17 my partner Annabel had committed suicide. She was an artist, she taught me about values and emotions, about art and music. One evening I came home after playing rugby and found her on the couch. She was six months pregnant with our baby. I thought that everything was a lie. I was not open to consolation. I decided to cut off my emotions. On Friday the funeral took place. After that I destroyed everything of hers in our flat. On Saturday I signed in to the army. I denied every emotion and closed myself off. I chose as my surviving strategy to have control over all relationships, over all my emotions, but I also chose the expression of controlled aggression. The army is all about control and aggression, as is rugby.

'In the army I studied accountancy. I passed exams, and with the help of a head hunter, got a job outside the army. I was ruthless in negotiations. I was promoted, but nobody wanted to mix with me socially. In a rugby match I met with a serious accident. I broke my pelvis. I was in a hospital for a month. To my astonishment the rugby team came to visit me. I thought that no one liked me. I believe this team visit opened the door to my emotions. When I went back to work I started hearing voices. I sat at my desk and somebody called me; there was nobody present, but it went on. It was a destructive voice. I left my desk, went to the pub, and drank. A lot! But the next day they were there again. Aggressive voices.'

RECOVERY

In Ron's book *Recovery: An Alien Concept* he says: 'Any recovery journey has a beginning, and for me the beginning was my meeting with Lindsay Cooke, my support worker. It was her who encouraged me to go to the hearing voices self-help group in Manchester at the start of 1991. It was her not me who believed that a self-help group would benefit me. It was her who saw beneath my madness and into my potential. It was her faith in me that kick-started my recovery.'

Other people

'There are other essentials required for a journey to be successful; one of these is the ability to be able to navigate to your desired destination. In this I was fortunate not to have one navigator but many. After Lindsay Cooke, the first is Anne Walton, a fellow voice hearer, who at my very first hearing voices group asked me if I heard voices and when I replied that I did, she told me that they were real. It does not sound much but that one sentence has been a compass for me showing me the direction I needed to travel.

'The second is Mike Grierson. Mike was the person who navigated me through my first contact both with my voices and with society. He encouraged me to go out and socialise with people who had nothing to do with the psychiatric system. Mike was also one of the people who helped me to focus on my voices in a way that allowed me to explore my experience.

'The third and fourth are Terry McLaughlin and Julie Downs. Terry and Julie were my navigators back to normality, they rekindled my interest in politics and took me into their family without reservation. It was with Terry that I developed much of my early thinking around training and mental health. My fifth person is Paul Baker. Paul, who brought the Hearing Voices Network to the United Kingdom, encouraged me to become involved in the network. To all these navigators I owe my sanity.

'Navigators require a map or a plan from which to navigate, and I have been fortunate in the people who were my mapmakers; Patsy Hage, Marius Romme and Sandra Escher. I do not believe that these three fully understand what they have done. Little did Patsy know that the questions she asked were going to affect so many people. Indeed it is because of her questions that the Hearing Voices Network and Resonance and other networks throughout the world exist today. Whether she wants it or not she has a premier place in the history of the hearing voices movement.

'Sandra Escher is without doubt the person who made sure that ordinary people could understand the maps that were being made. Her ability to put across the message in language that is accessible to everyone has meant that their work has not remained in the world of academia but has been used by voice hearers from the very beginning.

'The final mapmaker is Marius Romme, Marius who in his own words is a 'traditional' psychiatrist. When he listened to Patsy Hage and explored what she was saying, it was then, in my opinion, he stopped being a traditional psychiatrist. When he asserted in public for the first time that hearing voices was a normal experience and that voice hearing was not to be feared, he stopped being a traditional psychiatrist. For many years I had argued that there is no such thing as mental illness, this has led me into some interesting debates. One of these debates was with Marius Romme, and during this discussion it became clear that Marius was not arguing a case for biological illness. What he in fact was saying was that illness could be expressed as a person's inability to function in society. This I can accept as it means that recovery is no longer a gift from doctors, but the responsibility of us all. This raises the question of whether society is prepared to take any kind of responsibility for the recovery of people with mental health problems. For example, in the Aboriginal culture when someone goes mad the whole tribe comes together to discuss what the tribe has done to cause the person to be mad. Can you imagine this happening in our cultures? I think not. When someone goes mad in our culture it is off to hospital with them.'

Self

'If people are the building bricks of recovery then the cornerstone must be self. I believe without reservation that the biggest hurdle we face on our journey to recovery is ourselves. Recovery requires self-confidence, self-esteem, self-awareness and self-acceptance. Without this recovery is not just impossible, it is not worth it.

'We must become confident in our own abilities to change our lives; we must give up being reliant on others doing everything for us. We need to start doing these things for ourselves. We must have the confidence to give up being ill so that we can start being recovered. We must work at raising our self-esteem by becoming citizens within our own communities, despite our communities if need be. I am convinced that when we grow confident about who and what we are, we can then be confident about who and what we might become.

'For me these four selfs; self-confidence, self-esteem, self-awareness and self-acceptance, are the second stepping stone on the road to recovery.'

Choice

'The third step is closely related to the second and it is rooted in our own status. We can choose to remain victims of the system. We can also choose to stop being victims and become victors; we can choose to stop feeling sorry for ourselves and start living again. This for me is the third stepping stone: 'choice'. The recovery road however demands that we not only make our own choices but that we take responsibility for all our choices good and bad.

As we make choices we will make mistakes. We must learn to see the difference between making a mistake and having a relapse. For it is the easy option to go running back to the psychiatric system when we make mistakes. Rather than face our own weaknesses we fall into the trap of blaming our biology rather than our humanity.

Ownership
'Ownership is the key to recovery, we must learn to own our experiences whatever they are. Doctors cannot own our experiences, psychologists cannot own our experiences, nurses, social workers, support workers, occupational therapists, psychotherapists, carers, and friends. Even our lovers cannot own our experiences. We must own our experiences. For it is only through owning the experience of madness, can we own the recovery from madness. The journey through madness is essentially an individual one; we can only share part of that journey with others; most of the journey is ours and ours alone. It is within ourselves that we will find the tools, strength and skills that we require to complete this journey, for it is within ourselves that the journey itself takes place.

'Recovery has become an alien concept, yet nothing I have talked about so far is based on rocket science, rather it is based on common sense; it is not anything new, it is merely a reiteration of a holistic view of life. We need to realise that sometimes we, all of us, make things much more difficult than they need to be. It is almost as if we need life to be a rocket science that we can never understand. We seem to spend much of our time making the complexities of living even more complex through our appliance of scientific objectivity rather than exploring our lives through the simple mechanism of personal subjectivity. The time has come to have a close encounter with an alien concept, it is time for recovery.'

RONNY NILSON

INTERVIEW WITH GEIR FREDRIKSON

I am 21 years old. I completed primary school and some courses at secondary school. Since then, I have done some part-time jobs. Music is my greatest hobby and I play the guitar.

I remember clearly the first time I heard voices. I was 11 and was visiting a family member who was hospitalised in an institution for drug addicts. Out in the institution's garden there was a tree and for some reason I put a small coin into a crack in the tree's bark. Then, suddenly, I heard a voice inside my head saying, 'You will also end up here, sometime.' At that time I didn't give it much thought. The next time I heard voices was when a relative of mine was sent to a special school for children suffering from behavioural difficulties. The same voice once again appeared saying, 'One day you will end up here.' To begin with, the voice was not present very often. I didn't think of it as hearing voices but rather as my own thoughts speaking loudly to me. However, at the same time, I had this notion that the voices represented something outside me, something I could not control.

There was mainly one voice that spoke to me: a negative one of a man in his 40s. He told me his name was Bjørn. I heard the voice in my head. My voices increased when I left home to start school. I struggled a lot with anxiety and confusion. After a while I was sent to a psychiatric clinic where my psychiatrist asked me if I heard voices. I answered, 'No.' My psychiatrist was glad to hear that. 'Otherwise we would have to hospitalise you in a psychiatric institution', he said. I got scared and decided not to tell anyone about my voices.

At that time I met a girlfriend and the voices grew more troublesome. They told me I wasn't good enough for her and that she wasn't good enough for me. We moved in together and moved to another place, and the problems only got worse. The voices were more frequent and very aggressive. They criticised my girlfriend and spoke very negatively about me and others. They told me not to trust anybody, to hit people and to kill them, or myself. After a while the relationship between me and my girlfriend came to an end. I went into a period of heavy drinking, became very confused and suffered from a lot of anxiety. I tried to kill myself, which resulted in being taken into a psychiatric institution. During that period I was in and out of institutions several times. I was asked if I heard voices but no more than that. I received antipsychotic medication, but the voices were still there.

I was admitted to another psychiatric hospital where I received treatment for psychosis and depression. I was kept in isolation for periods of time because I was regarded as threatening and aggressive. Some therapists asked me a little about my voices but I refused to talk about them. I would only confirm that I heard voices. I now received huge doses of benzodiazepams, because, I believe, they wished to calm me down. When I was drugged I more or less didn't care about the voices.

The voices made me scared and depressed. They really tormented me at that time. They gave me orders to kill and hit people and if I didn't do it, they told me to take my own life. I never gave much thought about the reason why I heard voices. But I had one explanation: I believed it was brain damage, and I settled for that. It seemed logical and not so frightening. Today I don't believe it is brain damage but a consequence of the traumas I experienced whilst growing up. At that time I had little influence on the voices. I tried in vain to talk to them. I also shouted at them and asked them to disappear, but they only grew worse.

Antipsychotic medication has never helped with the voices. Sedatives helped to some extent as they enabled me to get some sleep and feel more indifferent towards the voices. When listening to music the voices disappeared.

Currently, I don't hear voices, but when I started to work with and to relate to them I mostly used coping strategies like answering the voices with 'Yes' or 'No' and I made appointments to talk to them. To begin with, this method did not prove especially effective, but my therapist encouraged me to carry on. Gradually I succeeded.

I learnt about the Hearing Voices Network when I was transferred to a department for young clients at the hospital. There, I met Mr Geir M. Fredrikson who became my therapist. He was dedicated to voices. At that time I was depressed and periodically psychotic but Geir's interest in my voices and the way he worked with them made me curious. He gave me a lot of information and told me about other people who heard voices who had recovered, among them Ron Coleman. This gave me hope. Working this way changed my view on hearing voices. He related to my voices as if they were real. The support from my cousin Hildegunn through this whole period was precious. I also received good support from my family.

During the work with Geir we talked a lot about voices in general. He told me about coping strategies which I tried out. After some time we started working with my life story. Whilst I was growing up I experienced threats and violence which made me very anxious. I was often bullied at school. We worked with what the voices were actually talking about and the way they talked. After I was hospitalised, against my will, I started hearing a new voice.

I named it Grandfather/God. This voice was critical of how I was but it was actually trying to be positive and make me become nicer.

One day during a therapy session, Geir said, 'Do you know what Marius Romme says about aggressive voices? He says that when a person hears aggressive voices one can presume that the person has unresolved issues with aggression.' I immediately recognised myself. I started to talk about my aggression, where I directed it and about my violent fantasies which frightened me. In fact, I spoke about my whole life and how anxious and angry I have been, which was reflected by my voices. We worked with my anxiety, anger and the traumas I had experienced. After a while, the voices started to change. They were not so angry any more. It was possible to talk to them and they would listen to me. For long periods of time they would be completely gone. My relationship to the voices changed and so did the voices; my life changed. I was released from hospital and am now living by myself. I take no medication – I don't need it and I feel much better. I have friends. I have become a father to twins, and I have a part-time job. In my spare time I occupy myself with music – I play in a number of bands. I have become really dedicated to the Hearing Voices Network, and would like more people to learn about this way of relating to voices. Together with Geir I facilitate a group for people that hear voices. Geir and I travel a lot around Norway where we give lectures and conferences about hearing voices.

Looking back at the problems I have had, it was essential for me to get them treated by someone who was interested in me as a whole person. That was the foundation for my recovery.

Translated from Norwegian by Mr. Thore Brevik

RUFUS MAY

My name is Rufus May, I am 39. I have a partner Rebecca and two children Gregory (8) and Nathan (6). When I was 18 I was treated as an inpatient in East London for my unusual beliefs and bizarre behaviour. I was diagnosed with hebephrenic schizophrenia. After fourteen months of treatment I stopped taking the neuroleptic drugs (against medical advice). I used drama, dance, art and part-time employment, as well as the support of a close friend, to recover. After a number of different jobs I eventually studied psychology and trained as a clinical psychologist. I now work as a clinical psychologist with people in adult mental health services. I did not find being given a diagnosis of schizophrenia helpful; it stopped many people trying to understand my experiences or see me as a full human being with abilities and potential.

For as long as I can remember I have had a good ability to daydream and this has helped me to develop creatively. It also meant during stressful times, I was able to separate off my consciousness and, to some extent, escape into a dream world of heroes, monsters and special powers. I was an expert daydreamer, filling boring moments with such dreams. Sometimes it was intentional but, at other times, I got lost in my own thoughts when people were trying to talk to me. The dream would grab me and, meanwhile, I would pretend to be listening to the other person, and guiltily nod in what I thought were the right places. I also dabbled with drug taking in my teenage years, smoking cannabis quite heavily from the age 15 to 17.

At the age of 18 I found myself in a boring job as an office junior. I was anxious about my future – I had failed in my education and I had failed to get into the advertising business. On top of this, emotionally, I was struggling to adjust to the fact that my first girlfriend, who I had been with for a year, had left me. This left a big hole in my life. In hindsight this emotional loss echoed an earlier experience of abandonment I'd had when I was 11 years old: my mother had had a brain haemorrhage and had suffered some brain damage. Although she recovered, she had some personality changes which I found difficult to adapt to. My educational achievement went markedly down after this event (and stayed low for the rest of my schooling). Also, I found myself socially isolated; my best friend was in Germany and I was trying to avoid my former dope-smoking friends. I felt socially 'left out in the cold'. My ex-girlfriend and all her friends were planning to go to university, while

I seemed to have chosen a very boring career as a trainee draughtsman. Instead of getting depressed I gradually entered an alternative reality that had spiritual undertones. My experiences also included the television and radio talking to me and beliefs that I was a spy, involved in a science fiction-like battle between Russia and England. I was eventually admitted to hospital after I complained that I had a gadget in my chest that was being used to control me.

I found psychiatric treatment very oppressive; the drugs I was being given slowed my thinking down and made me weak and impotent. Nobody talked to me about my experiences and ideas. They thought this would encourage them and make them worse. Because my grandfather and aunt had been given diagnoses of schizophrenia, doctors were convinced I had a condition they assumed was genetic. My parents were told I would have to take the drugs for the long term; I could not bear this idea and this put us into conflict. During my hospital admissions I started to pick up on the behaviours of the other patients. I would act very mad and seem dangerous in order to protect myself. During the first admission I felt very frightened and demoralised. However, during my second hospital admission my close friend Catherine returned from abroad and started to visit me almost every day. She showed me an acceptance that was deeply healing. She believed I would get through this 'breakdown' and make a recovery. Her positive and accepting approach had a dramatic effect on my attitude towards my situation. My rebellious nature was also helpful in that I refused to accept the schizophrenia diagnosis. I refused to accept that my 'madness' was a meaningless product of a brain disease. I felt my unusual experience and ideas were part of a spiritual journey and made sure I avoided people who treated me in a patronising way. I witnessed fellow patients being neglected while doctors focused on medicating away their unusual experiences. One friend took her life while on heavy doses of neuroleptics and I became determined to try and challenge this narrow-minded approach to her problems.

I had a strong story of hope in my own family. I had witnessed my mother making a strong recovery from her brain haemorrhage and resulting disability through a combination of her own will and determination and support from others. I think I used this as a blueprint for my own recovery. I sought out community centres, churches, drama classes and later dance classes as places to connect with others and express myself. I used prayer and chanting to try to heal myself. Being detained under the Mental Health Act made me feel I was being punished. I believed that I needed to change myself morally in order to climb out of the psychiatric system and back into society. I vowed to make myself useful to the community so that it would not lock me up in future. At the same time I was always convinced that my ideas and experiences made sense in some way. I gradually came to see them as an emotional reaction to the break-up of my relationship with my first girlfriend, which had triggered some deeper emotional conflicts. This realisation came through a number of conversations with different friends.

While I did not agree that I had a serious mental illness, I did believe I was emotionally exhausted and had to relearn social skills and new ways to express myself that would not get me locked up. I knew I had to keep occupied to help my mind get back on an even keel. I tried lots of things and, if they didn't work, I moved onto something else, refusing to give up. A pastor at a local church supported me to set up a youth club. When I ended up getting readmitted, he visited me and prayed with me. I started doing odd jobs as voluntary work in a community centre. I tried to exercise regularly, though I found this difficult on the medication I was on. I eventually managed to get a part-time job as a security guard in a cemetery. The job involved walking at night in the heavily wooded Victorian cemetery. I think this was a very healing activity, being close to nature and having to face my fears of the dark and the unknown. I did a lot of art work in hospital to try and express what I was feeling and thinking, and I used some of this to get into art college, where I went for a few months. I had been on a fortnightly injection for about six months due to my reluctance to take medication. I had a hand tremor that was affecting my painting. I also felt emotionally blocked. I asked the doctors to take me off the medication. They refused, so I did it independently. I had by this time left home and was living with friends in a fairly liberal squatting community. When I had some sleepless nights and a few unusual ideas, people were pretty tolerant, whereas my parents might have panicked and notified mental health services. I got a job as a motorcycle courier, which kept me occupied. After a couple of years, I decided to return to education so that I could eventually train to be a clinical psychologist. I was determined to try and be part of a movement that would try to change the way society approaches mental health problems. This quest to go back into the psychiatric system as a professional – and to show that there are alternatives to biological psychiatry that are more helpful – became an important source of meaning in my life.

I now live with my family in a small village in Yorkshire. I work in mental health services as a clinical psychologist, which I have done for the last nine years. Since my breakdown in my late teens, I have been pretty healthy, physically and emotionally. It was as if it released something for me and allowed me to make important changes to how I live my life. I did have a bit of a problem with sporadic anger outbursts in my twenties and early thirties which only my partner generally witnessed. I have largely resolved that problem in the last five years using mindfulness meditation practice. I still enjoy creative activities, including dance, drama and storytelling. Over the last eight years I have become quite involved in the hearing voices movement, setting up groups, doing individual work and training. I do not use psychiatric diagnosis when I am helping people but instead focus on helping them to develop a framework that respects their unique experiences and life story. I share the hearing voices movement's values that voice hearing, visions and unusual beliefs are meaningful experiences which need to be listened to and made sense of. In my work listening to people's accounts of their voices, I have learned a great deal. I see people's voices as messengers of meaning. The voices often have clues to, or information about, injustices the person has experienced that they have not been able to come to terms with. The difficult voices often seem to be a challenge to the person to gain a greater sense of authority and authorship in their lives. I spend some time on public education work, where I try to share stories of people's recovery journeys through various media. I believe that, if we can educate people to respect voice hearing and other unusual experiences, there will be a big pressure on psychiatry to change; to stop just trying to repress these experiences, rather than understanding them and helping people to live with them and get on with their lives.

RUTH FORREST

I am a 27-year-old woman in training to become a mental health nurse. When I was small I was never confident; I was bullied at junior school, emotionally rather than physically. I was always left out and made fun of. I wanted to be cool but other people would do things like pretend that I was invisible, then, when I picked something up, they would say it was floating, as if I wasn't there. They blamed me for everything: if something was missing, they would point at me and say that I'd stolen it. There was no way to fight back because whatever I said, they would turn it against me or make a joke of it, so I felt hopeless and out of control. My parents were supportive and helped to have me moved to a different class at school, but everyone knew about me, so it was just as bad. They encouraged me to be stronger but, although this was meant to help, I didn't know how to do it. I see junior school as the unhappiest time in my life – the bullying finished at the end of junior school. At secondary school, my life improved. On my first day, I met a popular girl who lived in the same street as me; she liked me and helped me to make friends. But I was still very unsure of myself and continued to feel I was left behind others I was friends with, and I felt this way in the short relationships I had with boys from then on. It always seemed that people would like me until they got to know me well, then they didn't want me anymore. I carried on feeling that people could only like me if they didn't really know me. Still as a student I was not sure about myself. I felt I was left behind.

I started hearing a voice six years ago, when I was 21 and in my third year of university studying psychology. Before the voices, I'd been sad for a long time. I had the idea that I let people down. I felt guilty about a lot of things. At the time the voice started, a boyfriend had just broken up with me, and I felt rejected and really upset about it. I felt nobody wanted me. I'd had other short relationships that had always ended with the other person breaking up with me. The first time I heard a voice I was in my room at night, it was a man's voice. He was saying that he could see me and would come and find me, he knew about all the bad things I had done and he threatened to tell other people. He sounded as if he was outside the room, so I barricaded myself in. I was really scared because he said that he was coming in, and then that he was in sight of me, although I could not see anything. The next day, when the voice had stopped, I thought I must be going mad, that I must have been drinking too much, that my life was too hectic. The next night the voice came back, always very loud and always at night. Over the following month, more voices came. I was afraid that my friends in other rooms would hear these voices because they were so loud. They were all men, insulting and threatening me, telling me that everyone was going to know what I was really like, that every time I was able to make friends they would see that I was a horrible person. I was always very sensitive about how I came across to other people. I accentuated the negative and was always apologising. However, since living in Sheffield, I have stopped apologising all the time. I now know that it make things worse and I have learnt to forget about small things.

After about a month of hearing voices, I took an overdose. It was not a suicide attempt but an attempt to get into hospital for some help. In hospital, I asked them to cut out part of my brain. I was desperate. I couldn't sleep anymore. They put me on a drip and I was quite drowsy, so I slept. Although I remembered telling them about the voices when I had arrived, they simply told me that I had been incoherent, so, when I woke up, I decided it would be better to go along with that and say that I had just been distressed and confused. They discharged me – I knew this was the best thing to say if I wanted to avoid being kept in hospital. They had been concerned about my weight but I was already seeing a psychologist about my eating and mood problems. When I came out of hospital the voices were as bad as when I went in. I then went home for the summer to Bristol, to my parents. The voices were less of a problem in Bristol. I didn't do much that summer and I slept better since I was doing a lot of exercise. Living at home and not being surrounded by too many people made life easier.

After the summer, I went back to Edinburgh to do the fourth and final year of my psychology degree. The voices got bad again as soon as I returned to university. I just got into a routine: woke at six; exercised until the voices stopped; studied at the library; found someone to have lunch with; returned to the library; met someone for coffee, then studied again until I could find someone to drink with and stay out as late as possible. I would find people to be with and get drunk; then I could go home and fall asleep because I was able to block out the voices through alcohol. In this way I managed to finish my psychology degree. I got a first, living two different lives.

I went to India after graduating. I wanted to get away from everything to do with how my life was in the UK, and the lifestyle I was somehow maintaining. In India I began to think about the voices in terms of voices of God. Having never been religious, I began to go to mass each day, and I became serene and happy. I gave a lot of meaning to the voices and wanted to stay but I had to earn money so, after nine months, I returned to England. Having earned enough money I returned to India, believing that I would become a nun, but, when I arrived, they didn't want me as a nun. After that, India seemed different. It had no meaning for me and the people didn't seem warm any more; I became frightened and reclusive. However, I stayed for six months as I was afraid to return home. When I finally did return, I moved to Sheffield to live with my long-term boyfriend. We had been friends for many years and we moved in together after a couple of months. I had not told him about the voices but I felt very safe having somebody in the same bed. I was less panicky and afraid of the voices.

When I told James (my boyfriend) about the voices he said that my behaviour seemed to make more sense. He did not have any prejudices or preconceptions. He was accepting and supportive of me and said I could always wake him up if I was afraid. He did not interpret the voices as weird, and when I heard singing and thought it was about me, he would explain that it was a football song, not about me at all. He normalised my experience. He also said nice things about me, the opposite of what the voices said, and that was also helpful. This gave me a better feeling about myself: I thought, 'He knows me and he likes me.' He stimulated me to do what I wanted to do, to work in mental health. I had had that in the back of my mind since the age of 15 and the depression experience. He encouraged me to believe that I was more than capable of becoming a mental health nurse. I didn't want to become a clinical psychologist because of the people I had met in the profession and it being too much theory-driven; neither, I thought, were the best setting for helping people.

So I started my nurse training. The voices were under control then. They were usually there only at six in the evening when I was tired. I would have a drink, just to feel more relaxed, not to go on drinking as I had at university. The voices would still wake me up. I would put on my Walkman, have a cup of tea, get up and go running. Then I started to think about why I felt stressed. Before the nurse training, when I had been working with old people, I had not been stressed, but now I was. I was stressed more because I was surrounded again with people of my own age telling me about voices and schizophrenia as if it were all facts.

RECOVERY

That was when I started to go to the hearing voices group. I wanted to train as a nurse, to be able to change, to do things differently.

The hearing voices group:
- gives me the vocabulary to talk about what I experience
- means that I can listen to others talking about things I can relate to
- has to do with feeling accepted and normalising the experience (it is not that weird anymore, it is experienced by all the others)
- is about being honest about yourself (like when you have a stressful week, how that is experienced emotionally
- understanding the relation between the stress and what the voices say)
- is like talking about the whole of my life, the whole of me, because others understand
- has stimulated me to gain more insight: my main voice is the voice of someone who treated me badly when I was young. I no longer feel myself so much a victim since becoming conscious that I was not in the wrong

REFLECTION

From a young age my confidence was low and I sought reassurance from other people, which I did not get because I was ignored and bullied at junior school. As I got older I still desperately wanted to be noticed and appreciated. When I had only just started secondary school and was at a vulnerable age, an older man began to pay me attention, and this made me feel more worthwhile. Other friends began to have boyfriends and this man was complimenting me and listening to me. So when he started wanting me to do things for him (sexually) he did not have to physically force me, but he persuaded and manipulated me. This was when he changed in his attitude towards me and started to make me feel guilty and responsible for what I was doing. As he had never physically harmed me, it was easy for him to convince me that it was all my fault and had been my choice. When I took the overdose I wanted to die because I believed that nobody else cared about me, that he was the only person who was interested; yet I knew what I was doing for him was wrong, and I had started to think that he hated me. However, after the overdose, I realised that my family and many of my friends did care a lot, but, of course, they did not know about all the terrible things I had been doing with this man. Therefore I assumed that they only loved me and cared for me because they didn't really know the truth about me. At the same time, this man was threatening to tell everyone about what I had been doing.

I think what I have taken from this is a continued belief that people can only like me if they don't know me and a fear that if they knew the truth about me they would not be able to like me. Yes, I think the reason that I got involved with the older man in the first place was because I was sensitive to people's opinions of me and desperately wanted to be liked. I have always felt unsafe around people of my own age as I care too much about what they think of me and am afraid of being unpopular. The voices (his voice in particular) began when I was around a lot of young people and still feeling very secretive about what had happened, so his threats that they would find out (or overhear) were very real and very frightening and made me worry that I would lose everything in my life. Even now he threatens to expose me and every bad thing I have ever done, not just my involvement with him. This includes small mistakes I have made and things that I think are wrong but other people tell me are not that significant. The other voices are similar but generally just talk about me negatively, rather than threatening me or talking to me directly.

I am beginning to come to the conclusion that not being as secretive about my past may be the way to defeat the voices. If I can come to terms with what happened and be honest about it, as well as recognising that it was not all my fault, then he will have nothing left to threaten me with. He can't expose me if I expose myself. This is not something I intend to do in a big dramatic rush, but I think that gradually exploring and accepting my experiences will help me to develop. I am hoping to find a way to do this with a person I trust, who will help me through this.

SASJA SLOTENMAKERS

MARIUS ROMME AND SANDRA ESCHER

Sasja lived in the same village as us and knew that we were involved in voice hearing. She came because of her voice hearing and after a short-term therapy she participated in the children's study, which was at the beginning of July. She had finished secondary school in Maastricht and in September she was going to read communication studies at the university in Nijmegen. Participating meant that she could keep in touch and do us a favour at the same time. Sasja lives with her parents; her older sister has already left home and lives in student accommodation in Nijmegen.

When she came to us, it was more as a fellow villager than a patient. However, a therapeutic relationship develops, since she is looking for help with her voices experience as it scares her. At that time she is 18 years old. She talks fairly easily and openly about her voices, and about her life, so much so that immediately during our first encounter, we make an appointment for an interview about her voices experience. In fact, she explicitly comes for this experience. Sasja has been hearing voices that others do not hear for the last three months. It started with one, but since last week, there is another one too. The voices come to her via her ears, i.e., from the outside and it feels as if somebody is standing very close to her. The voices belong to someone else, as they are male voices. She estimates that both men are about 35 years old. The second one has only been around since last week. The first voice has remained the same for the last three months. The voices talk about her, to her and with each other. The voices talk in a certain rhythm. Although she cannot comprehend the voices, Sasja describes them as very threatening. 'I get the impression that I have to do something. It's like they want something from me and they are urging me to do something.' Despite the fact that the voices are whispering, the tone is quite high, more or less like the voice of Sandra, who interviews her. The frequency of the voices varies; sometimes they are there for two weeks in a row, then not at all for three weeks.

At first she did not want to believe it was a voice. Although Sasja initially cannot pinpoint one incident which could have led to the voice appearing, during the course of the interview, she discovers that the first voice appeared at the time of the fatal moped accident of Peter Pieters, a boy who used to be in her class. She explains that his parents were standing in front of the church to accept condolences and she thought: 'I will just look up to the tree so that

I don't need to cry (I will have everything under control then). She also remembers now what the voice said the first time she heard it: 'Look at the tree.'

The voice is terrifying. The first voice usually presents early in the morning at around five o'clock. She is woken up by the voice and then it becomes scary. Sasja finds the voice mainly negative, not just because of the tone, but also because it seems like they are ordering her to do something. Sasja cannot comprehend what the voices are saying. However, the voices confuse her, since they are unknown and intangible. During the interview she wonders whether this big fear (she lies in bed as stiff as a board) may in fact stop her from hearing what the voices are saying. When Sasja hears voices, she knows where she is and what the time is.

Sasja believes that the voices are linked to a particular sensitivity. Lately she has been having portentous dreams. For example, she dreamt that she would pass her French exam with a 70% score, whereas that was rather unlikely, because earlier she had achieved a 50% score. To her amazement, she passed with an overall 70% score. It has not been that long since she has believed that she knows beforehand what somebody is going to say. There is no real relationship. The voices are a kind of tape that keeps on playing. There is no response to Sasja's questions. She experiences the voices as loss of control. Sasja has an extensive social network. It is only with two girlfriends, a guy at work and her sister that Sasja talks about her voices. Not with her parents, they already got upset when she started a Reiki course and associated that with a 'sect'. When asked about her childhood, she says that it was not particularly nice and not bad, too dependent. Her family all live in the same street and everybody knows everything about everybody. It does not feel like being free. Sasja sometimes does not feel wanted and she also has the impression that she never does anything right.

When Marius and I discuss Sasja's interview, it emerges that the voices appear instead of certain emotions. Sasja can feel scared, but, for example, does not dare to feel sad. In order to get to that emotion Marius encourages her to write a farewell letter to the boy who passed away.

A week later, Sasja has tried to write the letter and she has taken ample time for it. She was sitting in the attic and in response to her question to the voice to say something comprehensible, she heard him clearly. After half a sentence, her father came up to the attic to get something and he made such a noise, that she could not hear the voice any more. When we talk about the farewell letter and about the emotions, Sasja reasons: 'Who am I to feel sad about that boy?' She also adds that she could have had another reasoning: 'it could have been worse, for example, it could have been my sister who had the accident.' It is remarkable that instead of a feeling, Sasja has reasons and she recognises this. (Sexuality is reasoned away in a similar fashion). She is very clever in avoiding her own emotions. When we talk about emotions and the death of the fellow villager, she stated that she missed having to got to know him better. Related to this, she explains that when she walks past all these people in town, she also regrets not getting to know these people better. She walks past them and they remain strangers. Marius draws a parallel with relationships within her family, these are superficial too.

Marius recommends that she should not occupy herself too much with the voices, since they replace feelings and asks her to keep a diary about situations where feelings play a role.

Sasja states that she is keeping a diary. She notices that she is irritated by superficialities, for exampple, cleaning her mum's house when other people come to visit, whereas she has noticed that when she is alone she does the same. Other emotions apart from irritation do not surface. However, something else emerges from the three examples given by Sasja:

1. She works in a restaurant and washes dishes. Somebody puts a large pile of dishes that have not been pre-soaked in front of her and she does not dare to speak up, as she is concerned that the other person may not like her.
2. Sasja goes to the hairdresser who cuts her hair too short, but she does not dare to speak up for fear of him not liking her.
3. After having worked till 2am, Sasja still has to get up at 9am the next morning, because, according to her mum, 'we've worked all day too.'

It is interesting that Sasja blames herself. At the hairdresser, she probably has not been clear enough. She gets up because she thinks that her parents think that she is lazy etc. Sasja does not differentiate between what others do wrong and what she does herself, but she gets herself involved by taking the blame for things. Her mother's 'we' makes it seem as if they are all the same. The question whether her mother has her own identity, is, after some reflection, answered negatively by Sasja. She does not have a clue about how her father thinks.

The examples show that Sasja has not developed her own point of view. She has not learnt to differentiate between her parents' and her own point of view. She has the impression that her parents are not listening to her, but at the same time, she has to draw the conclusion that she does not know much, for example, about her father. He is German, but until recently she did not know where he was born in Germany.

At the next appointment, Sasja starts by informing us that she has read our 'hearing voices' book. She can identify with some of the experience stories and she concludes that these people, like her, were in a phase of their lives during which changes occurred. They found themselves in a development phase. That is true, as she is leaving a village with a very tight family control system to go to a reasonably far away city, where she will have her freedom, but will have to manage everything on her own, despite the fact that her sister is studying there too. Such transitions are often even more threatening for people with emotional problems.

The question remains: when did Sasja lose her emotions? What happened in her life that made a great deal of impact which has led to a form of emotional distancing? Therefore, we will go back in time to look for extreme emotional incidents.

After some reflection and reticence, she tells, that as a 10-year-old girl, she witnessed her father grabbing her mother by the throat during an argument in the bathroom and that at that point she believed he would kill her. This has remained an unspoken incident ever since. She can hardly believe that this could still lead to her suppressing emotions. Therefore, we decide to stick to the present, to the way in which she suppresses emotions. She will try and reflect on her emotions more.

During our next encounter, we mainly discuss Sasja's complicated way in which she reasons things away as soon as emotions get involved. Sasja keeps on reasoning: 'who am I to …' much the same as with the death of that boy. Sasja increasingly realises this and during the conversation she also recognises the point at which she starts her complicated reasoning again. Between the three of us we discuss whether Sasja can't just simply have emotions without doing anything with them: basically just acknowledging that the emotions are present. Sasja recounts that the guy who works in the kitchen of the restaurant likes her. He supports her in her anger regarding the criticism she receives. Subsequently, he tells her, that he has been to Bosnia and that one of his mates committed suicide. She finds that very difficult. With this example in mind we tell her: why don't you tell this guy: 'That's quite something that you're telling me' and nothing else. You acknowledge the emotion, allow yourself some time and at that point in time you do not have to do anything with it. This conversation takes place not long before Sasja leaves for Nijmegen to study there.

A year later, during the second interview as part of the children's study, Sasja tells us that, as she has started her studies, she has been living in student accommodation for a year now. She lives in the same house as her younger sister. Sasja goes home every weekend. She continues to hear two voices, compared to last year, this has not changed. According to her, other people do not hear these voices as they do not respond when Sasja hears them. She hears the voices via her ears. On the basis of the sounds, she hears that it is not her voice. Sasja hears the voices both during the day and the evening. She cannot talk with the voices. They are male voices which sound monotonous and neutral. Sasja estimates that they are about thirty years old. These voices do not sound like the voices of people she knows. The frequency with which she hears them varies from three times a day to once a week. This year she has been hearing them less often and they disappeared for a while. They started again around January/February, but Sasja does not know why. And then she says: 'I have a woman friend who told her psychiatrist about me hearing voices; she thought it was dangerous and that I needed medication, she tried to convince me to go to this psychiatrist. I thought about it briefly but decided not to go.

In the meantime Sasja has started to believe that the voices are related to her personally; her dealing with emotions. In the past year, her uncle who lived opposite her parents, had a fatal accident. She has not started hearing voices. Last year, the voices made Sasja sad, not this year, last year scared, not this year. Sometimes they still cause Sasja to have difficulty in concentrating. The relationship has changed over the past year. She is not really frightened of the voices any more, but she has more control over them. When Sasja pretends they are not there, they stop. Thinking about something else helps too. Starting to do something helps, visiting someone helps, looking for distractions helps.

At the time of the third interview, two years later, Sasja occasionally hears a voice. Last year there were two, now there is just one. She does not think that others can hear the voice. She hears the voice via her ear and she thinks that it is someone else because of the sound.

She hears a male voice of about 30 years old. He is negative. The frequency with which she hears him varies: about once every two months. He does not sound like someone she knows. The voice appears when Sasja is in doubt or when she feels insecure. Last year the voice appeared in situations with far more emotions. Sasja has become more open to emotions. She finds it easier to respond to things and finds that she feels well within herself.

However, she still finds decision-making difficult, even things like which sandwich filling to choose. She cannot explain the voice, but believes that the voice is related to her personally, with her actions and therefore with her feelings. The relationship has changed inasmuch as it has become even more unimportant. Sasja has changed, has found her niche in life and strangely enough after acknowledging her emotions more last year, she now has found a reasoning which suppresses her relationship with emotions again. She calls it 'dealing with' and when I tell her that 'dealing with' is based on emotions, she laughs and admits that that is right. She states that the people around her find she has changed, more spontaneous and less distant. Her parents have not changed. They are still scared of the voices and do not talk about them. Sasja says: 'I think they are concerned that the entire family will start to talk about it.'

During the fourth interview, she states that she has not heard voices for about a year now. She claims that it is due to the fact that she accepts herself more now. The voices were frightening because of the loss of control. They wanted to control the situation. That is not the case any more. She is less scared of people too now and she is surprised about her popularity. She does not suffer from concentration problems either any more. Sasja: 'You only realise the consequences of the fact that you hear voices much later. You are forced to change with it, whether you want it or not. I don't really cope well with changes. I have become a bit more philosophical now.'

It is six and a half years now since the last interview took place and now in 2006, she graduated from university quite a while ago, has a job in Maastricht and cohabits with a very creative, independent-minded man. She is doing well with or without voices – we did not talk about it any more.

SJON GIJSEN

WITH SANDRA ESCHER

This story is taken from a talk held at the congress on the occasion of the conclusion of the children's study on hearing voices. The talk was prepared in cooperation with Sandra Escher who had conducted the four annual interviews with him during the three-year follow-up study between 1996 and 1999. Sjon was 16 years old at the time of the first interview.

I am Sjon, 22 years old and an experience expert, I would like to tell you something about my experiences with regard to my voices. As long as I can remember I have been hearing voices that were positive. When I was 16 I realised they had turned negative and caused problems. Amongst other things, they interfered with my decisions. For example, each voice gave me a different piece of advice which confused me. The voices wanted to hurt me and do evil and that frightened me. I did not realise at the time what it was doing to me. I only felt that later.

At one stage I started to drink more and more, as a result of which I started to feel less and less and emotionally I became numb. In a drunken stupor I attempted suicide and ended up in a closed psychiatric ward of the local general hospital. I had just turned 17, they considered me too young to stay there and therefore I was transferred to the Vincent van Gogh (psychiatric hospital). Now I am going to tell you a bit about the psychiatric treatment.

During the first weeks of my stay I was made to talk to a battery of therapists. They did ask me what was wrong with me, but nobody asked about the voices. I had to fill in two questionnaires with a total of 600 questions and according to the therapists I was psychotic. The way in which the questions were asked made my problem an illness. For example: Do you hear or see things that others don't? Because of the way the questions were asked, the psychotic box was always ticked. In the meantime I had no privacy at all any more. I shared a room with a total of three people which impacted on the voices. The voices became more irritating and annoying and it was then that I started to group them in order to keep an overview. I believed that I heard psychotic voices and paranormal voices. The paranormal voices were linked to the emotional transfer of the people around me. I dealt with these by occupying myself a great deal with hobbies, for example, listening to and making music, but meditation helped a great deal too which I had learned from a paranormal healer.

After a month I was prescribed medication, which had no impact on the voices, but they did on the body. I calmed down, but at the same time I became more anxious, since I had the feeling that the drugs were destroying my nerve cords. That is why I stopped taking them.

After a number of months my father found that I had not improved sufficiently. He compared me to a plant without water. And the way my father is, this is a call to action. He had heard about this study and got in touch. The appointment was made, if I were to take part in the study the voices interview would be conducted and this with the advice of Professor Romme would be sent to my counsellors. My father insisted that the counsellors would use the information from the interviews. The interview was conducted in the presence of my parents. I had the feeling people were listening to me and I also felt understood. The strange thing that came out of the study was that I only experienced psychotic voices when I was on the ward of the psychiatric hospital. Not during the weekend at home.

My mother had been busy too and asked for advice from a paranormal healer. When I was about 5 years old, he had established that I had a paranormal gift. This man then visited me on the ward to see where I had ended up. He believed that I did not belong there. I agreed wholeheartedly with him.

My solution to get out of there as soon as possible was to behave in the way they expected of me. A few months later I was home again. I was in there for about eight months. I was allowed home on condition of my parents that I had to finish my schooling and that I stuck to the rules of the house, for example, no alcohol, to be home on time. Not long after discharge the psychotic voices disappeared.

On a daily basis I still heard two paranormal voices, one was negative and was more like a thought, the other positive and helped me keep the negative one away. The thing that really helped here was attending a meditation group every three weeks and I start with meditation daily so that I am increasingly working on positive things. This has led to a great deal of peace in my life too.

How am I doing now? I do not hear any voices any more, I have a job, a nice girlfriend, I play in a band and I am now able to tell you this story. To summarise everything:

- my parents have always understood and appreciated who I was and who I am now
- I have gained a more positive attitude to life
- I am now able to manage my emotions better (music is important here)
- I enforce certain disciplines upon myself
- I have learnt to talk about my problems, they have got a name now

I would like to leave at that, do you have any questions?

STEWART HENDRY

WITH MERVYN MORRIS

My name is Stewart. I am a 34-year-old single man whose journey as a voice hearer started around the age of 14 – a very difficult time for me. It was a time when so much happened. My parents were in the process of splitting up. At the same time, two grandparents passed away. I had been told my brother had about twenty-four hours to live, which really shook me, even though it turned out what he needed was an operation on a burst appendix. Separation and loss had become a big part of my life.

At the same time, a lot was going on at school. I had been hacking into computers and messing about and, when it was discovered, somebody else got the blame and expelled for what I'd done. I felt very guilty but unable to own up. In fact, I was generally feeling very unsure of myself; in particular, I didn't have a girlfriend and seriously wondered if I was gay. And to cap it all, I was being bullied by the Head Boy, which was difficult to deal with because I felt I had nowhere to turn. But things really came to a head one day when on my way to school, a kid from another school tried to rob me, pulling some kind of knife in the park. Fortunately, a grandparent of a kid from my school intervened. But I just went home and didn't tell anybody about that situation. I stopped going to school, and just said I was not feeling well.

Eventually mum took me to the family doctor and I was referred to a specialist. I had no idea that this was a psychiatrist. Afterwards he talked to my mum alone, and then prescribed some medication. Neither I nor mum knew at the time these were psychiatric drugs. When I first had that medication (I remember it was Chlorpromazine) I slept for a day, and when I woke up I just realised something was different. I experienced what I later learned are side effects; my tongue got swollen, and I couldn't stand up, and my eyes started rolling. And that day, about 11 a.m., I started hearing this real bad voice; it was very negative, and derogatory, calling me all sorts of names and telling me to do things. It told me I was a really bad person. I recognised the voice as the bully from school, the Head Boy. Also that day I heard my brother's voice (it sounded unclear, like it was in the background) and mum's voice, and then the following day, my nan's [grandmother's] voice. My mum and nan's were more helpful, saying things like I was a good person and shouldn't kill myself. Sometimes, mum's and nan's voice would talk to each other. The way I explain and always think of it, it was nan saying goodbye. I couldn't explain why the other voices though, I just responded to what they were saying.

I also started to hear my teacher's voice, a woman, and she was asking me about why I wasn't going to school, and that she knew I was 'wagging' it, and she was going to send in the truancy officers. I think the reason the teacher was there was that she taught me computing at school at the time I was hacking, and the person who got expelled was in her lessons with me. I heard another three voices, eight in all; one was my own, like an older me that was trying to be comforting, and two were like my brothers, less involving, on the periphery. And as it turned out, treatment never really stopped them, just me!

Anyway, I had real problems with the tablets, and it was my next-door neighbour, a nurse, who said they were psychiatric tablets. She told my mum to phone up the local psychiatric hospital. I was given an injection and the side effects went pretty much straight away, but not for long. I wasn't admitted, instead I was sent to a day centre for five days a week. The side effects persisted even though they changed my drugs. The voices also persisted, including at the day centre.

At the day centre I got a picture about expectations of what life was going to be like. I was then only 15 and I spent my day with older people, at least fifteen to twenty years older than me. I saw nurses and doctors and attended groups for exercise, relaxation, anxiety management, and also saw a psychologist once a week. One day my mum, dad and me went to see a psychologist, and she asked if we had any idea about my diagnosis. I mentioned schizophrenia because of what I'd learnt from talking to other patients. I was right, and different professionals – nurses and social workers, psychologists and psychiatrists – all gave the same sort of message, time and time again: my prospects for the future were not great; I shouldn't have expectations about school, or work, or having any relationships.

The voices really stayed all through this time and for many years. The first few years I was in quite a bad way, the voices were quite derogatory and it was a hard time to cope with them. I remember feeling so bad about my situation – the bully voice always making me even more depressed – that I decided one day to hang myself, but it was the comforting voices that stopped me. After that I realise now that I'd become so drugged-up and emotionally flattened that I couldn't really do much about me or them. The bully voice came whenever I was feeling insecure, which was a lot of the time, and particularly taunted me about my sexuality, saying I was gay and that sort of stuff. I was also being prepared for living away from my mum. Just before my 16th birthday they [at the day centre] suggested about me moving away from the 'problem environment' at home, and I ended up sharing a house as a lodger with no one else anywhere near my own age.

RECOVERY

During this time there was a social worker I'll always remember, who saw what it was like for me, and eventually found me somewhere more suitable. She also gave me an alternative idea of what my future would be like. She was much more informal and friend-like, and treated me more like a person. We talked about the future, about doing things and relationships, and she really started me on the road to doing something about what I wanted. I think that she was one of the reasons I am at this point now, one of the turning points in my life. It was important to have some hope at a time when I thought that my life was over and I couldn't be expected to recover.

Another important time for me was at the age of 18, when I met another service user who worked for a local charity, and who'd set up a user group at the day centre. It was a real eye-opener because she was also a user, but she had a job, a partner, a house, all the things I'd been led to believe I couldn't have, things that were beyond me. I thought if she can do that then maybe I can do it too. So that was the big turning point for me really. I started to work with her and got involved in being a 'user rep', then doing advocacy, and then organising user councils. It was the start of what I do a lot of now.

Another turning point for me was around eight years ago. I said to my psychiatrist that I wanted to go self-employed. I had already started doing bits of training at university. I had also done some work on a project, working part time with a regular amount of income, so I thought I could try and make a living out of the work I was doing. When I suggested this to my psychiatrist I was told that I wouldn't cope and that I should go to industrial therapy! I didn't go back to see that consultant psychiatrist.

In fact not seeing my psychiatrist led to another turning point. Six months later I went to the GP because I wasn't too good, I was a bit low. To be honest I was expecting to see the prescription pad and to be given more drugs, but he actually asked me what was going on, how I was feeling, that sort of stuff. I probably took up an hour of his time; he even swapped one of the patients he was supposed to see to another doctor. I just talked about the issues for an hour and then we started to do this about every couple of weeks, usually at the end of his surgery. He started reducing the medication I was on, and that was a really big thing for me because I started to feel things again, you know, feeling emotions and that sort of stuff. I came to realise that, before then, I hadn't really felt things, and it was from then when I started to feel more like a normal person.

A few things started to happen for me. I started to get more involved in talking to people as a user advocate, including getting involved in training courses for nurses and social workers. There were some things happening around hearing voices too; the University of Central England was starting a course that included the 'accepting voices' approach, and I particularly remember meeting Ron Coleman who talked about negotiating with the voices. I was already able to talk back to my voices with my thoughts, but I learnt to make a specific time of day, the evening, when I would focus, and simply tell the voices 'later' if they came at another time. And it worked!

And this was the time I decided to become self-employed. There was another person in particular who helped me with this, she worked for a local voluntary organisation running 'out of hours' services, and we used to have long talks. I used to do my part-time job 'out of hours' work with her, and we used to have talks afterward. She used to give me a lift and we used to chat in the car again for about an hour or so afterwards, and it seemed the right next step. I decided to take the risk of stopping my disability allowance. I started going to the Job Centre and had to sign on and, instead, got a Jobseekers Allowance. I got a loan and a grant from the Prince's Trust to set myself up as self-employed, firstly as a trial. Because I lost a lot of my benefits, my mum and other people helped me out to begin with.

And my experience and relationship with the voices changed. Once I'd started to make a bit more of my life and I began to work, that was a big thing for me as well, a sort of sense of worth. I think because my self-esteem started to rise a bit more, it gave me a purpose rather than just sitting around drinking cups tea! I think also because of my outlook on life and being a bit more positive, and also dealing with the issues that the voices used to attack me about. For example, sorting out my sexuality was a big thing for me, and I was able to deal with it because less drugs meant I got sexual feelings back, and it became clear that what I wanted was a girlfriend, and now the voices just don't get on to me about this at all.

So things have worked out and now I am on my feet. In the past it was a hard problem just to get out of bed; walking down the road was a big issue, thinking people were talking about me. Getting on the bus was a big problem, a major problem, but now I am really just getting on with day-to-day life. I sometimes think about time and opportunities lost, but generally I look forward. Although I talk about my experiences when I am working as a trainer, only my close family and friends know about my voices.

I am now discharged from psychiatric services, and if I need anything I go and see my family doctor. I still take small amounts of antipsychotics and an antidepressant, partly because I feel OK most of the time on them (sometimes my thinking feels slowed down or I can't get out of bed, but that might be tiredness from work). Partly I take them because they are like a psychological crutch, I don't know what I'd be like without them, but equally I have no idea what they do for me either.

Until quite recently, when I was having a bad patch the voices would sometimes come back, but now I have a separate relationship, so I can tell them to go away and come back a bit later when it's a bit quieter, and I can talk to them in my head and deal with them more like thoughts. I remember the first time I really had the experience that they had stopped; it was weird, like I could hear a pin drop. My good voice, the older me, has remained with me, though, in fact, I haven't heard a voice for a few months now. It usually comes around six in the evening, after a good day, and praises me, but it has occasionally even given me some helpful suggestions during my work!

When I got the diagnosis 'schizophrenia' I think in a way it did give me a sort of reason why things were happening. And for a time in a way it helped because I started to accept the diagnosis as the reason. Time and experience has changed my views, the diagnosis has meant less and less to me. I started feeling that this diagnosis, sort of, destroyed part of my life. It doesn't really relate to my experiences, I don't really see it as an illness, in fact I don't see it as an illness at all. I know why I started hearing voices, because of what was happening to me at the time, although I still don't know why those things came to me as voices. I just accept that this is me and, all in all, things have turned out OK.

SUE CLARKSON

I have at times perceived my voices to be through my ears, and also in my head. I have perceived them as being other people: the abuser, when I was a child; a woman who I perceive as being weak; and one inner voice who communicates, through feelings, as the Almighty Universal Force, or God. The voices sometimes seemed to be another entity, but when I later explored my voices I realised that this entity was in fact my human spirit within; so now I perceive it to be within me, part of me, and also part of the universal life force which is in us all. I had two voices at the onset: a male dominant voice, which evoked fear within me, and the weak, timid voice of a woman. Later, on exploration, I learned that the male voice was that of the abuser when I was a child; and the weak, timid voice was that of myself, the child, expressing how vulnerable I felt – how hurt, humiliated and worthless. *The voice was of a woman yet the feelings were of the child I was when the abuse took place.* I later learned that this was because those feelings were still with me. But, being a strong independent woman bringing children up alone, I could not express them. I had to be strong. So, in order for these extreme and powerful emotions to be expressed, they manifested themselves as a voice within.

HISTORY

I was 5 years old. The voice was kind, caring and comforting. I was being sexually and mentally abused at that time. The relationship with my voices has always been related to suppressed emotions and the identity of my human spirit. Whenever I have been through traumatic experiences in my life, the voices have always seemed stronger, yet they have led me through a time of personal growth and understanding of myself on a deeper level.

I had an unhappy childhood. There was abuse, neglect, long periods of separation from my mother, whom I loved dearly, and then there was the death of my best friend, Carol, at the age of 8. At 9, my older sister took her own life with an overdose and I was the one who found her. I never felt safe or loved (only by my mother). I never felt supported, apart from the odd teacher who showed concern. The voices talk of the abuse, self-doubt, insecurities, and my inadequacies. These voices would obviously cause me discomfort and sometimes extreme stress, according to how I was able to handle the powerful, strong emotions they would release.

Influence
The voices have made me commit violence; they have evoked strong feelings of suicide; they have depressed me; they have created changes to my lifestyle and my negative thinking.

Relationship
At first, I denied the voices were real. This brought utter conflict within me, and fear, extreme fear, which would result in panic attacks and physical ailments. Then once I had accepted that the voices were real, my relationship changed. They completely took over – I felt like a puppet, they were completely in charge. I felt like a robot controlled by them. Later, I learned how to gain control by having set times when they could talk with me.

Explanation
I believe *my voices are suppressed emotions that are denied within myself.* When this happens over prolonged periods they manifest themselves as having characteristics, my logical mind conjures up characters associated with these characteristics. Other people relate to these experiences, especially if they have experienced it personally, but, as yet, I have not met anyone who has actually accepted my explanation.

Coping
My coping strategies are; to make time to view my emotions daily; deal with my emotions through a series of explorations; to be mindful of what I am feeling and why. Most of all, to strive towards self-respect, self-worth and, more importantly, self-acceptance; to learn to acknowledge the good and bad inside myself and to bring change to the things which are negative – and to learn to accept who I am.

Mental health
I have never been labelled as a typical voice hearer, nor have I ever been given the label of 'schizophrenic'. If I had I would never have accepted it as it is a label that has nothing to do with the experience. I was, however, admitted to a psychiatric ward for three months through them being aware that I heard voices. I was diagnosed with another label: post-natal depression. During my stay there I didn't feel it was an environment where I could talk about my voices: voices were looked upon as delusional. I received Chlorpromazine and an injection which once resulted in a locked jaw. Medication was

eventually reduced and by the time of my discharge I was drug-free and have remained so for some thirteen years until the present day. I looked elsewhere because in my heart I knew the answer to finding out what the voices were lay elsewhere – not in the psychiatric system.

RECOVERY

The first time I came into contact with people who showed an interest in my voice-hearing experiences was the Hearing Voices Network in Manchester. The information they supplied was about advertising conferences, self-help group meetings, membership and events within the network. I used the information by going along to the meetings and conferences and actually becoming an active member of the network.

No one other than myself could help me recover from the problems I had with my voices. But there were people who helped support me; these were other voice hearers who shared their experiences with me during self-help group meetings where I was the leader of the group. I was just providing the opportunity and allowing voice hearers to explore experiences, myself included. We created an atmosphere of well-being and healing. We could relate to each other through our experiences.

Working together with other voice hearers I learnt a lot about my own voice-hearing experiences. Out of that I compiled focusing/self-help techniques to help other voice hearers to explore their voices and to find their own individual experience and meaning. There was no set background theory, only our own experiences. As part of the process of looking within ourselves and our voices, we naturally develop an understanding between our voices and our life histories. And so it starts to make sense, *the more we explore our voices the more we discover and start to understand*. With this I used my own strengths, priorities (children) and positive capacities to recover from my problems with my voices.

This process involved acceptance, change, and the future.

Acceptance
I attended the self-help group and became an active member of a voice-hearer organisation
I accepted my voices as real
I stopped trying to get rid of them, but accepted them as personal
I became conscious of my ownership of my voices
I stopped looking for a cause outside myself
I looked for solutions in myself

I explored what had happened in my life that might have a relationship with my voices

I accepted those emotions which I did not like and could not easily master

Change

I stopped suppressing my emotions

I am now able to reflect on my horrible experiences

I am able to acknowledge having problems which lead to the voice-hearing experience

I have reclaimed my personal power

I have created hope for the future

Future

I found a job and loyal friends

I relied on myself to change my life

I learned to be proud of myself

I proved myself in my job, with friends and in bringing up my children alone

I changed my attitude towards being abused. I stopped blaming myself, punishing myself and doubting my self-worth

Self-help groups

I have attended and led self-help groups. The following aspects were helpful in my recovery:

I had an opportunity to talk freely about my voices

My experience was accepted as real and not only negative

I learned ideas and coping strategies

It was a first step to coping better

I became less isolated with my voices

I no longer had to deny or keep quiet about my experiences

I felt supported

I came into a non-judgemental atmosphere

I gained positive reinforcement from small gains that I made

I learned about the relationship between my voices and what I had suffered in earlier life

I could cope better with my daily life

I started a job again

And most important *I found self-acceptance*

My life now

I do still hear voices but I can now cope with them. My experiences with my voices are not always positive but now I understand what makes them negative so they don't have the power they once possessed. I am more self-confident. I don't have a partner or intimate friends but this is through choice as I just want time to discover myself more. I have a job I enjoy: walking with the elderly as an activity organiser (for which I am paid monthly). I have lived in the same rented accommodation for the past twenty-five years. It is a lovely home with a beautiful garden. My finances could be better as I am not fully self-sufficient: I still receive family income supplement. I do have hobbies: walking, DIY and gardening, so I keep quite busy. I have friends whom I can call on when needed, as they can on me. I do have a purpose in life: to live every day to the full. I do not take medication. I am not dependent on others, only as one naturally is dependent on others for interaction. I have not used mental health professionals or mental health services since 1993 when I was sectioned. The only involvement I have had is as a professional mental health trainer. I was an active member of the hearing-voices movement, as a self-help group leader, mental health trainer and counsellor, right up to 2006. I now just concentrate on living each day to the full and taking it as it comes. It hasn't taken me into mental health circles for the past several months and, as a result, I have felt much more positive. Hearing voices and mental health environments do not mix – you just become restricted. Speaking on a personal level, I feel mental health environments are much more distressing and destructive than any voice-hearing experience. But one never knows where life will take one. I feel I have been on a remarkable journey of self-discovery with my voices – an ongoing journey.

APPENDIX

THE INVITATION TO PARTICIPATE IN THIS STUDY (2002)

INTERVOICE
Nat. Hearing Voices Network
19 Oldham Street
Manchester
M4 1LW

Intervoice asks for your co-operation

Intervoice would like to ask your co-operation in composing an anthology of fifty stories of people who hear voices or did hear voices and profited by the 'accepting voices' approach.

You may well know of us already, because most of you who we ask for co-operation we know personally. However for those we do not know so well we provide some details of the work of Intervoice.

Intervoice is a charity organising meeting possibilities like conferences, a website and a discussion forum for people hearing voices and professionals who like to work with voice hearers. Intervoice promotes accepting the voices and engaging with them. The purpose is that people change their relation with their voices in order to take their lives in their own hands again.

To promote this approach more widely Intervoice would like to publish a book with fifty stories of persons hearing voices who have profited from the 'accepting voices' approach. The reason for this is to give evidence-based motivation for other voice hearers and professionals to overcome their hesitation in trying it out.

The idea is that you write your own anthology and that we provide guidelines, which are enclosed with this letter in order to make the task easier for you, and also to collect well-organised information.

Furthermore, members of Intervoice have agreed to help you if you like, in writing your story. You will find their names and telephone numbers at the end of this paper. Naturally you can also ask a good friend or the professional that helped you in coping with your voices or changing your relationship with them. Below we have quoted from the UK Hearing Voices Network the benefits of the 'accepting voices' approach, published in 'Coping with Voices'.

In order to make this challenge easier, we enclose an example. It is not our idea that you follow the guidelines or example literally, because voice hearers are different from each other and also the book would become quite dull. If you don't want to complete all the parts of the information we ask for, because of the privacy or intimacy of it, feel free just skip that part - but please go on.

We hope you will co-operate and we hope you will like it to write about your experiences.

With warm regards,

Marius Romme

GUIDE FOR WRITING AN ANTHOLOGY ABOUT HEARING VOICES AND THE PROFITS GAINED

Part I Experience, history, influence

- Please describe briefly who you are, include your full name (or only first name), age, gender, marital status, main education (one), main activities (max. two), main hobbies (max. two). Start with 'I am …'
- Please describe some of the characteristics of your experience such as 'I hear most of my voices from outside through my ears, or in my head (say what is true for you)'. 'My voices are 'not me' (not my thoughts or feelings) but from somebody else or something else (when you think some voices are part of yourself self, tell so)'. Describe how many years you have been hearing voices; did they ever disappear for some time. How often did/have you hear(d) the voices (all day; sometimes; weekly; monthly etc).
- Could you give a short description of the characteristics of the five voices who are most important to you. Tell us their name(s) or the name(s) you give them or the symbol that characterises them (like aggression man; silverman; mother type; whatever you think is appropriate). Could you also provide information on the age; gender; the characteristic way of speaking to you like scolding or helpful etc. of each voice.
- Please tell your 'hearing voices' history. That is: I was x years of age when it started. For instance 'I remember that I was … (if you remember say where you were and what you were doing). Would you then describe what has happened to you since the voices started and/or changed, for instance when the voices became ugly or changed in being nice. The issue we want you to cover here is to describe what you think might be their relationship to your life history and your personal development.
- Could you give the most important triggers that provoked the voices during the time you were very much hindered by them. For instance: 'When I am in the kitchen' or 'when I am alone' or 'when I feel tired', or 'angry' or 'afraid of…'. Please don't make this too long, one or two most important situations and one or two most important emotions will do. If you need to expand feel free.
- Can you give two typical phrases or expressions the voices use, when they talk to you and if you think it made sense or not and why?
- What impact does or did the voices have on you when you were most hindered by them. Did they threaten you; blackmail you; made you afraid; hinder you in doing what you like to do, etc. Could you also say if this has changed and what impact the voices have now?
- Then we would like you to write down if you had any influence on the voices for instance did you have any control or no control at all over the voices when they most hindered you and how this feel now.
- Most people have an explanation for their voices. What was or is your explanation? How important was this explanation for you and is this still the case? Did others accept this?
- Perhaps you can also tell us what coping strategies you used when they were most hindering you. We would also like you to say how you reacted to your voices.
- The last issue in this part is to tell how you related to the voices when they most hindered you and how this has changed, if it has changed.

Part II Meeting the accepting voices approach and the benefits of it for you
Can you now tell us:
> How did you come into contact with the 'accepting voices' approach. Where was this?
> Who first talked to you about your voices and showed interest? How did you react?
> What did you do with this information and how did you work with this person?

We would like you to tell us about the people you met and had a positive experience with.

This might well be a number of different people and possibly a number of different attempts. Just describe them rather briefly and as clearly as possible. It does not only have to be directly related to the voices but might also include other empowering activities or assistance of any kind that helped you living a more satisfying or independent life, in spite of the voices or with the voices.

We now give you a list of benefits of the accepting voices approach partly quoted from 'Coping with Voices' published by the UK National Hearing Voices Network in Manchester.

- I had an opportunity to talk freely about voices or other sensations
- I had my experiences accepted as real and not necessarily negative
- I learned ideas and coping strategies
- It was the first step to coping better
- I became less isolated because of talking more freely about my voices
- I did no longer have to deny or keep quiet about my experience
- I felt supported
- I came in a non-judgemental atmosphere
- I gained positive reinforcement from small gains that I made
- I learned about the relationship between my voices and what I had suffered in earlier life
- I could better cope with my daily life
- I started a job again
- Other …

Can you tell us what helped you and if possible give some evidence for this like the activities you undertake now and were not able to do before. We would like to know from you what really helped you, not what could have been helpful.

Part III How is your life by now?
In this last part we would like you to describe, how your life is now, how you feel on average; do you still hear voices and can you cope with them? Or if don't you hear them anymore and possibly miss them; or are you afraid that they may come back or are you just more confident about yourself? We also like you to tell us how you live your life in the sense of having a partner, having a job and what kind of job. What kind of housing you enjoy, if you enjoy it, and whether your financial position is feeling reasonably safe. All in all giving a short picture of your life and how dependent or independent you are from other people, carers, professionals, institutes. Are you active in the 'accepting voices' movement and if yes in what way? That is it.

It is not necessary at all to keep the order of parts that are proposed in this guideline. You might well like to start with part III or II and end up with part II or I. Feel free to tell your story in your way. The only thing we would like that you check afterwards if most items are covered in your story and eventually put the missing ones in.

Thank you very much for your co-operation. In editing we might propose some changes. However we will always ask your permission. For the length of the book we must ask you to restrict your story to a maximum of 3000 words.

EXAMPLE

Alex's story

I can remember hearing voices from a very early age, but it was always associated with seeing a floating face that always seemed to be smirking, but this has now gone. However, I was about ten when the voices became aggressive and difficult to handle. Throughout my childhood and early adolescence, a member of my family sexually abused me. The voices were ever-present during this time, and I can recall them teasing, bullying and talking to me. At the age of 14, I was taken to see a child psychiatrist, and I was admitted to a large hospital, which had established a special unit for children. However, the reality was that I was admitted to an adult male ward. Here, my voices went on the rampage. I was diagnosed as schizophrenic and given Modecate injections. This actually removed my ability to cope with the voices; my emotions were flattened, and my mind could not help me engage the voices.

I was transferred from one hospital to another. At no time was I asked what I thought and felt, and as soon as I said that I heard voices, I was either told to pull my socks up or given different cocktails of chemicals.

Only once in 15 years of psychiatric intervention, and at the age of 36, was I able to find someone who was willing to listen. This proved a turning point for me, and from this I was able to break out of being a victim and start owning my experience. This nurse actually found time to listen to my experiences and feelings. She always made me feel welcome, and would make arrangements so we would not be disturbed. She would switch off her bleeper and take her phone off the hook, and sometimes, as there were people outside her room, she would close the blinds. These actions made me feel at ease. She would sit to one side of me instead of across a desk. She told me that what we said was confidential, but that there were some exceptions, so I could decide what to reveal. Slowly, as trust grew between us, I was able to tell her about the abuse, but also about the voices. Sometimes when I was describing what happened to me, she would tell me that it was hurting her and she needed a break. At last, I had found someone who recognised the pain I was feeling. She helped me realise that my voices were a part of me, and had a purpose and validity. Over a six-month period, I was able to develop a basic strategy for coping.

Thanks to the support this worker gave, I have been able to develop a range of coping mechanisms. One of these is that I give them a specific time each day when they can flow and I can engage with them. However, to allow this to happen, I must prepare myself; some things done in advance also help, like establishing a regular sleeping pattern. Even when I promise the voices a particular time, they still carry on, but they do not overwhelm me. One of the things that I have had to learn is to allow myself to be in touch with my emotions, and sometimes I get afraid of my feelings and the voices.

Here are my voices ... and their triggers
- *Voice one: the Silver voice.* This voice is softly spoken and usually whispers, often-fragmented phrases and comments about the people I meet or have relationships with. Triggers: talking to people over the telephone; meet new people.
- *Voice two and three: the Two Brothers.* These two voices speak to each other, as well as to me, in a rhythmic pattern. They are very aggressive and abusive and talk to me about the other voices. These two voices are the most difficult to cope with. Triggers: these voices often seem to be dominant after any sexual activity.
- *Voice four: the Mechanical Voice.* This voice usually comes in the night, and is dominant and active when it is dark. It usually repeats the same set of phrases – it often tells me that other beings, usually animals, can hear all the voices, and that cats hear the best. Triggers: darkness; the full moon.

Training the voices: Getting them balanced with my life
- *The Silver voice.* I often found that drawing pictures or even speaking out loud what the voice is saying helps to reduce its power (each session lasts about ten minutes).
- *The Two Brothers.* These are the most emotionally demanding. If they start, I have to find a place of sanctuary and let them go (lasts up to three hours).
- *The Mechanical Voice.* I usually talk back to this voice, asking it questions that I hope it will find difficult to answer. By allowing myself to be afraid, I am able to question the voice by asking, for instance: 'You cannot hurt me, can you?' By teasing the voice, I prove that I am stronger.

I have found that in order to live my life, I have had to take control and reject the notion of seeing myself as a victim. You may find that by talking about them with orders, your voice may play you up for a few days, doing all it can to distress you and disrupt your daily routine – don't give in. Once you have established a pattern, and you keep to it, then the voices will become less powerful.

Writing this has not been easy. The voices have told me that once this is read by others who hear voices, my voices will become stronger and return to me. This does scare me a bit, but I am alive. I am pleased that we are coming together to share our experiences and explanations, but we have to be careful not to lose control, and that any movement does not end up synthesizing our experiences and turn them into stereotypes.

As far as my life now is concerned I still hear voices, but I am much more in control than before. I have a fulltime paid job and live with my wife and kid in a nice, rather small house. I am not worrying much about finance. In my job I also organise self-help for voice hearers and I take interviews with them.

Do you have any questions or do you need more guidance, you might contact one of the following persons:

Paul Baker, Spain
Ron Coleman, Gloucester
July Downs, NHVN Manchester
Roddy Gordon, C.I.C. Scotland

Babs Johnston, Melrose, Scotland
Terence McLaughlin, Stockport
Mike Smith, Birmingham
Phil Thomas, Bradford

ACKNOWLEDGEMENTS
MARIUS ROMME

The stories in this book make it clear that the principles of *Accepting Voices* (1993) and *Making Sense of Voices* (2000) can be of great help in the recovery process. Having an idea is one thing, but spreading it across the world is another matter altogether. The idea, naturally, has to be useful, but even more important is finding people who will try to work with it, and people who will put their energy behind it to get the idea promoted. To these two main parties our acknowledgments are directed. To all the people who have become involved we are very grateful, and it is amazing just how many people there are, as well as how much energy they given.

First of all we thank those voice hearers who have tried out an alternative approach, and were so brave to tell their very personal stories. They have played the most important role by being so open and courageous in telling their very intimate experiences, and putting their pain and struggle into the public domain. They were all convinced that by publishing their stories they might contribute to changing the predominantly negative attitude towards voices within society and mental health services. Hearing voices is an experience that needs to be accepted and explored as it has a personal meaning. Each of the fifty voice hearers found the capacities and the power to change their own world. They stopped fighting their voices by, instead, learning to live with them.

The anthologies show the need and necessity for the emancipation of people with mental health problems. Too many people in our society and too many professionals working in the mental health field still see those amongst us with mental health problems as being different, as not being a normal person. It might be compared with the general attitude towards homosexuality many years ago. Homosexuals changed public opinion by organising themselves, using political pressure and the media in their fight for recognition. This battle is yet to be won by voice hearers who also need to go public and fight for their acceptance as full citizens. However, acceptance starts with accepting oneself and that is what becomes apparent from the stories in this book. People show that living with voices is about accepting oneself and also being accepted by others as emancipated full citizens. This means that much work still has to be done by voice hearers in our society, and others will have to support this process.

The hearing voices movement began in the eighties with Patsy Hage and me. In 1984 Patsy Hage was referred to me as a patient who was greatly hindered by her voices. Patsy was critical about my approach as a psychiatrist. I did not talk about her experience. I doubted the reality of her voices. However, after a year she convinced me of their reality, their intrusiveness and the disturbance they created in her life. It was because of her suicidality that I looked for another approach. Patsy is the one to whom I am grateful for stimulating me to think more critically about the generally accepted approach to hearing voices within psychiatry. She made me do something about it. The first step I took was to ask her to talk with other voice hearers who were also patients of mine about their experiences. They talked, recognised each other's stories, but did not know how to cope with their voices. I reasoned that if they could explain to each other what it is to hear voices clearly enough, then there must also be people in the world who have learned to cope with them. It thus became my task to get in touch with those individuals who could cope. And then I sought advice from

Sandra Escher who, at that time, was working as a science journalist in my department at the University of Maastricht, teaching young scientists how to write for publication. Sandra was a great help, in particular her idea that television provided a possibility to get into touch with many people, and would make it possible to call to voice hearers who could cope with their voices. However, to be invited by a media show we also needed a news headline, and Sandra thought that organising the first ever Congress for voice hearers might be that headline. And she was right. Imme Reichard as Director of Pandora, a patient information service, helped us to get in touch with the very famous – in Holland – talk show of Sonja Barend. On this programme Pasty and I presented our predicament, asked people to respond, and also announced the Congress. Sandra had prepared the questions that Sonja Barend would ask Patsy, so that Patsy would feel reasonably safe.

More than seven hundred people responded, with five hundred telling us they heard voices, and some also saying they could cope with them. It was impossible to contact all these people personally so we decided to develop a questionnaire to send to the people who had given their addresses.

Then we started preparing for the Congress, by inviting people who had returned the questionnaire for an interview, selecting voice hearers who were able to tell their story in a comprehensive way, and those voices hearers who could cope well and had not been psychiatric patient. Three hundred and fifty people attended the congress. It was also attended by Professor John Strauss, who helped us to write an article for the *Schizophrenia Bulletin* (1987), and to whom we are very grateful because it brought our idea to a global audience.

Meeting voice hearers who could cope well with their voices started our research interest. Sandra Escher became more involved, and we wrote a research proposal. We were supported by Professor Joop van London, a psychiatrist and Director General of the Ministry of Health and also Chair of the Committee of the Prevention Fund. He provided for the funding of a four-year research project to compare patients hearing voices with non-patients hearing voices, and also for an annual Congress. We are very grateful to Professor Joop van London as, at that time, it was quite an unorthodox research proposal. He has continuously been a great support, in particular later on with the financing of Sandra's research on children hearing voices.

During the next years we met many voice hearers who could cope well with their voices and who had never been a patient. We became more and more enthusiastic about the way people seemed to be able to take their lives back. We gained more knowledge about other roads that could be followed in living with voices. In Maastricht the enthusiasm wasn't great, but in Italy, in 1988, at a Congress celebrating the 10th anniversary of the 1978 Reform Act (of mental health law) we met Paul Baker, a social worker from Manchester; Alain Topor, a psychologist from Stockholm, and Professor Alec Jenner, head of the Department of Psychiatry at the University of Sheffield. Paul, Alain and Alec were the first three who were enthusiastic in quite uncertain times, and have since supported us over many years by inviting us for conferences and training sessions. We are very grateful to them and will further tell about them when we talk about their country. We will now tell the history of each country involved in the hearing voices movement and in that way thank all the people involved.

Holland

At the first congress for voice hearers, held in Utrecht at the School of Journalism (a non-medical setting), voice hearers directly became very enthusiastic in talking about their voices in a fully accepting atmosphere, and with everyone interested in their experience. We decided to start an association for those voice hearers who wanted to meet again, and also to have a support group because we could expect criticism; it is always wise to organise support if you want to change something in society. The association founded was called Resonance (Weerklank in Dutch).

In the first years we received a great deal of press coverage in many talk shows on TV. We organised congresses in different towns and we were telephoned by many people who would like to find a therapist working this way. That was the main problem in the beginning, and still now in Holland there are not enough therapists using our approach, and not enough groups available to refer voice hearers to. We are still in need of a full-time position to coordinate and stimulate self-help and training facilities.

Resonance has continued to run, keeping as its main role the spreading of information. We would like to thank Ans Streefland, Mieke Simons and Jeannette Woolthuis, all previously holding the same position as the present Chair Wilma Bouvink, putting great energy into Resonance over the past twenty years. We would also like to thank all the other voice hearers, board members and donors, and all those who joined Resonance to put their energies into groups and activities, especially the periodical that has been published four times a year, every year.

The first support group was started in Sittard by Resi Malecki, and she has kept it running for twelve years. Thereafter other groups started, such as a group still running in Roermond led by Flore Brummans and Riny Selder, and in Maastricht run by Jan Verhaegh and Marietje Lemmens. Two psychiatric hospitals also started support groups in the east of Holland, for which we thank dr Dick Brouwer and dr Frans van Hal, both psychiatrists. We would also like to thank drs. Ben Steultjens, who started a group in Amsterdam in the early days, and is still active in an outpatient setting.

We ourselves restricted our work to research and the rest of the world! In 1992 we started our comparative study of patients and non-patients who heard voices. We are grateful to Monique Pennings who did most of the interviews, and to Adriaan Honig, a psychiatrist, who collected the sample of 'patients' from the community mental health department and who, together with another psychiatrist Dirk Corstens, took care of the diagnostic component. We would like also to thank Bernardine Ensink who had completed her PhD (in 1992) in this area, and who was involved in analysing the research data. It was a pity this study is only very partly published (Romme, 1996, and Honig et al., 1998) because we didn't find the time. Financial pressures pushed us to start new studies. Sandra began a follow-up study on children hearing voices, and Alex Buiks joined her in this research. Monique Pennings started a study on support groups. This last study was recently re-edited by Ben Steultjens and published by Resonance (2007). In the period between 1996 and 2000 Monique, Sandra and I wrote *Making Sense of Voices* (1999), reporting a systematic way of working with people hearing voices.

We are very grateful to Dirk Corstens for his continued involvement since 1992, initially as a psychiatrist in training, undertaking the diagnostic component of the protocol. As a psychiatrist he has since remained involved, opening an outpatient clinic for voice hearers, and testing with us our system of making a construct of the relationship between voices and the voice hearers' problems in life. He is now completing his PhD, describing the construct method more extensively, evaluating training sessions and the effect of supervision sessions. From his outpatient clinic for voice hearers he has developed many contacts, so has been able and has found time to write a number of interviews for this book. Indeed there are many aspects of Dirk's work for which we are grateful. When we were invited abroad Dirk started to join us. He now has taken over a lot of the activity of both Sandra and I, doing more training sessions, especially in Scotland and Denmark, and also now in Palestine and England. I hope he will continue on from my relationship with Intervoice. We have had many nice and constructive talks. Dirk's wife Lien also followed a training in 'voice dialogue', and on occasions joins Dirk. Both of them have become friends.

Professor Dr Jim van Os has also been a great stimulus to our work from the start of his appointment as Head of the Psychiatry Department at the University of Maastricht. He very much supported our focus on psychotic experience, and became more and more critical towards the DSM system, especially regarding schizophrenia. He inspired and guided Sandra to do her PhD, and helped greatly with the publications that formed the basis of her thesis. He has also supported the 'First World Congress on Hearing Voices', to be held in 2009 in Maastricht, by sharing the financial commitment. We are also thankful to Philippe Delespaul who assisted Sandra with her research.

England

We have very good memories of our contacts with Alec Jenner, Professor of Psychiatry at the University of Sheffield who we first met in Italy in 1987. He was very much interested in our approach, and over the years has invited us to give presentations in Sheffield. He was especially interested in the user perspective and also published the journal *Asylum* (www.asylumonline.net).

In England it was Paul Baker who made the start with the hearing voices movement. We had met him at the same congress in Italy as Alec Jenner. He has a brother who was hearing voices, and he first discussed the concept with his brother. Thereafter he came to stay with us, bringing along four of his friends working in mental health in Manchester, mainly to see if we were trustworthy. We passed that test and were invited to England for a week, giving nine presentations in four days in Liverpool, Manchester, Leeds and Sheffield. The then chair of Resonance, Ans Streefland, accompanied us, a non-patient voice hearer whose talk provided the information that it was possible to live with voices. Paul Baker wrote a nice small book about the accepting voices ideas in very understandable language and it has since been translated into several languages. Paul is still active as the secretary of Intervoice, writing newsletters, and has set up the website of Intervoice, keeping it running and up to date.

We are also specially grateful to Paul because he set up the first hearing voices group in Manchester with four people (Anne Walton, Helen Heap, John Williams and Ron Coleman) who all became active in the movement in different ways.

Ron became the most famous voice hearer, a charismatic man who impresses many people with his intelligence, insight and his performances. He took many initiatives to promote the accepting voices movement, spreading the approach across the world, starting with other enthusiastic people in England, then supporting us in Europe with spreading the movement (especially in Denmark), and then to Palestine and over the oceans to New Zealand and, very successfully, to Australia. Ron is also a good networker and has very impressive colleagues such as Mike Smith, with whom he wrote several books, and his wife Karen Taylor, with whom he has set up a training centre.

We have known Ron for many years and we have many stories to tell, including the times Ron took us 'treasure hunting' as we called it; we would cross the UK from north to south, west and east, and then end up close to the city where we had been the previous week.

We were always wondering where we were going to give our next presentation as Ron did not inform us because, in between, he also had to see some people somewhere in a village or city we didn't know. Every day we would take him to the train and then meet later that day, or the next morning, in some hotel that we still had to find in some city miles away.

With Phil Thomas, a psychiatrist from Bradford, and Ron, we toured America. We met Ron at New York airport where he came out of the plane in his Scottish kilt, telling us that in this way people would recognise his body in case the plane crashed. It had been his first flight. His favorite hobby was to challenge psychiatrists in a competition for the interpretation of research findings. Ron reads a lot and knows a lot. We passed many evenings in cafés after a day's work making plans. Ron wrote a very fine book about his recovery process (Coleman, 1997).

Richard Bentall was the first person from an academic setting who invited us to give a presentation at Liverpool University in 1992. He introduced us to his group of research psychologists, most still studying Vaughn and Leff's concept of 'expressed emotions'. This group became active in cognitive behavioural therapy studies on hallucination and delusions. Richard Bentall has always been very stimulating to us. With Gill Haddock he developed 'focusing' which reduced anxiety about and frequency of voices by talking with voice hearers about their voices. In 1996, our 1992 presentation was published in a book edited by Gill Haddock and Peter Slade, alongside reports on a number of studies in this area undertaken by this research group. There are some differences between the 'accepting voices' approach and the cognitive approach, mainly regarding the illness concept. Richard has been on several occasions a guest in our house, was a keynote speaker at Congresses we organised in Holland, and was the external supervisor for Sandra's M.Phil, and member of the panel for her PhD. To us Richard is a special friend.

In 1993 we composed the Dutch book *Stemmen Horen Accepteren* (*Accepting Voices*) which is a combination of experience and science. It contains case studies of patients and non-patients hearing voices, and professional explanations for the experience. Then we came into touch with Anny Brackx, Publishing Director of Mind, who is not only a nice person, but also a good professional and important to us as she could read Dutch. She was very enthusiastic about our book, and so it was translated and published by Mind. After 15 years it is still a book that people buy. We are very grateful to Anny Brackx as, if not for her, our ideas would have been mainly confined to Holland. But we are grateful for more reasons because Anny promoted the book fiercely, and this enabled us to break through internationally. Over the years our contacts with Anny extended beyond the business side. We loved to have a good meal and a good chat in one of the wonderful London restaurants she knows. She also organised training days for us in England, and published our second book *Making Sense of Voices*, to which she gave a beautiful and impressive form, and made it a success.

In England many people were inspired and started to create a network, inspiring or setting up support groups for voice hearers, and because of them the hearing voices movement has grown the most in England, where about 180 groups are active. We are therefore first of all very thankful to the parents of the movement in England; Terence McLaughlin and Julie Downs. Regretfully, Terence died in 2007, but he has inspired and followed very intensively the development of the hearing voices movement in England, and completed his PhD in 2005, describing the philosophy by combining theory with practice. Julie Downs coordinated the English network from an office in Manchester, offering very many people the stimulation and contact they needed, organising congresses and training, finding the money for the network to survive, and starting support groups in prisons for example. She also did lots of different things that were necessary to develop new opportunites for voice hearers, which the movement clearly was. Without Terence and Julie I doubt if the movement would have got off the ground. However, as a result of their work, many more people in England took up the challenge.

One of the first psychiatrists to invite us to the UK was Phil Thomas, at the time still working in Wales. We thank him for all we did together, even joining up for trips to the USA and Japan, for the friendship with him and his wife Stella. He also wrote a chapter about our approach in his book: *The Dialectics of Schizophrenia* (1997).

As we have already described, the contacts started with Paul Baker and Ron Coleman, and extended by Terence and July, but we also learned to know the power, capacities and input of what we could call the younger generation.

Firstly we should mention Rufus May, who wrote many articles, influenced the psychology profession, and also started new initiatives and played a role in a beautifully intriguing film about the possibility to recover with voices in settings where there is a lot of antagonism toward these new ideas. We very much appreciate and are grateful for all his contributions.

A most powerful and charming person we would like to express our gratitude to is Jacqui Dillon, the current chair of the English Hearing Voices Network, a very gifted women, working hard to promote change in the approach to mental health problems in general, and specially hearing voices. She stimulated the formation of support groups in London, twenty-five in all, and she also developed a fine course in setting up and facilitating support groups for voice hearers. We are very lucky that she cooperated on this book because of her knowing many recovered voice hearers, and doing beautiful interviews with them.

Another of the younger generation is Peter Bullimore, a very fine man with a great working power and idealism, who started a paranoia support group. Although nobody thought this would be possible, it is working out fine. We are thankful to him and his wife Linda for the nice contacts, and we are still connected in developing a paranoia interview.

In England we also met the last editor of this book, Mervyn Morris, at a large Congress organised by Ron Coleman in Birmingham in 1996. At the University of Central England, (now BCU, Birmingham City University) he developed a postgraduate training course, initially for nurses, and then for other workers and also service users. This course is organised around accepting voices and making sense of them; it has also been evaluated, and this study is to be presented at the Maastricht Congress in September 2009. He also organised my invitation to become a Visiting Professor and, more importantly, as Supervisor, he guided Sandra Escher with her M.Phil; a three-year follow-up study of 80 children hearing voices. Mervyn and his wife Diana have become friends and are a continuing inspiration. Mervyn has also organised the publishing of this book with PCCS Books, and undertaken most of the editing.

It is hardly possible to recall everyone we've met in England, and by whom we've been invited, but we must mention Professor Ian Parker who invited us to Manchester, and guided Terence McLaughlin with his PhD about the hearing voices movement. We also want to thank Paul Hammersley from the same city with whom we wrote an article about abolishing the schizophrenia concept. He is very active with the CASL (Campaign for the Abolition of the Schizorphenia Label) initiative for abolishing the schizophrenia concept.

We'd also like to thank Adam Jones (2001) who wrote a book about the hearing voices movement entitled *Raising Our Voices* and, as a result became Mind Journalist of the Year 2001.

Many more voice hearers we met in England were very stimulating, including Louise Pembroke; Sue Clarkson; Eleanor Longden; Marion Aslan; Stewart Hendry, and professionals who started self-help groups, organised meetings, or were intellectually stimulating us, including; Mike Smith who wrote together with Marion Aslan (2007) a book about basic concepts in mental health; Lucy Johnstone (1989; 2000), who wrote *Users and Abusers of Psychiatry*; Dorothy Rowe, who wrote several books promoting the user perspective and principles of mental health, and Brian Martindale with whom we are composing a book on 'psychosis as a personal crisis', to be published by Routledge next year. We would like to thank them and many others in England very much for their contributions.

Scotland

In Scotland we would like to thank Professor Phil Barker who lives in Dundee, but we first met in Newcastle when he invited us to present at a very nice congress he organised. We also have good memories of Pat Webster and her son, who were the driving forces of the Scottish network at the time. They invited us as keynote speakers at their conferences. The Scottish network has become very active, and with their new coordinator Angy Much have even travelled to Australia with nineteen people, demonstrating their great organisational talents as well. We remember a nice invitation to Glasgow and to Aberdeen by Christine Brown, following up actions in Aberdeen with Dirk Corstens, and we also are grateful to Rodney Gordon for the conference he organised.

Wales

We are most grateful to Hywell Davies who invited us to Wales, and who after that started a support group and the network in Wales. Hywell wrote some very nice information leaflets about the hearing voices experience for the network in Wales. Later on he became a really great help, financially supporting the website of Intervoice, which otherwise would not have survived.

Finland

It was in the beginning of the 1990s that we were invited to Finland to present our first research results in a rather big psychiatric hospital by a very active director psychiatrist. He organised different visits for me and Sandra, Ron Coleman and Paul Baker. It was a very nice experience with great hospitality. The Finnish user movement is well organised. Every patient becomes a member and that is one of the reasons why it is possible in Finland to get finance for the user perspective. It was the first country to install a paid worker to organise the hearing voices support groups, and that person was Marja Vuorinen, who also took the initiative to translate the accepting voices book called 'Moniaaniset'. Kisse de Bruin took over from her and, with great energy, stimulated the 'onset hearing voices groups'. In 2005 there were twenty-three such groups spread all over the country. She reported very clearly about their activities in the Intervoice meeting of 2007, and we hope to see them again in Maastricht in 2009, and are very grateful to both her and Marja.

We must reflect here by looking at the variation in the development of the hearing voices movement in the different countries where a paid coordinator has proven to be an absolutely essential instrument to getting hearing voices groups started. Finland has twenty-three groups, England one hundred and eighty, and Denmark also quite a number, and these three countries are those with paid coordinators.

Austria

Austria was the second country that began to invite us to visit, also in the early nineties. Chuck Schneider, a psychologist, and Marleen Weiterschein, a psychiatrist, have been active throughout all the years since. They both worked at a social psychiatric ambulatory centre, organising a tour for us to give presentations in Linz, Gratz and Salsburg. At that time we had completed just a number of interviews for the accepting voices book, and we had made an inventory in our own social-psychiatric outpatients service, looking at how often people were hearing voices, and within what diagnostic categories. It showed that many patients had never talked about their voices, and many professionals did not know that a number of their patients heard voices. Like the Austrians, we only had just started a support group, so we exchanged our experiences.

As in Holland they had started their group with people with long-term psychiatric histories. They also noticed that those people liked to talk about their experience when they felt safe. They didn't want more medication as they said they still heard voices. In Austria they had the disadvantage that they had not met those people who could cope well with their voices and had not become a patient. We've kept contact since, and they have always attended our congresses, for example in 1996 they travelled with eight voice hearers to the Maastricht congress.

Later we were invited by Professor Heinz Katschnig, head of the psychiatry department of the University of Vienna, and have been invited back several times since. There we met Professor Michaela Amering, who also became an enthusiastic supporter of the accepting voices approach. She started a trialogue group. She had a very positive input in Vienna supporting voice hearers. She did not expect wonders, but offered the kind of support that made people feel more safe, and gave them a chance to develop. We have kept a very good contact and become friends. She published a book in German *Recovery* about the user perspective in 1997. Heinz Katschnig and Michaela Amering organised in July 2003 a huge congress, with 600 participants about the issue of hearing voices, and a report was published in 2005.

Italy

In Italy, Pino Pini, a psychiatrist from Florence working in Prato, took the initiative to have the book *Accepting Voices* translated into Italian (*Accettare le Voci*, 1997). Pino invited us many times to give presentations on conferences he organised in Prato and Florence. He started a support group in Prato, which continued for many years, and he followed the development of the movement by visiting the Intervoice meetings. He became, with Donatella Micinesi, very nice friends.

We also later met Marcello Macario, who was also a psychiatrist who started to work with voice hearers, and became a very inspiring person for the Italian national network together with Franco Angeli, who in 2006 translated Ron Coleman's book, and composed a book about hearing voices in a new style, with a chapter about our work. Together with the voice hearer Cristina Contini from Capri, they make a stimulating trio.

Portugal

In Portugal the movement started at the same time as in Italy. Professor Zagalo-Cardoso, a psychologist at the University of Coimbra, together with his friend Dr Cunha-Oliveira, a psychiatrist in Coimbra, translated the *Accepting Voices* book into Portuguese (*Na Companhia das Vozes*). They had heard about this approach from Professor Alec Jenner, and had visited our congress 'Developing Partnership between Professionals and Users' during August 1995 in Maastricht.

We are very grateful to them for the translation, which is a significant piece of work, as well as for their invitation to Coimbra. They were such nice hosts, and we had some lovely evenings, laughing a lot and eating the local specialities. We also thank Dr Zagalo for his invitation to the 20th anniversary of the psychological faculty at the University of Coimbra, with a presentation published in the book *Psicologia e Sociedade: Cyclo de conferencias;* Universidade de Coimbra (1998).

Japan

Wakio Sato became interested when he was working at the Richmond fellowship in London. When he returned to Japan, he promoted the 'accepting voices' approach by writing several articles in the journal of the Japanese Psychology Association. He then invited us for a tour in Japan, where we gave several presentations at well-organised meetings with a lot of very attentively listening people. Naturally it was all translated into Japanese, which took quite some time, but the attendees were very patient. We have the most fantastic memories of this journey; the great and warm and luxurious hospitality, the enormous crowded town of Tokyo with its beautiful modern buildings. Wakio and his friends introduced us to their fantastic cultural habits, that are such a contrast to the great technical development there. It is an astonishing difference between technology and culture; the very special food; the organised perfection of their train transport; the luxurious hotels, and then sleeping on a typical Japanese bed on the floor. We are grateful for the first invitation to Sandra and me, as well as for the second to Phil Thomas and me, presenting also at the congress of the World Psychiatric Association. Wakio and colleagues also started a self-help group in two different towns. Wakio Sato, Yotaka Fujimoto and Tsuyoshi Matsuo regularly report to Intervoice on what is going on, and we are happy we will meet up again in Maastricht in September 2009.

Germany

We are most grateful to many people in Germany for promoting in different ways the accepting voices approach. We were first invited by Klaus Walker who completed a doctorate thesis on this theme, and organised a number of presentations for us in various psychiatric hospitals in and around Berlin. Klaus was a very nice man, but the hospitals we visited were not very open to our approach. It was his supervisor, Mrs Dr Monika Hoffmann, a very warm, clever and highly skilled psychologist and psychotherapist, together with a woman friend psychiatrist, who promoted this approach, and who really were active in helping people hearing voices (see also the story of Antje Müller, the coordinator of the Berlin Network). Monika also stimulated many students to write their thesis about hearing voices, including Klaus Walker. She is a great friend to us and we have stayed many times at her flat. We were then invited by Dr Thomas Bock in Hamburg, who was promoting the interaction of professionals in mental health, users of mental health services and family members, to talk together about their experiences in so-called 'trialogue groups'. All over Germany there are 70 groups, meeting regularly. He introduced us to a number of meetings, which helped spread the ideas of accepting and understanding voices. He then promoted with the publishing company 'Psychiatrie Verlag' in Bonn, the translation of our *Accepting Voices* book into

German *Stimmen Hören Akzeptieren* in 1997. He also wrote with a journalist woman friend Irene Stratenwerth, a book *Hearing Voices* (*Stimmen Hören* in German, published by Kabel in 1998) and Irene Stratenwerth took the initiative to make a TV documentary on hearing voices for North West German Broadcasting (NWDR).

In the meantime in Berlin the network 'Stimmen Hören' was founded, intensively stimulated by Monika Hoffmann, and coordinated by Hannelore Klafki, a very special woman. Hannelore was a very energetic woman who fought for the interests of users of psychiatric care, and had the experience herself, which motivated her to make the world a better place.

The network runs a very nice website, and every two years they organise a congress in Berlin supported by a women politician and psychiatrist. As part of their regular activities they support individual voice hearers, run an ongoing hearing voices group, and a 'Trialogue' group. They also write newsletters and help to stimulate the formation of support groups in Germany. This enthusiastic group also organised a second edition of *Accepting Voices* in German with the cooperation of the first publisher. We would like to thank these publishers, and especially the Director Mrs Koch of Psychiatrie Verlag, for her outstanding support in also publishing *Making Sense of Voices* in German.

We've had many good times in Berlin with the network at conferences, and cafés too because meeting voice hearers outside official occasions is a wonderful way of getting to know each other. We are also especially grateful to Monika Hoffmann; Hannelore Klafki; Antje Müller and Caroline von Thysen for the nice times we had in Berlin with them. We were very much shocked when we heard in September 2005 that Hannelore had died very suddenly due to an aneurism in the brain.

In Berlin we also met Peter Lehmann, a very active publisher of anti-psychiatric books who, together with Peter Stastny, a New York psychiatrist, published a very positive and interesting book *Alternatives Beyond Psychiatry* (on alternatives in mental health care). We are glad to have been invited to talk about Intervoice and the hearing voices movement. Peter Lehmann has also composed a fine book of the texts of Hannelore Klafki (2006).

We would also like to thank others, especially the voice hearers we met in Berlin like Frank Dahmen and Andreas Gehrke. More recently we met Joachim Schnackenberg, a trained social worker and nurse of German origin, who worked in England and was trained by Ron Coleman when still in Gloucester; they worked together with voice hearers, making Joachim both enthusiastic and knowledgeable. He has since translated *Making Sense of Voices* into German (*Stimmenhören Verstehen*, 2008), and developed with us, and has since run, a training programme in Germany. Joachim Schnackenberg (2008) also wrote an article in German. We thank him for all this very much, and hope he will continue.

Switzerland

From Switzerland we first met Theresja Krummenacher, who came and visited the Intervoice meetings, mostly just looking at what was going on, and then coming forward as a very inspired promoter of user interests. She organised the translation of Paul Baker's book *The Voice Inside* and expanded it with stories of voice hearers she had met in Switzerland. This was the first publication in the French language about accepting voices. She is also the founder of a national network called REEV (Reseau déntraide des entendeur de voix: Source of self-help for voice hearers). In this organisation she started a self-help group in Geneva, ongoing now for many years.

Although Theresja is of our older generation, she is more active than a lot of young people. She organised two visits for us to present our work; one at a two-day course in Basel lead by Dr Jacob Christ; the other on a full-day course in Geneva lead by Dr Merlot, both part of postgraduate courses for psychiatrists, and we are grateful for these opportunities.

Sweden

After we had met Alain Topor in Italy, he wrote in Swedish an article about accepting voices, and after some years he became very active in promoting this approach.

He organised training sessions with therapists and voice hearers, and helped start the Swedish network. He translated *Understanding Voices* (1996) into Swedish (*Hora Röster*, 1998), our research report on the comparative study of patients and non-patients hearing voices. He was also the force behind the translation of our book *Making Sense of Voices* (1999) into Swedish (*Forsta och Hantera Röster*, 2003), in cooperation with the Swedish user association RSMH. He wrote a wonderful thesis 'Managing the Contradictions' (2001) on the process of recovery. Through Alain we also met Noella Bickham, who helped us publish an article about the children's research (Escher, 2005)

We are very grateful to him and to Liz Bodil for all their hard work and efforts to promote the accepting voices approach in Sweden. Liz Bodil (1999) because she started from her experience as a voice hearer and as a social worker, to work with voice hearers in a non-medical atmosphere, inviting them for a summer camp and, before that, giving presentations about accepting voices (see story of Ami Rohnitz). She also wrote a book about the accepting voices issue, *Inre Röster* (1999), and did her PhD on the subject. With her lies the root of the Swedish network, and she stimulated Ami Rohnitz to develop herself and become the coordinator of the Stockholm network, giving talks and training. Together with Siv Wetterberg, Ami keeps the network running.

In the very beginning of the nineties we also met Maths Jesperson, the secretary of an international users and ex-users society, who was also a great stimulus to promoting the accepting voices approach in the south of Sweden in Lund. We are thankful to him also because he was very good at formulating the essence of our own and others' thoughts and reasoning.

Norway

We met Siri Blesvik in Oslo, who'd had experience with a hearing voices group she had set up in Cambodia, and who has since become the professor at the nursing school in the University of Oslo. She has always been very positive about the approach of accepting voices and, like Marit Borg, has tried to introduce this approach to Norway's psychiatric services. We think that one of the reasons that not much has yet come off the ground there is the official psychiatric institutes, who find it very difficult to understand this approach, or to have an open mind. The reason we think Geir Fredrikson from Molde was more successful in working with voice hearers was because he was not so bound by the limitations of psychiatric thinking. We would like to thank all three of them for their efforts in promoting the accepting voices approach.

Denmark

We were first invited by Karl Bach, who was promoting the users' perspective in Denmark. It was quite a big congress in Aarhus, but at the time our talks seemed still too strange, but we got another invitation to Aarhus by a nursing-school teacher, but that also didn't fall on fertile ground. It took some years before a new stimulus came from Jorn Erikson, based near Copenhagen. He ran a clinic for very long term psychiatric patients, and was especially inspired by Ron Coleman and Mike Smith who started to work at their clinic, changing the approach, and they were successful in bringing about change. After this the contacts grew rapidly in Copenhagen and again in Aarhus the second largest city in Denmark, where Trevor Eyles, an English mental health nurse, took the lead. Together they found a publisher who translated *Making Sense of Voices* into Danish (*Giv Stemmerne Mening*, 2003). They also founded a national network, and a very inspiring woman voice hearer, Olga Runciman, became the coordinator. She organised an Intervoice meeting in 2007 with the help of the others. Thereafter the number of support groups started to rise in different places in Denmark, with Ron Coleman and Dirk Corstens often going there for training and conferences, and Dirk also starting his research there for his PhD. He gave training in making 'Constructs', a systematic method of relating voices to what has happened in the life of the voice hearer, and by doing so getting more insight into the meaning of voices. He also gave supervision in follow-up visits. The method was developed in Maastricht and published in *Making Sense of Voices*, but not much used because it needs training and supervision. Because of the work of Trevor Eyles and Jorn Erikson the network has become evermore successful in Denmark, and we are very thankful to them, and besides, they are also very nice people to meet regularly and have a friendship with. Jorn and his wife Ann will also be translating this book into Danish.

USA

Our first tour of the United States was organised by Phil Thomas. We visited Professor Ron Diamond in Massachusetts, Dr Loren Mosher in Washington, and Dr Dick Warner in Denver, all three modern psychiatrists focusing on the user perspective. They were very attentive listeners, but nothing came of it. Like elsewhere, contact with mainstream psychiatry did not easily happen. With psychosis, the way of working in psychiatry is mainly focused on the illness category, and there is no experience in orientation and working with the separate complaints. Hearing voices is seen as part of an illness, and therefore no one is trained or used to focusing on the hearing of voices, or on the delusions themselves. We have been supported by and worked with psychiatrists in Europe, but most of them were more independent from mainstream organisations, except in Vienna. Setting up support groups for voice hearers in Europe is hardly the work of psychiatrists, but rather psychologists, social workers, nurses, support workers or voice hearers themselves. We think the situation will not have been much different with accepting homosexuality, as they also were not organised by psychiatry, but by the group themselves as the main force in emancipation. And they too still have to fight for their own interests.

So it took some more years before the first support groups started in America, and that was set up by a voice hearer mental health activist Jenny Branks in Massachusetts. Now there is also a group in Orlando, also set up by voice hearers, and another in Massachusetts set up by Professor Gail Hornstein (2009). Gail is a psychologist who studied the literature of people's own mental health experiences for many years, and interviewed many users talking about their experiences. She has recently published an excellent and well-written book reporting these experiences.

Australia

Our first contact with Australia was with John Watkins who, after our article in the *Schizophrenia Bulletin*, responded with a booklet *Hearing Voices: A self-help guide*, published by The Richmond Fellowship of Victoria in 1993. He later wrote a very fine exploration with a wider scope (John Watkins, 1998). We did not meet during those times, but Ron Coleman later introduced the accepting voices approach in Australia and New Zealand, within the wider perspective of recovery.

Last year we held the Intervoice meeting in Perth, Australia, and there we had the pleasure to meet and thank those who had cooperated with great enthusiasm in the recovery congress and accepting voices approach, and had set up an Australian Network with many groups spread around Australia, and also New Zealand. It was great to see how well the congress on recovery and the Intervoice meeting were organised. We are specially grateful to Joe Calleja, director of the Richmond Fellowship West Australia in Perth, who organised the Recovery congress, and Lyn Mahboub and Marlene Janssen who organised the Intervoice meeting in Perth.

Spain

The first initiative in Spain was taken by Professor Manuel Gonzales de Chavez, who invited us to take part in his very well organised annual course on schizophrenia. He was a fabulous organiser, and the course attracted 800 participants. It was a great opportunity to introduce the accepting voices approach in Spain. He also organised the translation of the book *Making Sense of Voices* into Spanish (*Dando Sentido a las Voces*, 2005). The following year we were invited to take part and give a course at the ISPS triennial conference in Madrid, which he also organised as well as his course. It is also due to him that we have been invited to compose a book on hearing voices in the ISPS series to be published by Routledge next year. We are grateful to Manuel for all this, and to Brian Martindale, the series editor, who has supported us through the Routledge 'procedures'. We have not yet found an activist in Spain who might start a network and support groups.

Palestine

We have met some of those who picked up the attitude necessary to respond in another way, which is necessary with accepting voices. But it is Ron Coleman who, with the help of John Jenkins and WHO, have promoted this change in a psychiatric hospital in Bethlehem. We are thankful for the brave people in Bethlehem because it is not easy to live there and change things.

Eire and Northern Ireland

We've worked with Liz Ellis, who organised meetings in Dublin and Belfast, but at that time nothing more came of it. We've also regularly met nurses from Eire and Northern Ireland at UK conferences, but it has been others who took up the accepting voices approach in both countries. Goedele van Laake undertook a postgraduate follow-up study on Sandra's children research, and then moved to Eire and has become active there. Most active is Brian Hartnett, who as coordinator, will start a national network.

Russia

In 1998 the Geneva Initiative on Psychiatry organised the translation of the book *Accepting Voices*. The purpose of the Geneva Initiative on Psychiatry is to publish books and brochures which contribute to the creation of a civil society and development of science in Ukraine on a noncommercial basis. We are grateful for this initiative, but know nothing of any follow up. We neither speak Russian, nor know anybody in the Ukraine.

Greece

Greece, until now is the last country to became involved in the accepting voice approach. People from Greece attended the ISPS conference in Madrid, and thereafter attended some conferences in England. They invited Peter Bullimore to Athens to talk about the Hearing Voices Network, and he will soon be going back for a second visit. We will wait, hope and see.

And finally ...

During the last twenty-five years there have been a number of PhDs completed about the accepting voices approach and hearing voices movement, and we are very grateful for the ways they have included voice hearers' experiences, and for this reason they are also important, as well as for the very interesting results of the studies. Such theses were written up by Mike Grierson in 2003 at Manchester University; Lisa Blackman in 2001 at Goldsmith College in London; Terence McLaughlin in 2003 at Manchester University; Sandra Escher in 2005 at Maastricht University; Vanessa Beavan in 2006 at Auckland University in New Zealand; and Liz Bodil in 2007 at Stockholm University.

We are also thankful to those scientists who wrote a chapter or paragraph on the accepting voices approach in their book, including Phil Thomas (1997); Lucy Johnstone (2000); Ad Bergsma (2001), and Gail Hornstein (2009).

We would also like to thank those teachers and scientists who have invited us to write a chapter in their books, including Tom Heller (Heller et al., 1996a); Gillian Haddock and Peter Slade (1996b); Mary Copeland and Piers Allot (2005b); Heinz Katschnig and Michaela Amering (2005); Warren Larkin and Anthony Morrison (2006a); Jack Jenner (2006c); our chapter with Dirk Corstens in Andrew Moskowitz et al. (2008); Jos de Kroon (2008); Frank Laroi (2009); and Laurens Henkelman (2009).

When a new method is introduced there is much interest in training, and that in itself is right, and might well be what is missing; a proper training program for mental health professionals in using the approach of Accepting and Making Sense of Voices, including the possibility of supervision. There is now testing going on in Denmark by Dirk Corstens from Maastricht, Joachim Schnackenberg in Germany, and Mervyn Morris and Jim Chapman at Birmingham City University. Jacqui Dillon has also developed a training in setting up and facilitating hearing voices groups. We will become more active in this field after the 2009 World Congress in Maastricht.

REFERENCES

Adams, J (2001) *Raising Our Voices: An account of the Hearing Voices movement.* Gloucester: Handsell Publishing.

Al-Issa, I (1977) Social and cultural aspects of hallucinations. *Psychological Bulletin, 84* (3), 570–87.

Aleman, A & Laroi, F (2008) *Hallucinations: The science of idiosyncratic perception.* Washington, DC: American Psychological Association. [Authors are based at the University of Groningen, Holland]

Amering, M & Schmolke, M (1997) *Recovery: Das Ende der Unheilbarkeit.* Bonn: Psychiatrie Verlag.

Angeli, F (2006) Allucinazioni uditive Rivista Sperimentale di Freniatrie. *La rivista della salute mentale, CXXX,* (2).

Aslan, M & Smith, M (2007) *Thrive.* www.crazydiamond.org.uk

Baker, P (1999) *Entendre des Voix Guide pratique et Temoignages,* published by Movement 'Les Sans Voix' Case Postale 235 Ch – 1211 Geneve 17.

Baker, P (2003) *The Voice Inside.* Manchester: Hearing Voices Network.

Beavan, V (2007) *Angels at Our Table: New Zealanders experiences of Hearing voices.* PhD Thesis. University of Auckland, NZ.

Bentall, RP (1990) *Reconstructing Schizophrenia.* London: Routledge.

Bentall, RP (2003) *Madness Explained.* London: Penguin.

Bergsma, A (2001) *In Wat bezielt de psycholoog. Gesprekken met vooraanstaande psychologen: 'De stemmen van Marius Romme'* (pp 282–8). Amsterdam: Uitgeverij Nieuwezijds.

Bijl, RV, Ravelli, A & van Zessen, G (1998) Prevalence of psychiatric disorder in the general population. *Social Psychiatry Psychiatric Epidemiology, 33,* 587–95.

Blom, JD (2003) *Deconstructing Schizophrenia.* Amsterdam: Boom.

Boyle, M (1990) *Schizophrenia: A scientific delusion?* London: Routledge.

Chadwick, P (2006) *Person-Based Cognitive Therapy for Distressing Psychosis.* Chichester: Wiley.

Coleman, R (1999) *Recovery: An alien concept.* Gloucester: Handsell Publishing. (Order from the author: Isles of Lewis, Scotland. Email: ron@roncolemanvoices.co.uk)

Coleman, R & Smith, M (1997) *Working with Voices: Victim to victor.* Gloucester: Handsell Publishing.

Conway, T (2006) An experience of group work in a medium secure psychiatric hospital. *Voices Magazine,* Spring, 3–4.

Corstens, D, Romme, M & Escher, S (2008) Accepting and working with voices: The Maastricht approach. In A Moskowitz, I Schäfer & MJ Dohoray (Eds), *Psychosis, Trauma and Dissociation: Emerging perspectives on severe pathology* (pp 319–33). Chichester: Wiley.

Dallos, R & Johnstone, L (2006) *Formulation in Psychology and Psychotherapy: Making sense of people's problems.* London: Routledge.

De Jong, JTVM (1987) *A Decent into African Psychiatry.* Amsterdam: Royal Tropical Institute.

Downs, J (ed) (2001) *Starting and Supporting Hearing Voices Groups.* Manchester: The Hearing Voices Network.

Downs, J (2005) *Coping with Voices and Visions.* Manchester: The Hearing Voices Network.

Eaton, WW, Romanoski, A, Anthony, JC & Nestadt, G (1991) Screening for psychosis in the general population with a self-report interview. *The Journal of Nervous and Mental Disease, 179,* 689–93.

Ensink, BJ (1992) *Confusing Realities: A study on child sexual abuse and psychiatric symptoms.* Amsterdam: Free University Press.

Escher, S (2005a) *Making Sense of Psychotic Experiences.* PhD thesis. University of Maastricht.

Escher, S (2005b) Stimmenhören bei Kindern. In H Katschnig & M Amering (Eds) *Stimmenhören* (pp 45–54). Vienna: Facultas Verlag.

Grierson, M (1993) *Hearing Voices: A sociological study.* PhD thesis. Sociology Department, University of Manchester.

Herman, JL (1992) *Trauma and Recovery.* New York: Basic Books

Honig, A, Romme, MAJ, Ensink, BJ, Escher, SDMAC, Pennings, MHA, DeVries, MW (1998) Auditory hallucinations. A comparison between patients and non-patients. *Journal of Nervous and Mental Disease, 186,* 646–51.

Hornstein GA (2009) *Agnes's Jacket: A psychologist's search for the meaning of madness.* Rodale, NY: Macmillan.

James, A (2001) *Raising Our Voices: An account of the Hearing Voices Movement.* Gloucester: Handsell Publishing.

Johns, LC & van Os, J (2001) The continuity of psychotic experiences in the general population. *Clinical Psychology Review, l21* (8), 1125–41.

Johnstone, L (2000) *Users and Abusers of Psychiatry.* London: Routledge

Karlsson, L-B (Ed) (1999) *Inre Röster och Vad Man Kan Göra.* Stockholm: Vastra Stockholsomrade Bromma.

Karlsson, L-B (2007) *Berättelser om Inre Röster* [Narratives of Inner Voices: A phenomenological and communicative perspective]. PhD Thesis, Stockholm University.

Katschnig H & Amering, M (Eds) (2005) *Stimmenhören.* Vienna: Facultas Verlag.

Klafki, H (2006) *Meine Stimmen – Qualgeister und Schutzengel* [Texts of an engaged voice hearer]. Berlin: Peter Lehmann Anti-psychiatrie Verlag.

Laing, RD (1967) *The Politics of Experience and The Bird of Paradise.* London: Penguin.

McGuire, PK, Silbersweig, DA, Wright, I et al (1995) Abnormal monitoring of inner speech: A physiological basis for auditory hallucinations. *The Lancet, 346,* 596–600.

McLeod, T, Morris, M, Birchwood, M, Dovey, A (2007) Cognitive behavioural therapy-based group work with voice hearers (I). *British Journal of Nursing. 16* (4), 248–52.

Meddings, S, Walley, L, Collins, T, Tullett, F & McGowan, B (2006) The Voices don't like it. *Mental Health Today,* September, 26–30.

Morland, R (2003) How do people experience being part of a hearing voices group? *Voices Magazine,* Summer, 10–12.

Newton, E, Larkin M, Melhuish R & Wykes, T (2007) More than just a place to talk: Young people's experiences of group psychological therapy as an early intervention. *Psychology and Psychotherapy: Theory, Research and Practice,* 80, 127–49.

Pennings, M & Romme, M(1997/2007) *Gesprek groepen voor mensen die stemmen horen.* University of Maastricht. [Second edition, 2007, Foundation Resonance]

Read, J, van Os, J, Morrison, AP, Ross, CA (2005) Childhood trauma, psychosis and schizophrenia. *Acta Psychiatrica Scandinavica, 112,* 330–50.

Romme, MAJ (1996) *Understanding Voices: Report of comparative study of patients and non-patients hearing voices.* University of Maastricht and P&P Press; www.roncolemanvoices.co.uk

Romme, MAJ (1998) *Höra röster.* FoU-enheten/psykiatri; email fou@algonet.se [A translation of Understanding Voices 1996 University of Maastricht]

Romme, MAJ (2005) Stimmen hören was ist normal, was sit krank? In H Katschnig & M Amering (Eds), *Stimmenhören* (pp 14–22). Vienna: Facultas Verlag.

Romme, M & Escher, S (1989) Hearing Voices. *Schizophrenia Bulletin, 15* (2), 209–16.

Romme, M & Escher, S (1993) *Accepting Voices.* London: Mind

Romme, M & Escher, S (1996a) Rehabilitating voice-hearers. In T Heller, J Reynolds, R Gomm, R Muston & S Pattison (Eds) *Mental Health Matters: A reader* (pp 326–32). London: Macmillan, in association with the Open University.

Romme, M & Escher, S (1996b) Empowering people who hear voices. In G Haddock & PD Slade (Eds) *Cognitive Behavioural Interventions with Psychotic*

Disorders (pp 137–51). London: Routledge.

Romme, M & Escher, S (1997a) (with A Zagalo-Cardoso e JA Cunha-Oliveira) *Na Companhia Das Vozes*. Lisbon, Portugal: Coleccao Novos Rumos, Editorial Estampa.

Romme, M & Escher, S (1997b) *Accettare le Voci*. Milano, Italy: Giuffre.

Romme, M & Escher, S (1997c) *Stimmenhören Akzeptieren*, Bonn, Germany: Psychiatrie Verlag.

Romme, M & Escher, S (1997d) *Moniaaniset*. Vantaa, Finland: Printway Oy.

Romme, M & Escher, S (1998a) *Accepting Voices*. Geneva Initiative on Psychiatrie, Switzerland.

Romme, M & Escher, S (1998b) Understanding voices. In A Duarte Gomes & JM Pires Valentin (Eds) *20 Anos Faculdade de Psicologia e de Ciencias da Educacao* (pp 93–104). Universidade de Coimbra, Portugal.

Romme, M & Escher, S (1999) *Stemmen Hören Accepteren*. Baarn: Tirion.

Romme, M & Escher, S (2000a) *Making Sense of Voices*. London: Mind,

Romme, M & Escher, S (2000b) *Stimmenhören Akzeptieren, Neunplus 1*. Berlin: Edition Wissenschaft.

Romme, M & Escher, S (2003a) *Forsta och Hantera Röster. Fou enheten Psykiatrin Sodra & Riksforbundet for Social och Mental Halsa*. Stockholm, Sweden www.rsmh.se

Romme, M & Escher, S (2003b) *Giv stemmerne mening*. Systime Academic Arhus www.systime.dk

Romme, M & Escher, S (2004) *Stimmenhören bei Kindern und Jugendlichen*. In Thomas Bock et al (Eds) Anstösse: Zu einer anthropologischen Psychiatrie (pp 211–18) Bonn: Psychiatrie-Verlag.

Romme, M & Escher, S (2005a) *Dando Sentido a Las Voices Fundacion para la investigacion y el tratamiento de la esquizofrenia y otras psicosis*. Celebración del 50º Aniversario del ISPS, Madrid, Spain.

Romme, M & Escher, S (2005b) In ME Copeland (P Allott, Ed), *Wellness Recovery Action Plan* (pp 114–18). Liverpool: Sefton Recovery Group.

Romme, M & Escher, S (2006a) Trauma and hearing voices. In W Larkin & A Morrison (Eds) *Trauma and Psychosis* (pp 162–92). London: Routledge.

Romme, M & Escher, S (2006b) L'elaborazione di un diverso approccio sull'esperienza degli uditori di voci [The development of an approach based on the experience of voice hearers] In F Angeli Allucinazioni uditive Rivista Sperimentale di Freniatrie. *La rivista della salute mentale, CXXX*, (2).

Romme, M & Escher, S (2006c) Empowerment and making sense [Dutch]. In J Jenner (Ed), *Hallucinations* (pp 84–94). Assen, Netherlands: Van Gorcum.

Romme, M & Escher, S (2008a) *Stimmenhören Verstehen. Der Leitfaden zur Arbeit mit Stimmenhörern*. Bonn, Germany: Psychiatrie-Verlag.

Romme, M & Escher, S (2008b) Trauma en Psychotherapie. In J de Kroon

Zachte Landing (pp 167–81). Antwerpen, Belgium: Garant.

Schnackenberg, J, Romme, M, Escher, S (2008) Stimmenhören: Ein Phanomen emanzipiert sich. *Kerbe Forum fur Sozialpsychiaterie 26* (4), 4–7.

Stastny, P & Lehmann, P (2007) *Alternatives Beyond Psychiatry*. Berlin: Peter Lehmann Publishing [www.peter-lehmann-publishing.com].

Thomas, P (1997) *The Dialectics of Schizophrenia*. London: Free Association Books.

Tien, AY (1991) Distributions of hallucination in the population. *Social Psychiatry and Psychiatric Epidemiology, 26*, 287–92.

Topor, A (2001) *Managing the Contradictions: Recovery from severe mental disorders.* Stockholm University Department of Social Work.

Van der Hart, O (Ed) (1995) *Trauma, dissociatie en hypnose* [Trauma, dissociation and hypnosis]. Lisse, Netherlands: Swets & Zeitlinger.

Van Os, J, Hanssen, M, Bijl, RV et al (2001) Prevalence of psychotic disorder and community level of psychotic symptoms.' *Arch Gen Psych, 58* (July) 663–8.

Watkins, J (1993) *Hearing Voices: A self-help guide*. The Richmond Fellowship of Victoria.

Watkins, J (1998) *Hearing Voices: A common human experience*, Melbourne: Hill of Content. [2nd edition (2008) Michelle Anderson Publishing Pty Ltd. www.michellandersonpublishing.com]

Wykes T, Parr AM, & Landau S (1999) Group treatment of auditory hallucinations. Exploratory study of effectiveness. *British Journal of Psychiatry, 175,* 180–5.

Zammit, S, Spurlock, G, Williams, H et al (2007) Genotype effects of CHRNA7, CNR1 and COMT in schizophrenia: Interactions with tobacco and cannabis use. *British Journal of Psychiatry, 191*, 402–7.

CONTRIBUTORS

Marius Romme, MD, PhD, was Professor of Social Psychiatry at the Medical Faculty of the University of Maastricht (Netherlands) from 1974 to 1999, as well as Consultant Psychiatrist at the Community Mental Health Centre in Maastricht. He is now a Visiting Professor at the Centre for Community Mental Health, Birmingham City University. His research over the past twenty-five years has focused on the voice-hearing experience.

Sandra Escher, MPhil, PhD, was a science journalist and worked as a senior researcher at the University of Maastricht, focusing on children hearing voices. She is now an Honorary Research Fellow at the Centre for Community Mental Health, Birmingham City University.

Jacqui Dillon is the Chair of the National Hearing Voices Network, England, a user-led charity which works to promote acceptance and understanding of the experiences of hearing voices, seeing visions, tactile sensations and other sensory experiences. She is an international speaker and trainer specialising in hearing voices, 'psychosis' and trauma. She is a published writer.

Dirk Corstens is a social psychiatrist and psychotherapist working at the RIAGG (community mental health service) in Maastricht. He has worked with Marius and Sandra since 1992, and now leads a treatment facility for voice hearers in Maastricht. Dirk is also currently preparing a PhD on courses for voice hearers and professionals and the voice-dialogue method for voice hearing.

Mervyn Morris is Professor of Community Mental Health and Director of the Centre for Community Mental Health at Birmingham City University, focusing on service redesign and developing alternative approaches through user expertise, particularly in the area of psychosis. He has run a practice-based university-accredited training on the *accepting voices* approach since 1999.

NAMES INDEX*

A
Aleman, A 39
Al-Issa, I 23
Allot, Piers 337
Amering, Michaela i, ii, 331, 337
Ami 14, 20, 21, 30, 43, 48, 49, 58, 63, 68, 96, 99, **104**, 334
Andreas 19, 80, 98, **108**, 333
Annat, Pia 150
Antje 11, 15, 19, 21, 28, 31, 33, 44, 49, 56, 70, 71, 78, 92, 93, 100, **112**, 332, 333
Aslan, Marion **238**, 330
Audrey 16, 18, 28, 29, 87, 98, **118**

B
Bach, Karl 334
Baker, Paul 49, 73, 74, 286, 325, 327, 329, 330, 333
Barend, Sonja 325
Barker, Phil 330
Beavan, Vanessa 337
Bentall, Richard 25, 328
Bergsma, Ad 337
Bickham, Noella 334
Bijl, RV 24
Blackman, Lisa 337
Blake, William 23
Blesvik, Siri 334
Blom, JD 25
Bock, Thomas 177, 332
Bodil, Liz 14, 48, 49, 334, 334, 337
Borg, Marit 334
Bosman, Denise **134**
Bouvink, Wilma 326
Boyle, Mary 25, 184
Bracken, Pat 16, 49, 143, 144
Brackx, Anny 328
Bramley, Sally 269

Branks, Jenny 335
Brevik, Thore 291
Brink, Jeanette 18, 20, **198**
Brouwer, Dick 326
Brown, Christine 330
Brummens, Flore 13, 18, 20, 21, 42, 48, 57, 80, 96, 99, **157**, 277, 326
Buiks, Alex 326
Bullimore, Peter 14, 17, 18, 19, 28, 96, **267**, 329, 337

C
Calleja, Joe 336
Carlyn, Karina 13, 18, 19, 46, 48, 49, 55, 67, 69, 97, **230**
Caroline 28, 40, 89, **124**
Chadwick, Paul 92, 338
Chapman, Jim 337
Chappin, Fernand 79, **153**
Christ, Jacob 334
Clarkson, Sue 13, 15, 18, 21, 28, 51, 56, 76, 79, **314**, 330
Coleman, Ron 2, 7, 8, 9, 11, 12, 15, 28, 32, 33, 51, 74, 78, 87, 93, 96, 117, 121, 123, 178, 183, 223, **283**, 312, 327, 329, 330, 333, 335, 336
Contini, Cristina 331
Conway, Terry 76, 85
Cooke, Lindsay 285
Copeland, Mary 337
Corstens, Dirk 5, 31, 52, 89, 134, 135, 158, 186, 326, 330, 335, 337, 342
Cunha-Oliveira, JA 331

D
Daan 14, 15, 46, 66, 69, **126**

---

* The voice hearers' stories are indexed by surname (where given) and also by first name. The page where their story begins is printed in **bold**.

Dahmen, Frank 18, 28, 41, 43, 66, 80, 96, **161**, 333
Dallos, R 54
Davies, Hywell 330
Davies, Peggy 28, 31, 88, 97, **265**
Debra 3, 12, 17, 18, 19, 32, 33, 34, 82, 96, 99, 100, **130**
de Bruin, Kisse 330
de Graaf, Frans 35, 41, 44, 96, 97, **163**
de Jong, JTVM 23
de Klerk, Lisette 14, 15, 18, 42, 51, 56, 68, 90, **234**
de Kroon, Jos 337
Deegan, Patricia 183
Delespaul, Philippe 327
Denise **134**
Diamond, Ron 335
Dillon, Jacqui 5, 14, 16, 26, 28, 47, 94, **188**, 329, 337, 342
Don 10, 28, 31, 33, 98, **139**
Downs, Julie 14, 73, 75, 78, 84, 85, 286, 328
Dugger, Don 10, 28, 31, 33, 98, **139**

E
Eaton, WW 24
Eleanor 10, 12, 14, 15, 16, 17, 20, 27, 28, 29, 32, 34, 35, 44, 49, 50, 71, 98, 99, **142**, 330
Elisabeth 82, 99, **147**
Ellis, Liz 336
Ensink, Bernardine 8, 40, 326
Erikson, Jorn 334, 335
Escher, Sandra 1, 8, 13, 25, 48, 49, 51, 52, 54, 59, 70, 72, 73, 92, 134, 144, 234, 281, 284, 286, 325, 329, 337, 342
Exell, John 53, 80, **212**
Eyles, Trevor 5, 49, 52, 56, 103, 150, 151, 223, 335

F
Fernand 79, **153**
Fisher, Daniel 183

Flore 13, 18, 20, 21, 42, 48, 57, 80, 96, 99, **157**, 277, 326
Forrest, Ruth 81, 97, **296**
Frank 18, 28, 41, 43, 66, 80, 96, **161**, 333
Frans 35, 41, 44, 96, 97, **163**
Fredrikson, Geir M 5, 103, 291, 290, 334
Fujimoto, Yotaka 332

G
Gavin **169**
Gehrke, Andreas 19, 80, 98, **108**, 333
Ghandi, Mahatma 23
Gijsen, Sjon 28, 34, **307**
Gina 14, 15, 20, 28, 33, 46, 49, 56, 67, 89, **171**
Gold, Betty 101
Gonzales de Chavez, Manuel 336
Grierson, Mike 286, 337, 344

H
Haddock, Gillian 328, 337
Hage, Patsy 56, 69, 71, **260**, 286, 324
Hammersley, Paul 329
Hannelore 3, 11, 14, 17, 20, 28, 34, 49, 52, 71, 80, 99, 115, **176**, 333
Hartnett, Brian 336
Heap, Helen 48, 74, 232, 285, 327
Helen 31, 42, 47, 52, 100, **180**
Heller, Tom 337
Hendry, Stewart 3, 10, 11, 16, 18, 19, 20, 27, 28, 29, 45, 52, 71, 98, 99, **309**, 330
Henkelman, Laurens 337
Herman, Judith Lewis 14, 82, 94, 184, 190
Hoffmann, Monika 177, 332, 333
Holloway, Jan 13, 28, 48, **194**
Honig, Adriaan 8, 326
Hornstein, Gail 335, 337
Huisman, Robert **280**
Hutten, Mrs 3, **186**

J

Jacqui 14, 16, 26, 28, 47, 94, **188**, 329, 337
Jan 13, 28, 48, **194**
Janssen, Marlene 336
Jeanette B 18, 20, **198**
Jeannette W 3, 17, 18, 28, 53, 91, 96, 178, **203**, 326
Jenkins, John 336
Jenner, Alec 325, 327, 332
Jenner, Jack 337
Jesperson, Maths 334
Jesus 23
Jo 41, 52, **209**
Joan of Arc 23
John E 53, 80, **212**
John R **218**
Johns, LC 24
Johnstone, Lucy 54, 330, 337
Jones, Adam 329
Johnny 3, 14, 16, 28, 29, 33, 46, 49, 52, 55, 67, 71, 78, 151, **222**
Jolanda 18, 28, 57, 60, 61, 62, 64, 65, 70, **225**

K

Karina 13, 18, 19, 46, 48, 49, 55, 67, 69, 97, **230**
Katschnig, Heinz 331, 337
Klafki, Hannelore 3, 11, 14, 17, 20, 28, 34, 49, 52, 71, 80, 99, 115, **176**, 333
Koch, Ute 333
Krummenacher, Theresja 333

L

Laing, Ronnie D 241
Lampshire, Debra 3, 12, 17, 18, 19, 32, 33, 34, 82, 96, 99, 100, **130**
Landau, S 85
Landman, S 127, 128
Larkin, Warren 337
Laroi, Frank 39, 337
Lehmann, Peter 176, 333
Lemmens, Marietje 326
Lisette 14, 15, 18, 42, 51, 56, 68, 90, **234**
Longden, Eleanor 10, 12, 14, 15, 16, 17, 20, 27, 28, 29, 32, 34, 35, 44, 49, 50, 71, 98, 99, **142**, 330

M

Macario, Marcello 331
Mahboub, Lyn 336
Malecki, Resi 326
Marion **238**, 330
Marsman, Daan 14, 15, 46, 66, 69, **126**
Martindale, Brian 330, 336
Matsuo, Tsuyoshi 332
May, Rufus 28, 30, 33, 44, 183, **292**, 329
McGuire, PK 39
McLaughlin, Terence 48, 78, 232, 286, 328, 329, 337
McLeod, Terry 76, 85
Meddings, Sara 75, 85
Merlot, Paul 334
Micinesi, Donatella 331
Mieke 28, 46, 50, 55, **244**, 326
Mien 12, 14, 16, 18, 30, 42, 50, 51, 53, 66, 68, 69, 81, 82, 91, **248**, 277
Miller, Alice 117
Milligan, Spike 241
Mohammed 23
Morland, Rebecca 76, 85
Morris, Mervyn 329, 337, 342
Morrison, Anthony 337
Mosher, Loren 335
Moskowitz, Andrew 337
Müller, Antje 11, 15, 19, 21, 28, 31, 33, 44, 49, 56, 70, 71, 78, 92, 93, 100, **112**, 332, 333

N

Newton, Elizabeth 77
Nilson, Ronny 27, 28, 32, **289**

O
Odi 28, 32, **251**
Olga 28, **253**, 335
Oquosa, Odi 28, 32, **251**

P
Parker, Ian 329
Patsy 56, 69, 71, **260**, 286, 324
Peggy 28, 31, 88, 97, **265**
Pembroke, Louise 330
Pennings, Monique 74, 85, 155, 326
Perkins, Rachel 183
Perretta, Lorraine 216
Peter B 14, 17, 18, 19, 28, 96, **267**, 329, 337
Peter R 28, 76, 79, 97, **273**
Pini, Pino 331
Plog, Ursula 177

R
Read, John 8, 25, 40, 51, 184
Reichard, Imme 325
Reid, Audrey 16, 18, 28, 29, 87, 98, **118**
Reynolds, Peter 28, 76 79, 97, **273**
Rilke, Rainer Maria 23
Riny 18, 81, **277**, 326
Robert **280**
Robinson, John **218**
Rohmit, Gina 14, 15, 20, 28, 33, 46, 49, 56, 67, 89, **171**
Rohnitz, Ami 14, 20, 21, 30, 43, 48, 49, 58, 63, 68, 96, 99, **104**, 334
Romme, Marius 1, 8, 13, 25, 48, 49, 51, 52, 54, 59, 72, 73, 74, 85, 89, 144, 234, 260, 284, 326, 342
Ron 2, 7, 8, 9, 11, 12, 15, 28, 32, 33, 51, 74, 78, 87, 93, 96, 117, 121, 123, 178, 183, 223, **283**, 312, 327
Ronny 27, 32, 34, **289**
Rose, Nigel 49, 232
Rufus 28, 30, 33, 44, 183, **292**, 329

Runciman, Olga 28, **253**, 335
Ruth 81, 97, **296**

S
Saint Paul 23
Saint Teresa 23
Sasja 13, 22, 35, 45, **301**
Sato, Wakio 332
Schnackenberg, Joachim 333, 337
Schneider, Chuck 331
Schumann, Robert 23
Selder, Riny 18, 81, **277**, 326
Simons, Mieke 28, 46, 50, 55, **244**, 326
Sjon 28, **307**
Slade, Peter 328, 337
Slotenmakers, Sasja 13, 22, 35, 45, **301**
Smith, Mike 15, 87, 93, 117, 243, 327, 335
Socrates 23
Sonnemans, Mien 12, 14, 16, 18, 30, 42, 50, 51, 53, 66, 68, 69, 81, 82, 91, **248**, 277
Sparvang, Johnny 3, 14, 16, 28, 29, 33, 46, 49, 52, 55, 67, 71, 78, 151, **222**
Stastny, Peter 333
Steultjens, Ben 326
Stewart 3, 10, 11, 16, 18, 19, 20, 27, 28, 29, 45, 52, 71, 98, 99, **309**, 330
Stowers, Chris 75
Strauss, John 325
Streefland, Ans 326, 327
Sue 13, 15, 18, 21, 28, 51, 56, 76, 79, **314**, 330
Svanholmer, Elisabeth 82, 99, **147**
Swedenborg, Emanuel 23

T
Taylor, Karen 327
Thomas, Phil 5, 31, 103, 265, 283, 328, 329, 332, 335, 337
Tien, AY 8, 24
Topor, Alain 325, 334

V

Van der Hart, O 167
van Hal, Frans 326
van Hoeij, Jolanda 18, 28, 57, 60,
    61, 62, 64, 65, 70, **225**
van Laake, Goedele 336
van London, Joop 325
van Os, Jim 24, 327
Verhaegh, Jan 326
von Thysen, Caroline 333
Vuorinen, Marja 330

W

Waite, Terry 241
Wallcraft, Jan ii
Walker, Klaus 332
Walton, Anne 12, 74, 78, 286, 327
Warner, Dick 335
Watkins, John 23, 335, 336
Webster, Pat 330
Weiterschein, Marleen 331
Wetterberg, Siv 334
Williams, John 74, 327
Woolf, Virginia 23
Woolthuis, Jeannette 3, 17, 18, 28,
    53, 91, 96, 178, **203**, 326
Wykes, Til 75, 85

Y

Young, Gavin **169**

Z

Zagalo-Cardoso, Antonio 331
Zammit, S 39

Also available from PCCS Books – www.pccs-books.co.uk

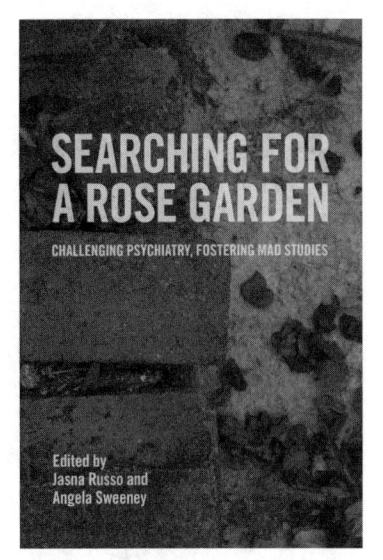

Searching for a Rose Garden:
challenging psychiatry, fostering mad studies

Edited by Jasna Russo & Angela Sweeney
(PCCS Books, 2016)

SEARCHING FOR A ROSE GARDEN is an incisive critique of all that is unhelpful about sanestream understandings of and responses to mental distress. Drawing on world-wide survivor activism and scholarship, it explores the toxicity of psychiatry and the co-option and corruption of survivor knowledge and practice by the mainstream. Chapters on survivor research and theory reveal the constant battle to establish and maintain a safe space for experiential knowledge within academia and beyond. Other chapters explore how survivor-developed projects and practices are cultivating a wealth of bright blooms in the most hostile of environments, providing an important vision for the future.

Referencing Joanne Greenberg's book *I Never Promised you a Rose Garden*, this collection demonstrates the challenge, determination and successes of the authors in working towards a paradigm shift in the understanding of madness and distress.

'… an exceptionally insightful collection in which contributors reflect on the successes, setbacks, and ongoing challenges in contesting and supplanting psychiatry… The transformative effects of the collective knowledge woven together in this book will reverberate for decades to come.'
Dr Richard Ingram, Independent Mad Studies Researcher

'… a vital contribution to the building of Mad Studies as a discipline grounded in activist scholarship [and] a comprehensive and accessible must-read for those interested in building real alternatives to the limited, and often damaging, approaches to madness and distress that dominate today.'
Dr Brigit McWade, Sociology Department, Lancaster University

'A profoundly important volume and a herculean effort. Comprehensive, modern, bold, accessible, survivor-produced research, knowledge and practice. *Searching for a Rose Garden* offers concrete examples of people rejecting and altering "mental health" systems around the world. This is a must-read for anyone who has ever heard the word "psychiatry".'
Lauren J Tenney, PhD, MPhil, MPA, Psychiatric Survivor

Also available from PCCS Books – www.pccs-books.co.uk

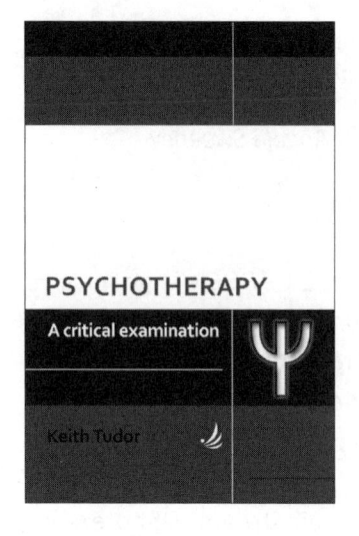

Psychotherapy: A critical examination

Keith Tudor

Part of the Critical Examinations Series

pp. 275

PCCS Books, 2018

www.pccs-books.co.uk

In the latest addition to the PCCS Books Critical Examination series, psychotherapist, academic, teacher and supervisor Keith Tudor focuses his spotlight on psychotherapy. Drawing on the philosophies and practices of myriad disciplines, traditions, modalities, cultures, eras and civilisations, the book aims to fuel continued critical reflection on psychotherapy as a practice, discipline and profession. Its breadth, depth and sharpness of scrutiny will appeal to practitioners, academics and educators at every level, including students and those considering psychotherapy as a career.

Keith Tudor is Professor of Psychotherapy at Auckland University of Technology, an Honorary Senior Research Fellow of the University of Roehampton and a Fellow of The Critical Institute, with a long and varied career in the psychotherapy profession as a practitioner, teacher, supervisor and academic. He trained originally in gestalt therapy, and subsequently in transactional analysis and person-centred psychology. He is also a teaching and supervising transactional analyst.

'Keith Tudor's remarkable *tour de force* marks a historical turning point in the evolution of the psy therapies. No therapist can afford not to read this book.'
Dr Richard House, chartered psychologist, left-green political activist and writer

'This important book teaches clinicians to think carefully and to question everything about psychotherapy: its doctrines, its institutional training, its assumptions, its practices, its aims, its views of the human. Keith Tudor is training us to be practising philosophers, for the benefit of those whom we serve. A valuable and challenging read.'
Donna Orange, Assistant Clinical Professor (Adjunct) and Consultant/Supervisor for the New York University post-doctoral program in psychotherapy and psychoanalysis